Laryngeal Evaluation

Indirect Laryngoscopy to High-Speed Digital Imaging

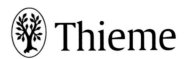

Laryngeal Evaluation
Indirect Laryngoscopy to High-Speed Digital Imaging

Editors

Katherine A. Kendall, MD
Director, Voice Clinic
Otolaryngology Section
Minneapolis VA Medical Center
Associate Professor, Department of Otolaryngology–Head
   and Neck Surgery
University of Minnesota
Minneapolis, Minnesota

Rebecca J. Leonard, PhD
Clinical Director, Voice, Speech and Swallowing Center
University of California–Davis
Professor, Department of Otolaryngology–Head and Neck Surgery
University of California–Davis Medical Center
Sacramento, California

Thieme
New York • Stuttgart

Thieme Medical Publishers, Inc.
333 Seventh Ave.
New York, NY 10001

Managing Editor: Dominik Pucek
Executive Editor: Timothy Hiscock
Editorial Director, Clinical Reference: Michael Wachinger
International Production Director: Andreas Schabert
Production Editor: Grace R. Caputo, Dovetail Content Solutions
Vice President, International Sales and Marketing: Cornelia Schulze
Chief Financial Officer: James W. Mitos
President: Brian D. Scanlan
Compositor: Thomson Digital
Printer: Gopsons Papers Ltd.

Library of Congress Cataloging-in-Publication Data

Laryngeal evaluation : indirect laryngoscopy to high-speed digital imaging / edited by
Katherine A. Kendall, Rebecca J. Leonard.
    p. ; cm.
  Includes bibliographical references.
  ISBN 978-1-60406-272-4
  1. Larynx—Radiography. I. Kendall, Katherine. II. Leonard, Rebecca.
  [DNLM: 1. Laryngeal Diseases—diagnosis. 2. Laryngoscopy—methods.
  3. Larynx—anatomy & histology. 4. Larynx—physiology. 5. Stroboscopy—methods.
  WV 505 L336 2010]
  RF512.L37 2010
  616.2'207572—dc22
                                    2009052790

Important note: Medical knowledge is ever-changing. As new research and clinical experience broaden our knowledge, changes in treatment and drug therapy may be required. The authors and editors of the material herein have consulted sources believed to be reliable in their efforts to provide information that is complete and in accord with the standards accepted at the time of publication. However, in view of the possibility of human error by the authors, editors, or publisher of the work herein or changes in medical knowledge, neither the authors, editors, nor publisher, nor any other party who has been involved in the preparation of this work, warrants that the information contained herein is in every respect accurate or complete, and they are not responsible for any errors or omissions or for the results obtained from use of such information. Readers are encouraged to confirm the information contained herein with other sources. For example, readers are advised to check the product information sheet included in the package of each drug they plan to administer to be certain that the information contained in this publication is accurate and that changes have not been made in the recommended dose or in the contraindications for administration. This recommendation is of particular importance in connection with new or infrequently used drugs.

Some of the product names, patents, and registered designs referred to in this book are in fact registered trademarks or proprietary names even though specific reference to this fact is not always made in the text. Therefore, the appearance of a name without designation as proprietary is not to be construed as a representation by the publisher that it is in the public domain.

Printed in India

5 4 3 2 1

ISBN 978-1-60406-272-4

To my husband, J.R.: I often marvel how lucky I am to have
found my true soul mate. And to my coeditor, R.J.L., who has been a source
of mentorship, inspiration, and friendship for my entire career.

Katherine A. Kendall

Contents

Contents

Foreword

The twentieth century has been known as the era of human communications; at the center of this development has been the human voice. The principal organ of voice production, the larynx, requires supervision in health and disease, which in turn calls for imaging of the vocal organ.

On my return from the U.S. Naval Service after World War II, I settled in Chicago. In my work at Northwestern University, I faced a challenge of inadequate visualization of the vibrating larynx. My wife and I assisted in the restoration of the famous Lyric Opera, and I had an opportunity to assist a number of singers with vocal problems. During these examinations, I became concerned that my laryngeal mirror was not sufficient to present a clear and accurate view of the vocal margins during the vibratory cycle. On reflection, I realized that the blurred movements of the vocal folds were actually the result of the high vocal frequency of the singers' voices. In other words, my eyes were limited to the perception of eight or ten images per second, while the vocal cords of my patients vibrated perhaps a thousand times a second. Consultations with distinguished colleagues in Philadelphia, Boston, and New York failed to offer a solution to my quandary.

At this stage of my research on the vibrating vocal cords, I remembered an experience during my Naval service in which we examined a rapidly moving engine with ultra-high speed photography at about 5000 frames per second. It occurred to me that perhaps we could use similar equipment for the study of vocal fold movements in slow or ultra-slow motion. Why not apply the same principle to the vibrations of the pathologic larynx? After considerable searching, I discovered that Northwestern University *did* have such a camera tucked away in the corner of an old coal cellar in the basement of a campus building. We also had a skilled voice pathologist, Professor Paul Moore, who was able to adapt this equipment to examinations of the human larynx. Our medical school was ready to support our work with the essential space, and some of my patients were willing to provide the necessary financial assistance.

We started our imaging with motion pictures of a normal larynx at ultra-high speeds of 2000 frames per second, which, on normal playback, translated into slow motion pictures. As it happened, our first major film, "The Function of the Normal Larynx," won a first prize for the United States at the famous film festival in Venice, Italy, in 1957. Subsequent ultra-high speed motion pictures of "The Function of the Larynx under Daily Stress" and on "The Function of the Pathologic Larynx" won similar awards at international film exhibitions in Milan, Vancouver, Padua, San Francisco, and other international meetings. Even our more doubtful colleagues were impressed with these results and were willing to admit the scientific and clinical value of this new type of laryngeal examination. Over the next 25 years, our educational motion pictures on the larynx and voice were used for teaching and research at some 120 universities and colleges in the United States and abroad. (I have just learned that in some locations, they still are used for that purpose.)

Unfortunately, our equipment and several hundred thousand feet of research film were stolen during a move from our research institute in Los Angeles to a new medical facility. It was, of course, clear to us that this expensive and time-consuming examination was ill-suited for clinical practice in the office of the laryngologist or voice pathologist. That is one of the main reasons why I am so pleased to support Dr. Kendall's work with ultra-high-speed laryngeal imaging as is demonstrated in this book. Interested readers will note the necessary preparations and requirements for a successful study of the larynx in ultra-slow motion.

In an effort to prepare better clinical diagnostic equipment we worked with a German scientist, Dr. Rolf Timcke, who joined our Institute at Northwestern University. During his time with us, Dr. Timcke designed and fabricated the first practical electronic synchron-stroboscope for laryngeal imaging. On his return to Germany, Dr. Timcke established a factory that was designed for the production of stroboscopic imaging equipment, and which supplied stroboscopes for laryngeal examinations to most major European universities. We had an awful time with U.S. Customs officials, who were not familiar with this high-tech equipment and could not find any description of it in their manuals.

The American Academy of Oto-Rhino-Laryngology was equally suspicious, but for different reasons. During an annual meeting of our Academy in Chicago about 1960, we attempted to demonstrate our new electronic synchron-stroboscope to our colleagues. The Academy sent two distinguished professors (F.L. and P.H.) to our booth to evaluate this newfangled device. The two official examiners listened to our brief explanation, performed a short examination, and came to the conclusion that they did see some strange vibratory motions. They also reported back to their colleagues that this type of equipment would never be of help to the practicing laryngologist.

Some 40 years later, Part III of this book on laryngeal imaging confirms that video stroboscopy has "arrived." Numerous chapters of this textbook elaborate the value of a stroboscopic examination for the clinician in practice. Dr. Kendall and her associates have described the manifold diagnostic and clinical applications of laryngeal stroboscopy that are recommended for current day practice. Pertinent chapters discuss the indications and techniques of this procedure. Specific disorders are reviewed and paired with the appropriate stroboscopic evaluations.

These observations are equally true for the development of flexible endoscopy, which has become a routine procedure for the imaging of the larynx by both the practicing laryngologist and the skilled voice pathologist. The chapters on flexible endoscopy cover the range of this valuable examination for normal and pathologic evaluations of the laryngeal interior, and discuss the special applications of flexible endoscopy for in-office procedures. Needless to say, this technique has proved of great importance for the intralaryngeal evaluations of patients with a disruptive gag reflex.

While Dr. Kendall and her fellow authors have presented an excellent review of past and present techniques for laryngeal imaging, what is to be said about the future of this critical diagnostic tool? Some years ago, my colleague Dr. Yasuo Koike and I envisioned the use of computer techniques to assist in the early detection of laryngeal disease. Frankly, I am surprised that, in our computer age, this potential has not been fully explored. I am hopeful that Dr. Kendall and her team will continue their scientific explorations into further imaging of the human larynx and provide new opportunities for physicians, voice pathologists, and patients in the care of the human voice.

Hans von Leden, MD, ScD
Professor of Biocommunications (Emeritus)
University of Southern California
Los Angeles, California

Preface

Advances in imaging technology have improved our ability to examine the larynx. As a result, clinicians can identify subtle mucosal lesions while performing a detailed analysis of vocal fold vibratory characteristics. A thorough understanding of imaging technology combined with experience in examination interpretation is required to use these techniques effectively in laryngeal evaluation. In addition, a variety of imaging modalities are available, and one or more of these techniques may be employed for a laryngeal exam. Understanding the unique indications and limitations of each imaging method is vital to making an accurate assessment of the larynx.

Current laryngeal examination and imaging techniques, including indirect laryngoscopy, flexible laryngoscopy, videostroboscopy, and high-speed laryngeal imaging, are the central topics of *Laryngeal Evaluation: Indirect Laryngoscopy to High-Speed Digital Imaging*. This text is intended to emphasize the interpretation of studies and to serve as both a reference for practicing clinicians and a textbook for clinicians in training. It is written from the point of view of both otolaryngologists and speech pathologists, with the aim of enhancing interdisciplinary communication. Optimal patient management requires collaboration between these specialists, integrating the findings of the laryngeal examination with recommendations for treatment.

A working knowledge of laryngeal anatomy and the physiology of sound production is essential to the interpretation of laryngeal imaging. The laws of physics explain the phenomena, both normal and pathologic, observed during examination of the larynx. The chapters in Section I, The Basics, review anatomy and physiology and form the foundation for an understanding of laryngeal imaging that is furthered in Section II, Flexible Laryngoscopy.

The next three sections focus on videostroboscopy. Section III addresses the background of videostroboscopy, its performance, and interpretation of results, as well as covering what normal findings look like. Section IV focuses on the differential diagnosis of abnormal vibratory characteristics, and Section V describes how specific laryngeal pathology affects vocal fold vibration. The differential diagnosis of vibratory abnormalities is integrally linked to how vocal fold pathology affects vocal fold vibratory characteristics. By presenting the interpretation of the videostroboscopic examination from both perspectives—how specific laryngeal pathology can affect vocal fold vibration and how a specific vibratory abnormality is related to the clinical diagnosis—there is some inherent information overlap. This, however, has been done to provide a useful reference with a comprehensive discussion of the topic.

Section VI, Pediatric Imaging, is a detailed consideration of how laryngoscopic imaging in children diverges from that in adults, from anatomic differences to dealing with nervous parents. Numerous illustrations provide a good overview of what one might encounter in pediatric patients.

Section VII covers the latest technological advance in the field of laryngeal imaging—high-speed digital imaging. High-speed imaging promises to increase our ability to observe closely laryngeal function and to improve our understanding of laryngeal physiology and pathology. In addition, high-speed imaging has the potential for quantified measurement of vocal fold vibratory characteristics, increasing diagnostic accuracy and allowing the comparison of imaging exams for the purposes of tracking treatment outcomes and gathering research data. This will ultimately lead to advances in the treatment of laryngeal diseases.

The text is accompanied by a DVD that contains a collection of video clips from laryngeal imaging examinations. These examples are intended to illustrate the concepts discussed in the text, and references throughout the book chapters indicate which video clips are pertinent to specific topics. Readers will benefit maximally if they read chapters within reach of a computer to allow them to view the accompanying video illustrations. The book's appendix contains a detailed explanation of each video clip.

It is our hope that readers find this text a useful adjunct to their clinical practice and that the information takes their clinical abilities to a higher level. We are grateful for the contributions from so many individuals who are among the worlds most knowledgeable in the field of laryngeal imaging.

Katherine A. Kendall

Contributors

Mona M. Abaza, MD
Department of Otolaryngology
University of Colorado Health Sciences Center
Aurora, Colorado

Ronda E. Alexander, MD
Assistant Professor
Department of Otorhinolaryngology–Head
    and Neck Surgery
University of Texas Medical School at Houston
Houston, Texas

Kenneth W. Altman, MD, PhD, FACS
Director, Eugene Grabscheild MD Voice Center
Associate Professor
Department of Otolaryngology–Head
    and Neck Surgery
Mount Sinai School of Medicine
New York, New York

Gerald S. Berke, MD
Professor and Chief
Division of Head and Neck Surgery
Department of Surgery
Ronald Reagan UCLA Medical Center
UCLA Center for Esophageal Disorders
UCLA Voice Center for Medicine and the Arts
Los Angeles, California

Steven Bielamowicz, MD
Professor and Chief
Division of Otolaryngology
George Washington University Medical Center
Washington, D.C.

Andrew Blitzer, MD, DDS
Professor
Department of Clinical Otolaryngology
Columbia University College of Physicians
    and Surgeons
Director, New York Center for Voice
    and Swallowing Disorders
St. Luke's–Roosevelt Hospital Center
New York, New York

Heather Shaw Bonilha, PhD
College of Health Professions
Department of Health Sciences and Research
Medical University of South Carolina
Charleston, South Carolina

Lauren C. Cunningham, MD
Department of Otolaryngology–Head
    and Neck Surgery
Ohio State University Medical Center
Columbus, Ohio

Seth H. Dailey, MD
Assistant Professor
Department of Surgery
University of Wisconsin–Madison
University of Wisconsin Hospital
Madison, Wisconsin

Alessandro de Alarcon, MD
Assistant Professor
Department of Otolaryngology–Head
    and Neck Surgery
University of Cincinnati College of Medicine
Director, Center for Pediatric Voice Disorders
Pediatric Otolaryngology
Cincinnati Children's Hospital Medical Center
Cincinnati, Ohio

Dimitar Deliyski, PhD
Associate Professor
Director, Voice and Speech Laboratory
Communication Sciences and Disorders
University of South Carolina
Arnold School of Public Health
Columbia, South Carolina

Lisa B. Fry, PhD
Associate Professor
Communication Disorders
College of Health Professions
Marshall University
Huntington, West Virginia

Glendon M. Gardner, MD
Senior Staff Otolaryngologist
Department of Otolaryngology–Head
    and Neck Surgery
Henry Ford Health System
Detroit, Michigan

Murtaza T. Ghadiali, MD
Associate Physician
Department of Head and Neck Surgery
Kaiser Foundation Medical Center
Fontana, California

Nazaneen N. Grant, MD
Assistant Professor
Department of Otolaryngology–Head
    and Neck Surgery
Georgetown University School of Medicine
Georgetown University Hospital
Washington, D.C.

Edie R. Hapner, PhD
Assistant Professor
Department of Otolaryngology
Emory University School of Medicine
Director of Speech-Language Pathology
Emory Voice Center
Atlanta, Georgia

Yolanda D. Heman-Ackah, MD
Associate Professor
Department of Otolaryngology–Head
    and Neck Surgery
Drexel University College of Medicine
Philadelphia, Pennsylvania

Robert E. Hillman, PhD
Co-Director and Research Director
Surgery and Health Sciences and Technology
Harvard Medical School and Massachusetts
    Institute of Technology
Center for Laryngeal Surgery and Voice
    Rehabilitation
Massachusetts General Hospital
Boston, Massachusetts

Cristina Jackson-Menaldi, PhD
Adjunct Professor
Department of Otolaryngology–Head
    and Neck Surgery
Wayne State University Medical Center
Co-Director, Lakeshore Professional Voice
    Center
Lakeshore Ear, Nose and Throat Center
St. Clair Shores, Michigan

Katherine A. Kendall, MD
Director, Voice Clinic
Otolaryngology Section
Minneapolis VA Medical Center
Associate Professor, Department of
    Otolaryngology–Head and Neck Surgery
University of Minnesota
Minneapolis, Minnesota

Mario A. Landera, MA
Speech Pathologist
Department of Otolaryngology
University of Miami
Miami, Florida

Rebecca J. Leonard, PhD
Clinical Director, Voice, Speech
    and Swallowing Center
University of California–Davis
Professor, Department of Otolaryngology–Head
    and Neck Surgery
University of California–Davis Medical Center
Sacramento, California

Donna S. Lundy, PhD
Associate Professor
Department of Otolaryngology
University of Miami
Miami, Florida

Nicolas E. Maragos, MD
Associate Professor
Department of Otorhinolaryngology–Head
 and Neck Surgery
Mayo Medical School and Mayo Clinic
Rochester, Minnesota

J. Scott McMurray, MD
Associate Professor
Division of Otolaryngology–Head
 and Neck Surgery
Department of Surgery
University of Wisconsin School of Medicine
 and Public Health
Madison, Wisconsin

Daryush D. Mehta, SM
Harvard–MIT Division of Health Sciences
 and Technology
Massachusetts Institute of Technology
Center for Laryngeal Surgery and Voice
 Rehabilitation
Massachusetts General Hospital
Boston, Massachusetts

Claudio F. Milstein, PhD
Associate Professor
Department of Surgery
Cleveland Clinic Lerner College of Medicine
 of Case Western Reserve University
The Voice Center, Head and Neck Institute
The Cleveland Clinic
Cleveland, Ohio

Natasha Mirza, MD
Veterans Administration Medical Center
Hospital of the University of Pennsylvania
University of Pennsylvania
Philadelphia, Pennsylvania

Adam D. Rubin, MD
Adjunct Assistant Professor
Department of Otolaryngology–Head
 and Neck Surgery
University of Michigan Medical Center
Ann Arbor, Michigan
Co-Director, Lakeshore Professional Voice Center
Lakeshore Ear, Nose and Throat Center
St. Clair Shores, Michigan

Cesar Ruiz, SLPD, CCC-SLP
School of Nursing and Health Sciences
LaSalle University
Philadelphia, Pennsylvania

C. Blake Simpson, MD
Professor
Department of Otolaryngology–Head
 and Neck Surgery
University of Texas Health Science Center
 at San Antonio
San Antonio, Texas

Joseph C. Stemple, PhD
Professor
Rehabiliation Services
University of Kentucky College of Health
 Sciences
Lexington, Kentucky

Lucian Sulica, MD
Associate Professor
Department of Otorhinolaryngology
Director of Voice Disorders/Laryngology
Weill Cornell Medical College
New York Presbyterian–Weill Cornell
 Medical Center
New York, New York

Melin Tan-Geller, MD
Laryngology Fellow
Department of Otolaryngology–Head
 and Neck Surgery
The Mount Sinai School of Medicine
New York, New York

Hans von Leden, MD, ScD
Professor of Biocommunications (Emeritus)
University of Southern California
Los Angeles, California

Gayle E. Woodson, MD
Professor and Chair
Division of Otolaryngology
Department of Surgery
Southern Illinois University School
 of Medicine
Springfield, Illinois

Steven M. Zeitels, MD, FACS
Eugene B. Casey Professor of Laryngeal
 Surgery
Director, Center for Laryngeal Surgery
 and Voice Rehabilitation
Department of Surgery
Massachusetts General Hospital
Harvard Medical School
Boston, Massachusetts

I

The Basics

1

The History of Laryngeal Imaging

Steven M. Zeitels and Alessandro de Alarcon

The origin and development of laryngeal imaging chronicles the initiation of the field of laryngology, and improved imaging continues to provide the foundation for a majority of the developments in our specialty today. Observing the larynx with high resolution and great precision allows for our understanding of normal/abnormal anatomy and function, which is the basis of designing treatment strategies.

A primary focus of 19th century laryngology was mirror-guided management of laryngeal airway obstruction, primarily from infectious diseases of the upper aerodigestive tract.[1] This continued into the early 20th century when Kirstein, Killian, and Jackson popularized direct laryngoscopic surgery, which was invaluable for treating cancer, stenosis, and a spectrum of benign phonatory lesions. Later in the 20th century, the key imaging advancements were stereoscopic magnified laryngoscopy in the operating room as well as office-based flexible laryngoscopy and stroboscopy. Today, researchers are exploring the value of high-speed imaging of vocal fold vibration.

◆ The Origin of Mirror Laryngoscopy and the Field of Laryngology

The origin and growth of laryngology is inextricably linked to the development of endoscopic laryngeal imaging and laryngoscopic surgery. Phillip Bozzini (1773–1809) was the first individual to suggest that image-controlled endoscopic surgery was possible and is therefore considered to be the father of minimally invasive surgery (**Fig. 1.1**).[2] In 1807, at the age of 34, he described the Lichtleiter ("light conductor"), which was composed of a universal handle that incorporated a candle and a reflector as an extracorporeal light-source (**Fig. 1.2**). He attached a variety of cannulae to the handle to facilitate the examination of accessible orifices (i.e., throat, urethra, rectum). This concept was a revolutionary advancement in medical and surgical science, but his work continues to be largely unrecognized. The laryngeal cannula consisted of an additional mirror that allowed for visualization of the lower pharynx and larynx. Unfortunately, the medical community did not embrace Bozzini's method, and he died in 1809 before the validity of his approach could be established.

There were several other reports of mirror laryngoscopy in the first half of the 19th century; however, none were widely acknowledged or accepted.[3–9] Most notable were the descriptions by Babington, Liston, and Avery.[3,4,7] Babington first used the term *glottoscope* (1829) for his instrument, which consisted of a variety of mirrors as well as a retracting spatula to distract the tongue base. By retracting the tongue base out of the visual field, Babington's glottoscope became the first device to employ

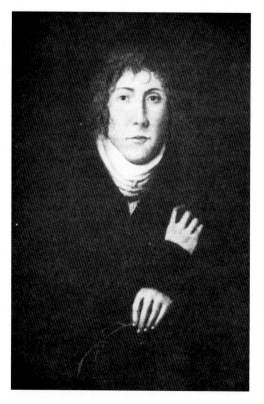

Fig. 1.1 Phillip Bozzini (1773–1809).

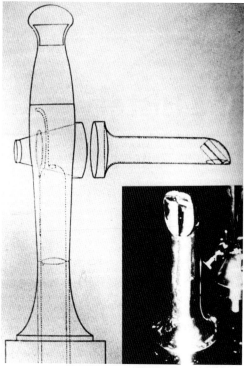

Fig. 1.2 Bozzini's Lichtleiter ("light conductor"). Note the line drawing displaying a universal handle with a candle as a light source; the laryngeal speculum is seen in the inferior right in the inset photograph. Courtesy of American College of Surgeons.

internal distension of supraglottal tissues to enhance visualization of the glottis.[10,11] Liston's brief description of mirror laryngoscopy (1837) for the assessment of laryngeal edema was important because he introduced the concept of heating the mirror to avoid condensation on the reflecting surface.[7] Avery (1844) designed a laryngeal cannula similar to Bozzini's, however he employed an artificial light source separate from the device in the form of a headlight.[3] This remarkable device employed a perforated concave mirror to reflect the illumination into the oropharynx to facilitate visualization of the larynx.

Manual Garcia (1805–1906), the renowned vocal pedagogist, reported auto-laryngoscopy to the Royal Society of London in 1855 (**Fig. 1.3**).[12] This investigation was catalyzed by his desire to better understand singing phonation. In his paper entitled "Observations on the Human Voice," Garcia made important contributions to the understanding of laryngeal sound production especially with regard to rhythmic pulsation of the expiratory airstream. Clerf believed that Garcia's emphasis on observations and deductions regarding laryngeal physiology led to the subsequent widespread adoption of mirror laryngoscopy by physicians, which had not occurred as a result of prior 19th century descriptions of the technique.[13]

There is little debate that laryngology was born from the imaging investigations of the acclaimed classical voice teacher. In addition to inspiring the genesis of this new field in medicine, Garcia maintained active engagement with laryngologists as the field developed from its infancy. This is evidenced in Mackenzie's text, *The Hygiene of the Vocal Organs*.[14] The tremendous esteem that laryngologists held for Garcia was vividly illustrated in Mackinlay's description of the celebration for the maestro's 100th birthday (1906).[15] Laryngologists commissioned John Singer

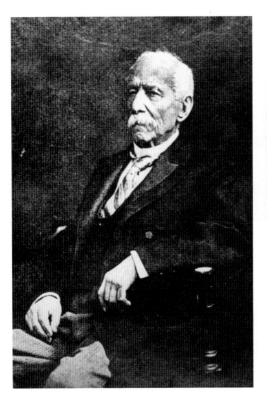

Fig. 1.3 Manuel Garcia (1805–1906) at approximately 80 years old. Courtesy of Rhode Island School of Design.

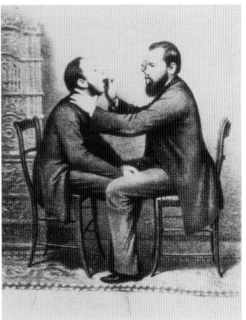

Fig. 1.4 Johann Nepomuk Czermak (1828–1873).

Sargent to paint Garcia for his centennial birthday. It appears that Garcia was too frail to remain stable for the entire process. Sargent is reported to have used a photograph as a model for the majority of the painting, whereas the head and hands were derived from the live sitting.

In 1857, Turck explored, but then abandoned, the clinical application of mirror laryngoscopy.[16] He could not obtain a reliable image because, like Garcia, he was depending on the sun for illumination, and unfortunately it was often overcast in Pesth in the autumn. Shortly thereafter, his colleague Czermak borrowed the same mirrors and commenced further investigations, which were highly successful (**Fig. 1.4**).[17] Czermak reintroduced the artificial light source and the perforated concave mirror. A feud developed between Czermak and Turck over priority for the medical application of mirror laryngoscopy. The most important aspect of the dispute between Turck and Czermak was that the bitter quarrel fueled attention in the Western world toward the fledgling field of laryngology. Both pioneers immediately concentrated on educating physicians in the technique of laryngoscopy by convening clinics throughout Europe. This dissemination of knowledge led to the development of a watershed of instruments and contributions (**Fig. 1.5**).

Stoerk (1859) reported the first laryngoscopically controlled manipulation of the laryngeal tissues, which involved the topical application of silver nitrate to the larynx.[18] Lewin (1860) was the first to report on the laryngoscopically guided management of laryngeal tumors.[19] In his series of 50 neoplasms, he excised three and applied caustics to four others. Mackenzie introduced mirror laryngoscopy to Great Britain after attending Czermak's clinic.[20] He acquired acclaim as a surgical innovator and a prolific author.[21,22] In 1886, Fraenkel published the first report of a transoral resection of a laryngeal cancer.[23]

In the United States, laryngoscopy and laryngology were initially slow to develop due to the concurrent outbreak of the U.S. Civil War. Near the end of the conflict, Louis Elsberg (1837–1885), who attended the Jefferson

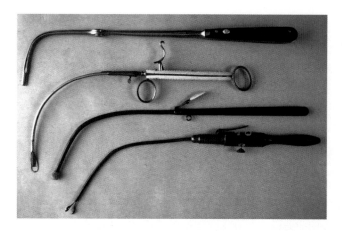

Medical College in 1860, published the first formal American book (1864) in laryngology and endolaryngeal treatment.[24] Soon thereafter, he received the Gold Medal from the American Medical Association for his publication entitled *Laryngoscopal Surgery Illustrated in the Treatment of Morbid Growths within the Larynx.*[25]

Similar to virtually all laryngologists of the day, Elsberg was a physician and not a trained surgeon. Yet Jacob da Silva Solis-Cohen (1838–1927), at the conclusion of his Civil War service as a surgeon in the Union Navy and Army, was influenced to become a laryngologist by his boyhood friend and medical-school classmate—Elsberg. To the best that the authors can document, Solis-Cohen became the first formally trained surgeon to become a laryngologist, which was based on mastering mirror-guided imaging. This imaging skill allowed for surgical procedures, which fueled the progress of laryngology. Solis-Cohen's professional development became a critical turning point in the history of laryngology, laryngeal surgery, and ultimately phonosurgery. He combined his newly acquired laryngoscopic skills with rigorous surgical training and wartime experience to the fledgling medical specialty of laryngology. Most likely, he is the first specialist head and neck surgeon in history and was probably the first individual to cure a laryngeal cancer, which was done by means of a laryngofissure and hemilaryngectomy.[26,27]

Solis-Cohen realized and taught that precise management of the upper aerodigestive tract disorders required both endoscopic and open surgical skills. This philosophy was vividly displayed in his magnum opus (1872), *Diseases of the Throat: A Guide to the Diagnosis and Treatment*, which was the benchmark for textbooks of its kind for decades.[28] As a young man, Chevalier Jackson personally borrowed Solis-Cohen's texts. It is likely that his compendium, *Peroral Endoscopy and Laryngeal Surgery*, is modeled after Solis-Cohen's text.[29]

◆ The Origin of and Development of Direct Laryngoscopy and Endolaryngeal Surgery

The isolated reports of mirror laryngoscopy in the early 19th century arose from the need to image the airway. Infectious diseases were a formidable problem that could cause membranous laryngeal airway obstruction.[30,31] Horace Green (1802–1866) dedicated his career to this problem and spent time with Trousseau and Belloc in Europe. He became the first specialist for throat and respiratory diseases in the United States (**Fig. 1.6**). Green described blind transoral application of caustics to the larynx to treat infectious inflammatory disorders of the laryngeal membranes, as reliable laryngeal imaging was yet to be discovered.[32–34] However, he was maligned by his contemporaries, who did not believe that his transoral interventions were possible.[35–37] Later, Green resolved this skepticism by placing a whalebone probang transorally through the glottis of a patient who had a tracheotomy

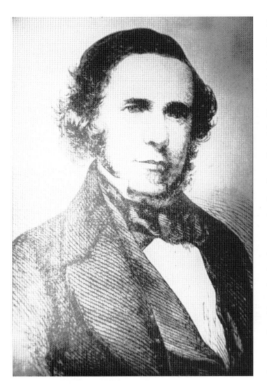

Fig. 1.6 Horace Green (1802–1866).

until the probang could be observed through the tracheotomy site.

In 1852, Green made his most seminal contribution to laryngology by describing the first direct laryngoscopy and visually controlled excision of a laryngeal neoplasm. He was managing a child with obstructive sleep apnea. He excised her tonsils, which did not resolve the problem. Subsequently, he inserted a bent tongue spatula (similar to a Macintosh laryngoscope) and was able to observe a ball-valving fibroepithelial polyp obstructing the glottal aperture. Using sunlight for illumination, he was able to successfully observe and resect the lesion due to the favorably cephalad position of the child's larynx. He reported the case in detail in his landmark textbook, *On the Surgical Treatment of Polypi of the Larynx, and Oedema of the Glottis*.[38] The book contained a drawing of what the artist could view during the procedure.

Both Bozzini and Green were courageous figures in medical history, as their work was not accepted by their contemporaries, who could not replicate their techniques. They were both branded as charlatans by the general medical establishment. Although Bozzini died shortly after his book was published, Green lived through the initial period of the origin of laryngology and he was vindicated. Louis Elsberg, the first president of the American Laryngological Association, dedicated that organization's first meeting in 1879 to Green and referred to him as the father of American laryngology because of his brilliant skill and courageous contributions.[37]

No attempt to repeat Green's 1850s work with direct laryngoscopy occurred until the end of the 19th century. Unaware of Green's accomplishment, Kirstein reintroduced direct laryngoscopy (autoscopy) in 1895 (**Fig. 1.7**).[39,40] Kirstein, who was in private practice, was visionary in his appreciation of the value of his technique, yet he was fully aware of the potential academic resistance both to a different approach for visualizing the larynx and to a new technology. He therefore called his procedure autoscopy and avoided calling it laryngoscopy. He wisely concluded in the preface of his text, "Of course, many a laryngologist is convinced that the laryngological technique needs no additions; others may think differently. Only the future can decide this question." Kirstein's success in precipitating a paradigm shift in endolaryngeal surgery was due to his careful and patient approach to change and to the fact that there was great academic interest in the field of laryngology. This allowed for enough open-minded inspection to embrace the advantages of direct endolaryngeal surgery, which has served us well in the 20th century. In 1895, Kirstein even predicted the enhanced value of autoscopy if it were to be married to improved imaging techniques, which could be provided by magnification and stroboscopy.

Killian (1860–1921), who was an academic surgeon, was initially incredulous of Kirstein's claims regarding direct laryngeal imaging. After viewing Kirstein's demonstration, however, Killian became absorbed with the new technique. Not to be outdone, Killian perfected rigid bronchoscopy by 1897, thereby demonstrating direct examination of the airway distal to the larynx.[41] Killian was destined to make other major contributions to direct laryngoscopy in the early 1900s.

All substantive improvements in endoscopic surgery of the larynx during the 20th century have enhanced precision. Increased precision is

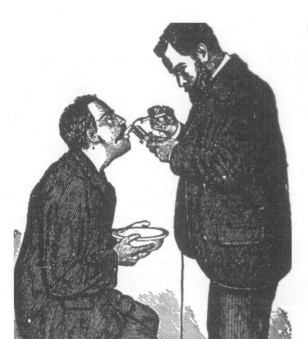

Fig. 1.7 Alfred Kirstein (1863–1922).

inevitably linked to better exposure of the operative field and in turn improved visualization. The important innovations enhancing laryngeal exposure had been introduced by 1925. Jackson employed Kirstein's head and neck position for direct laryngoscopy in the supine position (**Fig. 1.8**).[42] Killian introduced the inverted V laryngoscope blade to conform to the anterior glottal commissure and designed the laryngeal suspension that facilitated bimanual surgery (**Fig. 1.9**).[43–46] Internal distension in the anteroposterior dimension was reintroduced by Haslinger (initially by Babington) with his bivalve laryngoscope and in the mediolateral dimension by Jackson with his laryngostat.[47,48] Although previously used by Czermak, external counterpressure was formally described by Brunings (**Fig. 1.10**).[49] All laryngologists use one or more of these concepts; recently, however, Zeitels and Vaughan combined them together while using *elevated vector suspension*.[10]

Most surgeons throughout the world employ torsion-fulcrum laryngoscope holders to maintain the laryngoscope in position for endolaryngeal surgery. They mistakenly refer to this as suspension laryngoscopy. This misconception appears to have evolved from an article in the early 1950s that referred to a gear-powered

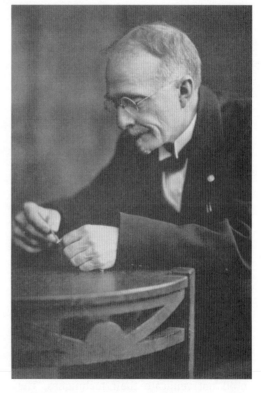

Fig. 1.8 Chevalier Jackson (1865–1958).

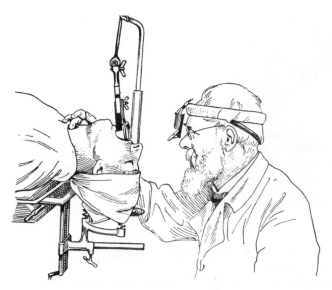

Fig. 1.9 Gustav Killian (1860–1921).

torsion-fulcrum holder as a suspension device.[50] Remarkably, there were no references indexed in this report. Prior authors and scientific reports discussing these types of devices referred to them using terms such as "fulcrum-lift," "self-retaining," and "stabilizer."[51–54]

The development of torsion laryngoscope holders arose from functional necessity, but their popularity today largely persists due to habit and custom rather than anatomic science and engineering principles. Because Killian's disciples had difficulty using the suspension gallows on patients who are awake with marginal non-endotracheal anesthesia, they designed the precursors of current laryngoscope holders. Bruning's laryngoscope system pushed off the larynx, whereas Seiffert's instrument used the chest wall as a means of support (**Figs. 1.10 and 1.11**). Remarkably, chest-support torsion-holder systems were used exclusively for spatula laryngoscopes until the late 1940s, at which point they were retrofitted for use with tubular laryngoscopes.[50–54]

The introduction of general endotracheal anesthesia to direct laryngoscopic surgery in the 1960s should have catalyzed a rebirth in the use of true elevated vector suspension.[55] Detailed discussions of the forces required for optimal exposure of the larynx advocate the use of a suspension-type device from which the patient is hanging. This information was well known to Strong and Vaughan when they fathered the Boston University Suspension Gallows (Pilling Co., Research Triangle Park, NC).[56] Unfortunately, this suspension gallows did not gain wide acceptance and has remained primarily in use among the trainees of two generations of surgeons trained by Strong and Vaughan. Zeitels designed a substantially more robust suspension gallows and academically resurrected the value of true suspension laryngoscopy so that now this philosophy is gaining more widespread adoption.[57]

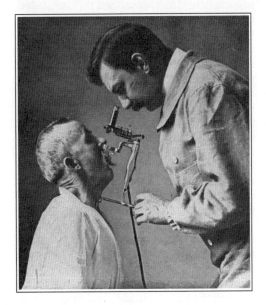

Fig. 1.10 Wilhelm Brunings (1876–1958).

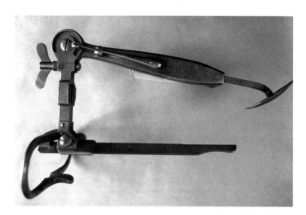

Fig. 1.11 Seiffert's direct laryngoscope.

The justification for a return to a suspension gallows is that the most precise endolaryngeal procedure will be accomplished with the widest endoscopic surgical field, which requires the largest laryngoscope that can be placed between the lips and the larynx. Placement of the largest-lumen laryngoscope requires hanging the patient by the soft tissues adjacent to the lower jaw with accompanying general endotracheal anesthesia and muscular paralysis.[10,11,58-60] It cannot be achieved by using the maxilla as a fulcrum and the laryngoscope as a lever.

Around 1960, the surgical microscope was introduced to endoscopic laryngeal surgery by Scalco and colleagues, Jako, and Kleinsasser.[61-64] Jako also designed the first set of microlaryngeal hand instruments.[65] Kleinsasser designed hand instrumentation as well and became preeminent in educating surgeons throughout the world in microlaryngoscopic technique.[66] At the same time, Priest introduced the concept of general endotracheal anesthesia to laryngoscopy.[55] These innovations led to a new era of precision because of the stable magnified surgical field. In the early 1970s, Polanyi worked with Jako, Strong, and Vaughan and coupled the carbon dioxide laser to the surgical microscope.[67-72] The laser provided precise hemostatic cutting as well as a delivery system that consisted of a joystick and a foot-pedal. This in turn allowed for precise bimanual surgery under high magnification, which was problematic for those who had difficulty controlling their nondominant hand in a magnified field.[73]

◆ Laryngeal Stroboscopy

The aforementioned history reflects the inseparable linkage and interdependence of laryngeal imaging, performing vocal arts, laryngeal physiology, and laryngeal surgery.

The laryngeal stroboscope, which was fundamental for understanding and teaching the physiology underlying laryngeal sound production, was introduced initially by Oertel in 1878.[74] In this brief communication, Oertel outlined the concept; however, the device functioned poorly due to the lack of a consistent adjustable power source to regulate the rotating perforated disks (**Fig. 1.12**). His landmark article (1895) described the use of electricity for this purpose, which facilitated the feasibility of the laryngeal stroboscope.[75] Furthermore, Oertel ingeniously fitted the stroboscope with a magnifying telescope. There were several incrementally improved rotating disk devices in the early 20th century. However, in the 1950s, laryngeal stroboscopy became substantially more feasible with acoustically synchronized light flashes illustrated by Timcke's device.[76,77] His coauthors, von Leden and Moore, demonstrated that the electronic laryngo-synchro-stroboscope was clinically more valuable compared with the predecessor devices of the prior 50 years.[78,79]

Hans von Leden's career and voluminous scientific contributions serve as the foundation for modern *phonosurgery*, a term he developed (1963).[80-83] His seminal contributions have retained their heuristic value through the past 4 decades, and he continues to contribute into the present. Over the past

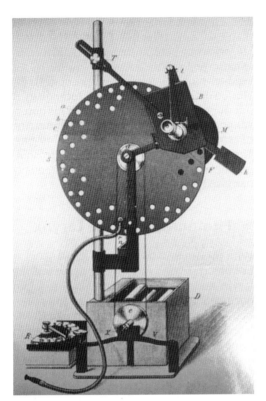

Fig. 1.12 Oertel's laryngeal stroboscope.

Broncho-Esophagological Association in 1962.[86,87] About the same time, the additional light provided by the surgical-microscope enhanced the self-contained illumination of the direct laryngoscopes. There has not been dramatic change since then.

◆ Magnified Laryngoscopy

A magnified view of the larynx was first reported in 1895 by Oertel in his description of the mirror-guided stroboscope (**Fig. 1.12**).[79] Brunings also used a magnified ocular and was the first to employ magnification to enhance direct laryngoscopy (**Fig. 1.10**).[88] Haslinger designed a tubular laryngoscope with accompanying telescopic magnification. Kahler's panelectroscope probably had magnification capabilities as well.[89] In the early 1950s, Albrecht used a colposcope for magnified indirect vocal fold examination and for photodocumentation of keratosis.[90] The first published report of the use of the surgical microscope during laryngoscopy was by Scalco, Shipman, and Tabb in 1960; they employed the Lynch spatula suspension laryngoscope for the task.[61,91] The surgical microscope was a monumental innovation for enhancing the precision of endolaryngeal surgery because it provided high-power magnification with a three-dimensional stereoscopic field.

Jako (in the United States) and Kleinsasser (in Europe) perfected surgical microlaryngoscopy.[62–66] Jako introduced the first set of microlaryngeal hand instruments, and Kleinsasser introduced the 400-mm lens. The latter innovation increased the working distance between the microscope lens and the proximal lumen of the laryngoscope, which facilitated the placement of the long-shafted otologic instruments. Both surgeons designed wide-bore examining tubes to accommodate the optical characteristics of the surgical microscope.

Kleinsasser designed his own hand instrumentation and established the foundations for cold-instrument microlaryngoscopic technique, which has recently enjoyed renewed enthusiasm as phonomicrosurgical procedures have increased in popularity. Today, most phonomicrosurgical procedures should be performed under high magnification to

2 decades, use of an acoustically synchronized laryngeal stroboscope in the management of routine voice disorders has become commonplace and has established the value of laryngeal stroboscopic imaging for any surgeon treating hoarseness and voice disorders.

◆ Illumination

Initial illumination for direct laryngoscopy was sunlight.[38] As a result of the introduction of electricity, Kirstein used a headlight with his initial autoscope spatula.[84] Subsequently, he designed an electrified handle with a proximal incandescent bulb and a prism to direct the light distally. Later, Jackson introduced distal illumination by means of detachable electrified light-carriers.[85] Holinger explained that little changed until "Broyles first demonstrated the advantage of fiberoptic light transmission in peroral endoscopes. . . ." during his address as the guest of honor of the American ensure maximal preservation of the vocal folds' layered microstructure (laminae propria and epithelium).

◆ Rigid Telescopic Laryngoscopy

Although Nitze introduced the concept of a rigid telescope to view the bladder in 1879, Harold Hopkins initiated the modern era of rigid telescopic imaging in the late 1960s.[92] Hopkins was approached by the urologist J.G. Gow asking if Hopkins could develop a better cystoscope, and he invented the rod-lens system to allow better light transmission from the bladder cavity. For the urologist, this provided a 50-fold improvement in the light level. A prototype cystoscope using rod-lenses and a camera was made at Imperial College in 1961. The British and American manufacturers were not interested, but after Hopkins lectured in Dusseldorf in 1963, Karl Storz combined this rod-lens with his cold light. The Storz cystoscope was produced in 1967, and similar rigid fiber endoscopes have since been used throughout the body. In turn, the Hopkins rod has been a key platform technology for laryngoscopic imaging.

◆ Flexible Laryngoscopy

In 1951, Hopkins developed the idea of using a bundle of optical fibers for transporting an optical image and began experiments in 1952. By 1953, he and his research student N.S. Kapany had produced a coherent fiber bundle in which the fibers were of precisely the same order at the distal and proximal ends.[93] Hirschowitz was later to collaborate with C. Wilbur Peters and Lawrence Curtiss to develop a permanent insulated glass coated optical fiber, making it possible to build the first fiberoptic gastroscope in 1957.[94] The first commercial gastroscope based on the prototype was produced by American Cystoscope Makers Inc. (Southborough, MA) in 1960, leading on to flexible fiberoptic endoscopes to inspect, biopsy, and intervene throughout the gastrointestinal tract.

In 1968, Sawashima and colleagues first reported flexible fiberoptic laryngoscopy.[95] This was a profound innovation in laryngology as many patients tolerated flexible transnasal laryngoscopy substantially better than transpharyngeal laryngoscopy with a mirror or rigid telescope. Unfortunately, the optical resolution of flexible laryngoscopic technology is inferior to that of rigid telescopes. This observation is especially dramatic when comparing telescopic with flexible stroboscopic imaging. The recent development of distal-chip technology for flexible laryngoscopes has substantially narrowed this deficit in resolution.

◆ Photography of the Larynx

With the origin of laryngology (late 1850s), it became clear that the striking images of the larynx and its associated pathology required documentation. However, detailed color photography was not readily available until the late 20th century. This required advances in cameras and print media, illumination, as well as rigid and flexible endoscopes.

Laryngoscopic image documentation served to define and describe pathology for identification of disorders, development of management strategies, follow patients' progress, enhance communication between clinicians, and provide a foundation for education. For the first 25 years of laryngology, image documentation required detailed drawings, which were elegantly depicted in laryngological texts of that era and beyond.[25,96,97]

The seminal effort in laryngoscopic photography was made by Stein in collaboration with Czermak and perfected by French (**Figs. 1.13 and 1.14**).[98,99] Although photographs of the larynx culminated from a series of elegant innovations, these images lacked optimal resolution, were cumbersome to obtain, and required exceptional equipment and skill. Apart from the obvious constraints of obtaining high-resolution photographic images of a small structure (larynx and vocal folds) in a dark chamber (pharynx), color was an invaluable missing component of the early laryngeal images. Contributions by Garel, Clerf, Holinger, Berci, Yanigasawa, and Benjamin provided the foundation for our current clinical paradigms of easily obtained photodocumentation in the office and the operating theater.[100–107]

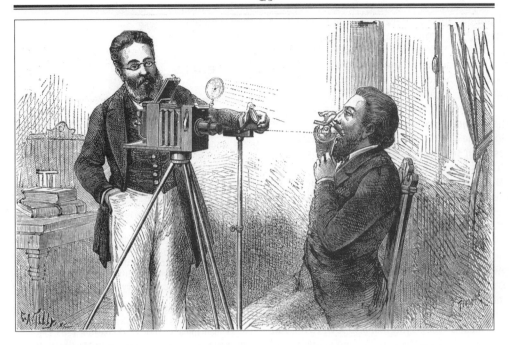

Fig. 1.13 Stein's laryngeal photography technique.

◆ Laryngeal Cinematography and High-Speed Imaging

Motion picture imaging of the upper respiratory tract has evolved substantially in the past 70 years. Farnsworth from Bell Laboratories was the first to use a high-speed motion picture camera to film the vocal folds in 1937.[108] During this same time period, stroboscopy was being developed for assessing patterns of vocal fold vibration.[109-111] The technology for capturing these moving images in a practical way had

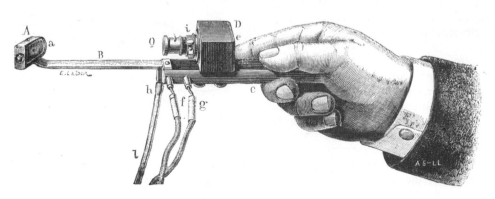

Fig. 1.14 Stein's laryngeal photographic device.

not yet developed. Brubaker and Holinger in the 1940s developed a motion camera for intraoperative use during bronchoscopy.[112] Although this camera produced excellent images, the camera was not widely adopted due to the expense of the device. Von Leden and Moore advanced these research efforts and developed a method of capturing normal and pathologic vocal fold vibration.[82,113] The results of this work raised more questions regarding the physiology of vocal fold mechanics. During this time period, cinematography remained a research tool and was impractical for use in clinical laryngology. For the most part, in the 1970s, motion picture filming of vocal fold mechanics remained in the research realm despite multiple investigators developing more effective techniques.[114-116]

The routine clinical use of color motion picture capturing devices became a reality in the 1980s and 1990s. Yanagisawa and others explored the practical use of videography and photography for laryngeal imaging.[117,118] The development of new video cameras, tape-based video systems, and low-cost color printers allowed the established widespread employment of motion pictures in the clinical setting during the past 3 decades. Yanagisawa championed the use of this readily available equipment for several reasons including (1) peer and trainee education, (2) patient education, and (3) treatment evaluation. In the past decade, the development of digital imaging and storage has made it feasible, economical, and practical for the practicing laryngologist to use motion-picture video. These motion pictures are an invaluable education and training instrument and are often incorporated into clinical research. Today, color ultrahigh-speed imaging of vocal fold vibration has become the new research frontier.

Despite these substantial advances in motion-picture laryngeal imaging, new ethical issues have arisen. How much information should be captured and at what resolution, as digital storage may have constraints? Are there different considerations for recording office visits compared with recording surgical procedures? Is the information officially a component of the medical record, and do surgeons want to explain/review details of surgery with patients? Laryngeal surgeons and speech-language pathologists must address these issues carefully, wisely, and responsibly while maintaining the highest level of care for their patients.

References

1. Zeitels SM. Preface. In: Atlas of Phonomicrosurgery and Other Endolaryngeal Procedures for Benign and Malignant Disease. San Diego: Singular; 2001:xi–xii
2. Bozzini P. Der Lichtleiter oder Beschreibung einer einfachen Vorichtung, und ihrer Anwendung zur erleucht ung inherer Hohlen, und Zwischenraume des lebenden animalischen Korpers. Weimar; 1807
3. Avery J. 1844 [Cited in Mackenzie M. The Use of the Laryngoscope in Diseases of the Throat. Philadelphia: Lindsay and Blakiston, 1865:25]
4. Babington BG. Description of the glottiscope. London Medical Gazette 1829;3:555
5. Baumes. Compte Rendu des Travaux de la Societe de Medecine de Lyons 1836–1838;19:18
6. Cagniard de Latour C. [Cited by Fournie: Physiologie de la Voix.] Journal L'Institut 1825;350
7. Liston R. Practical Surgery. London: J. & A. Churchill; 1837:350
8. Selligue AF. 1832 [Cited in Mackenzie M. The Use of the Laryngoscope in Diseases of the Throat. Philadelphia: Lindsay and Blakiston; 1865:17]
9. Senn of Geneva. 1829 [Cited in Mackenzie M. The Use of the Laryngoscope in Diseases of the Throat. Philadelphia: Lindsay and Blakiston; 1865:11]
10. Zeitels SM, Vaughan CW. "External counterpressure" and "internal distention" for optimal laryngoscopic exposure of the anterior glottal commissure. Ann Otol Rhinol Laryngol 1994;103:669–675
11. Zeitels SM. A universal modular glottiscope system: the evolution of a century of design and technique for direct laryngoscopy. Ann Otol Rhinol Laryngol 1999;108(Suppl 179):1–24
12. Garcia M. Observations on the human voice. Proc R Soc Lond 1855;7:397–410
13. Clerf LH. Manuel Garcia's contribution to laryngology. Bull N Y Acad Med 1956;32:603–611
14. Mackenzie M. The Hygiene of the Vocal Organs, 8th ed. New York: Edgar S. Werner; 1899
15. Mackinlay MS. Garcia the Centenarian and His Times: Being a Memoir of Manuel Garcia's Life and Labours for the Advancement of Music and Science. New York: D. Appleton and Company; 1908
16. Turc L. On the laryngeal mirror and its mode of employment, with engravings on wood. Zeitschrift der Gesellschaft der Aerzte zu Wien. 1858;26: 401–409
17. Czermak JN. Ueber den Kehlkopfspiegel. Wien Med Wochenschr 1858;8:196–198
18. Stoerk C. On the layrngoscope. Zeitschrift Der Gesellschaft Der Aerzte Ze Wein 1859;46:721–727
19. Lewin G. Allgemeine Medizinische Central-Zeitung 1861;30:654
20. Mackenzie M. The Use of the Laryngoscope in Diseases of the Throat with an Appendix on Rhinoscopy. London: J. & A. Churchill; 1865
21. Mackenzie M. Growths in the Larynx. London, UK: J. & A. Churchill; 1871

22. Mackenzie M. Diseases of the Pharynx, Larynx, and Trachea. New York: William Wood & Co.; 1880

23. Fraenkel B. First healing of a laryngeal cancer taken out through the natural passages. Langenbecks Arch Klin Chir Ver Dtsch Z Chir 1886;12:283–286

24. Elsberg L. Laryngoscopal Medication or the Local Treatment of the Diseases of The Throat, Larynx, and Neighboring Organs, Under Sight. New York: William Wood & Co.; 1864

25. Elsberg L. Laryngoscopal Surgery Illustrated in the Treatment of Morbid Growths within the Larynx. Philadelphia: Collins; 1866

26. Zeitels SM. Jacob Da Silva Solis-Cohen: America's first head and neck surgeon. Head Neck 1997;19: 342–346

27. Solis-Cohen J. Clinical history of surgical affections of the larynx. Med Rec. 1869;4:244–247

28. Solis-Cohen J. Diseases of the Throat: A Guide to the Diagnosis and Treatment. New York: William Wood; 1872

29. Jackson C. Peroral Endoscopy and Laryngeal Surgery. St. Louis: Laryngoscope Co.; 1915

30. Ehrmann CH. Histoire des Polyps du Larynx. Straasbourg; 1850

31. Trousseau A, Belloc H. Phthisie Laryngie. Paris: Chez and Bailliere; 1837

32. Green H. A Treatise on Diseases of the Air Passages. New York: Wiley and Putnam; 1846

33. Green H. Observations on the Pathology of Croup. New York: John Wiley; 1849

34. Green H. On the subject of the priority in the medication of the larynx and trachea. American Medical Monthly 1854;1:241–257

35. Dr. Horace Green and his method. Harper's Weekly 1859;5:88–90

36. Donaldson F. The laryngology of Trousseau and Horace Green. Trans Am Laryngol Assoc 1890;12: 10–18

37. Elsberg L. President's address: laryngology in America. Trans Am Laryngol Assoc 1879;1:30–90

38. Green H. Morbid Growths within the Larynx. In: On the Surgical Treatment of Polypi of the Larynx, and Oedema of the Glottis. New York: G.P. Putnam; 1852

39. Kirstein A. Autoskopie des Larynx und der Trachea (Laryngoscopia directa, Euthyskopie, Besichtigung ohne Spiegel). Archiv fur Laryngologie und Rhinologie 1895;3:156–164

40. Kirstein A. Autoscopy of the Larynx and Trachea (Direct Examination Without Mirror). 1897

41. Killian G. Ueber direkte Bronchoskopie. Munch Med Wochenschr 1898;45:844–847

42. Jackson C. Position of the patient for peroral endoscopy. In: Jackson C, ed. Peroral Endoscopy and Laryngeal Surgery. St. Louis: Laryngoscope Co.; 1915:77–88

43. Killian G. Die Schwebelaryngoskopie. Archiv fur Laryngologie und Rhinologie 1912;26:277–317

44. Killian G. Suspension laryngoscopy and its practical use. J Laryngol Otol 1914;24:337–360

45. Killian G. Suspension laryngoscopy. In: Jackson C, ed. Peroral Endoscopy and Laryngeal Surgery. St. Louis: Laryngoscope Co.; 1915:133–154

46. Killian G. Die Schwebelaryngoskopie und ihre praktische Verwertung. Wien, Austria: Urban & Schwarzenberg; 1920

47. Israel S. The Directoscope of Haslinger in diagnosis and surgery of the larynx. Laryngoscope 1923; 33:945–948

48. Jackson C, Tucker G, Clerf LH. Laryngostasis and the laryngostat. Arch Otolaryngol Head Neck Surg 1925;1:167–169

49. Brunings W. Direct laryngoscopy: autoscopy by counter-pressure. In: Brunings W, ed. Direct Laryngoscopy, Bronchoscopy, and Esophagoscopy. London: Bailliere, Tindall, & Cox; 1912:110–115

50. Lewy RB. Suspension fixation gear power laryngoscopy (with motion pictures). Laryngoscope 1954;64:693–695

51. King NE. Direct laryngoscopy aided by a new laryngoscope "stabilizer." Arch Otolaryngol Head Neck Surg 1951;53:89–92

52. Roberts SE, Forman FS. Direct laryngoscopy, a simplified technique; an aid to the early detection of laryngeal cancer. Ann Otol Rhinol Laryngol 1948; 57:245–256

53. Roberts SE. A self retaining dual distal lighted laryngoscope with screw driven fulcrum lift. Laryngoscope 1952;62:215–221

54. Sommers KE. Direct laryngoscopy and description of a self-retaining attachment for the laryngoscope. Arch Otolaryngol Head Neck Surg 1952;55:484–488

55. Priest RE, Wesolowski S. Direct laryngoscopy under general anesthesia. Trans Am Acad Ophthalmol Otolaryngol 1960;64:639–648

56. Grundfast KM, Vaughn CW, Strong MS, de Vos P. Suspension microlaryngoscopy in the Boyce position with a new suspension gallows. Ann Otol Rhinol Laryngol 1978;87(4 Pt 1):560–566

57. Zeitels SM, Burns JA, Dailey SH. Suspension laryngoscopy revisited. Ann Otol Rhinol Laryngol 2004; 113:16–22

58. Hochman II, Zeitels SM, Heaton JT. An analysis of the forces and position required for direct laryngoscopic exposure of the anterior vocal folds. Ann Otol Rhinol Laryngol 1998;108:715–724

59. Hochman II, Zeitels SM. Exposure and visualization of the glottis for phonomicrosurgery. Oper Tech Otolaryngol Head Neck Surg 1998;9:192–195

60. Zeitels SM. Premalignant epithelium and microinvasive cancer of the vocal fold: the evolution of phonomicrosurgical management. Laryngoscope 1995;105(3 Pt 2, Suppl 67):1–51

61. Scalco AN, Shipman WF, Tabb HG. Microscopic suspension laryngoscopy. Ann Otol Rhinol Laryngol 1960;69:1134–1138

62. Jako GJ. Microscopic laryngoscopy. Presented at: New England Otolaryngological Society; 1964

63. Jako GJ, Kleinsasser O. Endolaryngeal micro-diagnosis and microsurgery. Presented at: Annual Meeting of the American Medical Association; 1966

64. Kleinsasser O. Mikrochirurgie im Kehlkopf. Arch Ohren Nasen Kehlkopfheilkd 1964;183:428–433

65. Jako GJ. Correspondence documents between Geza Jako and the Stuemar Instrument Company. 1962

66. Kleinsasser O. Microlaryngoscopy and Endolaryngeal Microsurgery. Philadelphia: W.B. Saunders; 1968

67. Polanyi T, Bredermeier HC, Davis TW Jr. CO2 laser for surgical research. Med Biol Eng Comput 1970;8: 548–558

68. Jako GJ. Laser surgery of the vocal cords. An experimental study with carbon dioxide lasers on dogs. Laryngoscope 1972;82:2204–2216

69. Strong MS, Jako GJ. Laser surgery in the larynx. Early clinical experience with continuous CO2 laser. Ann Otol Rhinol Laryngol 1972;81:791–798

70. Strong MS. Laser excision of carcinoma of the larynx. Laryngoscope 1975;85:1286–1289

71. Vaughan CW. Transoral laryngeal surgery using the CO_2 laser: laboratory experiments and clinical experience. Laryngoscope 1978;88(9 Pt 1):1399–1420

72. Vaughan CW, Strong MS, Shapshay SM. Treatment of T1 and in situ glottic carcinoma: the transoral approach. Otolaryngol Clin North Am 1980;13:509–513

73. Zeitels SM. Laser versus cold instruments for microlaryngoscopic surgery. Laryngoscope 1996;106(5 Pt 1):545–552

74. Oertel M. Ueber eine neues laryngostroboskopische. Untersuchungsmethode des Kehlkopfes. Centralblatt Medizinischen Wiss 1878;16:81–82

75. Oertel M. Das laryngo-stroboskop und die Laryngo-Stroboskpische Untersuchung. Archiv fur Laryngologie und Rhinologie 1895;3:1–16

76. Timcke R. [Synchronous stroboscopy of the vocal cords in man and analogous sources of sound and the duration of opening.] J Laryngol Rhinol Otol (Stuttg) 1956;35:331–335

77. Timcke R. [Laryngostroboscopy with a new synchronizing stroboscope.] Arch Ohren Nasen Kehlkopfheilkd 1956;169:539–543

78. von Leden H, Moore P, Timcke R. Laryngeal vibrations: measurements of the glottic wave: part III. The pathological larynx. Arch Otolaryngol Head Neck Surg 1960;71:16–35

79. von Leden H. The electronic synchron-stroboscope: its value for the practicing laryngologist. Ann Otol Rhinol Laryngol 1961;70:881–893

80. von Leden H. Plastic surgery of the larynx. Revista Panamerica de Otorrinolaringologia y Broncoesofagologia 1963;1:7–11

81. von Leden H. Surgery for the improvement of vocal function. Revista Panamerica de Otorrinolaringologia y Broncoesofagologia 1969;3:137–143

82. Isshiki N, von Leden H. Hoarseness: aerodynamic studies. Arch Otolaryngol Head Neck Surg 1964;80:206–213

83. Hirano M, Koike Y, Von Leden H. Maximum phonation time and air usage during phonation. Clinical study. Folia Phoniatr (Basel) 1968;20:185–201

84. Kirstein A. Preface. In: Autoscopy of the Larynx and Trachea (Direct Examination Without Mirror). Philadelphia: F.A. Davis Co.; 1897:vii

85. Jackson C. Instruments. In: Tracheo-Bronchoscopy, Esophagoscopy and Gastroscopy. St. Louis: Laryngoscope Co.; 1907:15–34

86. Holinger PH. Presentation of instruments. Fiber-optic laryngoscopes, bronchoscopes and esophagoscopes. Ann Otol Rhinol Laryngol 1965;74:1164–1167

87. Broyles EN. Address of the guest of honor. Presented at: Annual Meeting of the American Bronchoesophagological Association; 1962

88. Brunings W. Direct Laryngoscopy, Bronchoscopy, and Esophagoscopy. London: Bailliere, Tindall, & Cox; 1912

89. Jackson C. Instruments. In: Jackson C, ed. Peroral Endoscopy and Laryngeal Surgery. St. Louis: Laryngoscope Co.; 1915:11–51

90. Albrecht R. Uber den Wert koloskopischer Untersuchungsmethoden bei Leukoplakien und Carcinomen des Mundes und Kehlkopes. Arch Ohren Nasen Kehlkopfheilkd 1954;165:459–463

91. Lynch RC. Suspension laryngoscopy and its accomplishments. Ann Otol Rhinol Laryngol 1915;24:429–446

92. Nitze M. Eine neue Beleucht Untersuchungsmethode fur die Harnohre, Harnblase und Rektum. Wien Med Wochenschr 1879;24:649

93. Hopkins HH, Kapany NS. A flexible fiberscope using static scanning. Nature 1954;173:39

94. Hirschowitz BI, Curtiss LE, Peters CW, Pollard HM. Demonstration of a new gastroscope, the fiberscope. Gastroenterology 1958;35:50–53; discussion 51–53

95. Sawashima M, Hirose H. New laryngoscopic technique by use of fiber optics. J Acoust Soc Am 1968;43:168–169

96. Jackson C, Jackson CL. Cancer of the Larynx. Philadelphia: W.B. Saunders; 1939

97. Turck L. Atlas zur Klinik der Kehlkopfkrankheiten. Wein, Austria: Wilhelm Braumuller; 1866

98. Stein T. Photographing the larynx. Sci Am 1885;21:179–180

99. French T. Photographing the larynx. Arch Laryngol 1882;3:221–222

100. Garel J. Nouvel appariel perfectionee pour la photographie stereoscopique du larynx sur le vivant. Rev Laryngol Otol Rhinol 1919;40:249–253

101. Clerf LH. Photography of the larynx. Ann Otol Rhinol Laryngol 1925;34:101–107

102. Holinger PH. Endoscopic photography in otolaryngology and broncho-esophagology. Proc Inst Med Chic 1948;17:138

103. Berci G, Caldwell FH. A device to facilitate photography during indirect laryngoscopy. Med Biol Illus 1963;13:169–176

104. Yanagisawa E, Eibling DE, Suzuki M. A simple method of laryngeal photography through the operating microscope. "Macrolens technique." Ann Otol Rhinol Laryngol 1980;89(6 Pt 1):547–550

105. Yanagisawa E, Yanagisawa R. Laryngeal photography. Otolaryngol Clin North Am 1991;24:999–1022

106. Benjamin B. Technique of laryngeal photography. Ann Otol Rhinol Laryngol 1984;109(Suppl):1–11

107. Benjamin B. Eighteenth Daniel C. Baker, Jr, Memorial Lecture. Art and science of laryngeal photography. Ann Otol Rhinol Laryngol 1993;102(4 Pt 1):271–282

108. Farnsworth D. High-speed motion pictures of the human vocal cords. Bell Laboratories Record 1940;18:203–208

109. Kallen LA. Laryngostrobscopy in the practice of otolaryngology. Arch Otolaryngol Head Neck Surg 1932;16:791–807

110. Perlman HB. Laryngeal stroboscopy. Ann Otol Rhinol Laryngol 1945;54:159–165

111. Powell LS. The laryngostroboscope. Arch Otolaryngol Head Neck Surg 1934;19:708–710

112. Brubaker JD, Holinger PA. An endoscopic motion picture camera for otolaryngology and broncho-esophagology. J Biol Photogr Assoc 1947;15:171–192

113. Von Leden H. Laryngeal physiology. Cinematographic observations. J Laryngol Otol 1960;74:705–712

114. Gould WJ, Jako GJ, Tanabe M. Advances in high-speed motion picture photography of the larynx. Trans Am Acad Ophthalmol Otolaryngol 1974;78: ORL276–ORL278
115. Koike Y. High speed photography of the larynx and film data processing. Can J Otolaryngol 1975;4: 800–806
116. Yoshida Y, Hirano M, Nakajima T. A video-tape recording system for laryngo-stroboscopy. J Jpn Bronchoesophagol Soc 1979;30:1–5
117. Yanagisawa E. Videolaryngoscopy using a low cost home video system color camera. J Biol Photogr Assoc 1984;52:9–14
118. Yanagisawa K, Shi JM, Yanagisawa E. Color photography of video images of otolaryngological structures using a 35 mm SLR camera. Laryngoscope 1987; 97(8 Pt 1):992–993

2

Laryngeal Anatomy

Katherine A. Kendall

The interpretation of laryngeal imaging in the evaluation of patients with voice problems requires a strong foundation in the anatomy and physiology of the larynx. Practitioners interested in maximizing the information obtained from laryngeal imaging must be familiar with laryngeal anatomy. To that end, this chapter reviews basic laryngeal anatomy with an emphasis on structures seen from a superior view of the larynx, as that is the view typically obtained from imaging techniques currently in use.

The larynx is a structure supported by a cartilage framework, lined by mucosa, and suspended from the hyoid bone (**Fig. 2.1**). The primary purpose of the larynx is to act as a sphincter. It is designed to protect the distal airway from ingested material and saliva and to regulate airflow into and out of the airway. The larynx is also designed to maintain airway patency. The cricoid cartilage is the only complete cartilaginous ring supporting the airway (**Fig. 2.2**). Lastly, the larynx functions in voice production.

◆ Laryngeal Cartilages

The laryngeal cartilages not only provide structural support for the larynx but also move relative to one another to control vocal fold position, length, and tension. The thyroid cartilage is shaped like a shield with a right and left lamina fusing in the midline (**Fig. 2.3**). The thyroid and cricoid cartilages interdigitate at the cricothyroid joint, which is located at the inner surface of the inferior-posterior aspect of the thyroid cartilage. The cricoid cartilage sits inside the posterior aspect of the thyroid cartilage. It projects below the thyroid cartilage anteriorly (**Figs. 2.1 and 2.4**). The cricothyroid joint is a synovial articulation allowing the thyroid cartilage to rotate forward and backward on the attachment to the cricoid cartilage. The cricoid cartilage is shaped like a signet ring with the wide lamina located posteriorly (**Figs. 2.2 and 2.4**).

Sitting on the superior surface of the posterior cricoid lamina are the paired arytenoid cartilages. The arytenoid cartilages are pyramidal in shape with the vocal processes located anteriorly and the muscular processes located laterally. The vocal ligament of the vocal folds attaches to the vocal processes of the arytenoids cartilages (**Figs. 2.5 and 2.6**). The intrinsic laryngeal muscles that act to open and close the vocal folds attach to the muscular processes of the arytenoid cartilages laterally. The arytenoid cartilages articulate with the cricoid cartilage through a joint that allows the arytenoids to both swivel and slide relative to the cricoid cartilage. Their movement is responsible for adduction and abduction of the vocal folds. Finally, the epiglottis is a

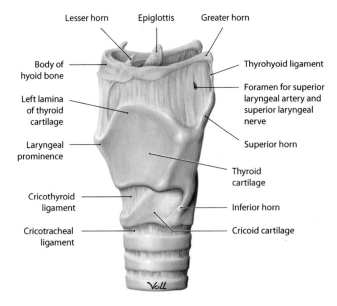

Lesser horn   Epiglottis   Greater horn

Body of
hyoid bone

Left lamina
of thyroid
cartilage

Laryngeal
prominence

Cricothyroid
ligament

Cricotracheal
ligament

Thyrohyoid ligament

Foramen for superior
laryngeal artery and
superior laryngeal
nerve

Superior horn

Thyroid
cartilage

Inferior horn

Cricoid cartilage

Fig. 2.1 Anterior-oblique view of the larynx. Note laryngeal cartilages are suspended from the hyoid bone via the thyrohyoid membrane. The cricoid cartilage is inferior to the thyroid cartilage along the anterior aspect of the larynx. The cricothyroid membrane spans the space between the two cartilages. (From THIEME Atlas of Anatomy, Neck and Internal Organs, © Thieme 2006. Illustration by Markus Voll.)

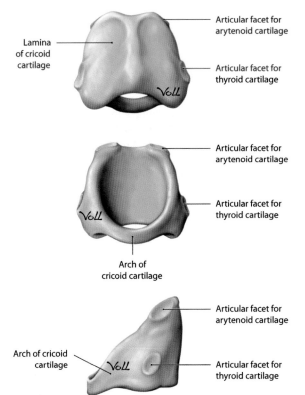

Lamina
of cricoid
cartilage

Articular facet for
arytenoid cartilage

Articular facet for
thyroid cartilage

Articular facet for
arytenoid cartilage

Articular facet for
thyroid cartilage

Arch of
cricoid cartilage

Articular facet for
arytenoid cartilage

Arch of cricoid
cartilage

Articular facet for
thyroid cartilage

Fig. 2.2 Cricoid cartilage. **(A)** Posterior view, **(B)** anterior view, **(C)** left lateral view. (From THIEME Atlas of Anatomy, Neck and Internal Organs, © Thieme 2006. Illustration by Markus Voll.)

2 Laryngeal Anatomy

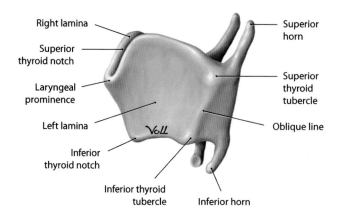

Right lamina

Superior thyroid notch

Laryngeal prominence

Left lamina

Inferior thyroid notch

Inferior thyroid tubercle

Inferior horn

Superior horn

Superior thyroid tubercle

Oblique line

Fig. 2.3 Thyroid cartilage, left lateral view. (From THIEME Atlas of Anatomy, Neck and Internal Organs, © Thieme 2006. Illustration by Markus Voll.)

leaf-shaped, elastic cartilage that is attached to the inner surface of the thyroid cartilage just above the anterior attachment of the vocal folds. This attachment is known as the petiole or thyroepiglottic ligament. The epiglottis flips down to cover the entry to the larynx during swallowing.

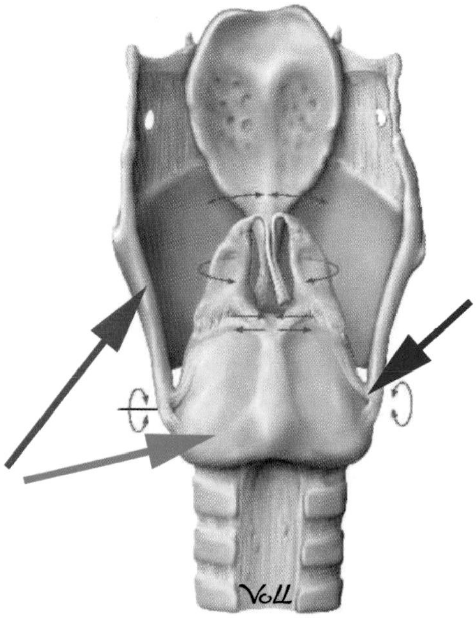

Fig. 2.4 Posterior view of the larynx. Note the relationship of the thyroid cartilage (*red arrow*) to the cricoid cartilage (*green arrow*). The purple arrow indicates the location of the cricothyroid joint. (From THIEME Atlas of Anatomy, Neck and Internal Organs, © Thieme 2006. Illustration by Markus Voll.)

◆ Laryngeal Membranes

The larynx is suspended from the hyoid bone by the thyrohyoid membrane. The thyrohyoid membrane is pierced by the superior laryngeal nerve and artery. The cricothyroid membrane runs between the anterior inferior margin of the thyroid cartilage and the anterior superior margin of the cricoid cartilage (**Fig. 2.1**).

◆ Laryngeal Intrinsic Musculature

The intrinsic laryngeal musculature attaches to the laryngeal cartilages, moving them relative to one another and thereby controlling the position, tension, and the length of the vocal folds (**Figs. 2.7 to 2.9**).

The lateral cricoarytenoid muscle is the primary adductor of the vocal folds. The fibers of this muscle attach to the muscular process of the arytenoid cartilages and run anteriorly and inferiorly to insert in the superior aspect of the cricoid cartilage. Muscle contraction pulls the muscular process of the arytenoids cartilages forward (and slightly downward), which, in turn, rotates the vocal processes of the arytenoids cartilages medially, closing the vocal folds (**Figs. 2.7 and 2.8**).

Abduction of the vocal folds results from contraction of the posterior cricoarytenoid muscles. These muscles also attach to the muscular process of the arytenoid cartilages and then run posteriorly to fan out and insert near the midline on the posterior aspect of the cricoid lamina. Shortening of the posterior

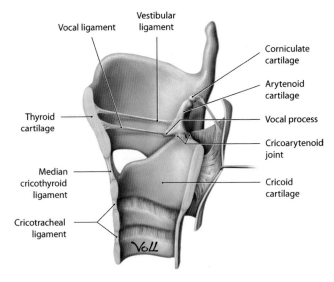

Vocal ligament

Vestibular ligament

Corniculate cartilage

Arytenoid cartilage

Thyroid cartilage

Vocal process

Cricoarytenoid joint

Median cricothyroid ligament

Cricoid cartilage

Cricotracheal ligament

Fig. 2.5 Sagittal view of the interior of the larynx illustrating the relationship of the arytenoid cartilage to the cricoid cartilage. Note that the vocal ligament runs between the vocal process of the arytenoid cartilage and the inner surface of the thyroid cartilage. (From THIEME Atlas of Anatomy, Neck and Internal Organs, © Thieme 2006. Illustration by Markus Voll.)

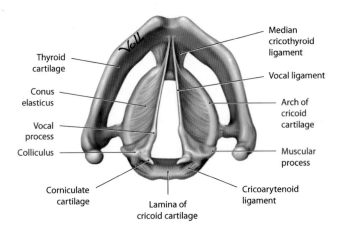

Thyroid cartilage

Median cricothyroid ligament

Conus elasticus

Vocal ligament

Vocal process

Arch of cricoid cartilage

Colliculus

Muscular process

Corniculate cartilage

Cricoarytenoid ligament

Lamina of cricoid cartilage

Fig. 2.6 Superior view of laryngeal cartilages. Note the position of the muscular process of the arytenoid cartilage.(From THIEME Atlas of Anatomy, Neck and Internal Organs, © Thieme 2006. Illustration by Markus Voll.)

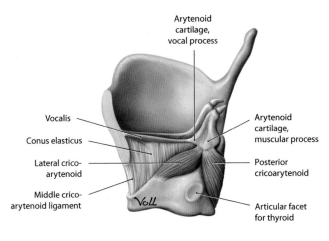

Arytenoid cartilage, vocal process

Vocalis

Arytenoid cartilage, muscular process

Conus elasticus

Lateral crico-arytenoid

Posterior cricoarytenoid

Middle crico-arytenoid ligament

Articular facet for thyroid

Fig. 2.7 Lateral view of the arytenoid and cricoid cartilages with the thyroid cartilage cut away. Note the lateral cricoarytenoid muscle runs from the muscular process of the arytenoid cartilage to the superior border of the cricoid cartilage. The posterior cricoarytenoid muscle runs from the muscular process of the arytenoid to the midline of the posterior lamina of the cricoid cartilage. (From THIEME Atlas of Anatomy, Neck and Internal Organs, © Thieme 2006. Illustration by Markus Voll.)

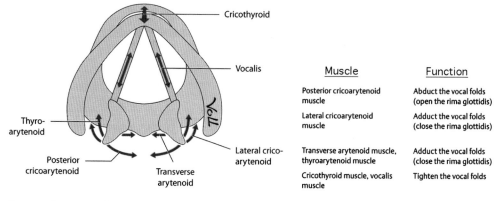

Muscle	Function
Posterior cricoarytenoid muscle	Abduct the vocal folds (open the rima glottidis)
Lateral cricoarytenoid muscle	Adduct the vocal folds (close the rima glottidis)
Transverse arytenoid muscle, thyroarytenoid muscle	Adduct the vocal folds (close the rima glottidis)
Cricothyroid muscle, vocalis muscle	Tighten the vocal folds

Fig. 2.8 Illustration of how the intrinsic laryngeal muscles act to move the laryngeal cartilages as viewed from above. (From THIEME Atlas of Anatomy, Neck and Internal Organs, © Thieme 2006. Illustration by Markus Voll.)

cricoarytenoid muscle fibers moves the muscular process of the arytenoid cartilages posteromedially. This results in movement of the vocal processes laterally and abduction of the vocal folds (**Figs. 2.7 to 2.9**).

The thyroarytenoid muscles attach to the anterior surface of the arytenoid cartilages and insert into the inner surface of the thyroid cartilage. They make up the "body" of the true vocal folds and are responsible for control of "tension" in the folds. In other words, contraction of these muscles results in greater resistance to airflow through the glottis during phonation allowing the buildup

of subglottic pressure and subsequent increases in vibratory amplitude and vocal volume. These muscles are also likely involved in pitch regulation as their contraction may lead to "shortening" of the vocal fold length (**Fig. 2.7**). The medial belly of the thyroarytenoid muscle is also known as the vocalis muscle (**Fig. 2.7**).

The muscles considered the most important in pitch regulation are the cricothyroid muscles. These muscles attach to the outer surface of the inferior margin of the thyroid cartilage and insert on the anterior and superior aspect of the cricoid cartilage. Contraction

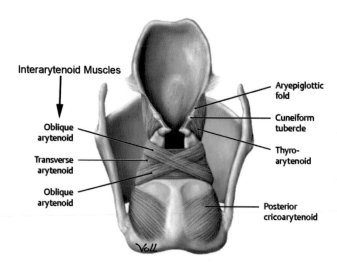

Fig. 2.9 Posterior view of the larynx illustrating the medial attachment of the posterior cricoarytenoid muscle. (From THIEME Atlas of Anatomy, Neck and Internal Organs, © Thieme 2006. Illustration by Markus Voll.)

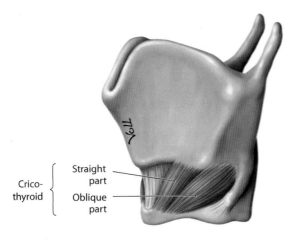

Fig. 2.10 Cricothyroid muscle. (From THIEME Atlas of Anatomy, Neck and Internal Organs, © Thieme 2006. Illustration by Markus Voll.)

Crico-thyroid
{
Straight part

Oblique part
}

of the cricothyroid muscles causes the thyroid cartilage to rock forward on the cricoid cartilage. This movement increases the distance between the vocal processes of the arytenoid cartilages and the thyroid cartilage, lengthening and tensing the vocal folds (**Figs. 2.10 and 2.11**).

The interarytenoid muscles run between the arytenoid cartilages and help to close the posterior glottis during voicing. Contraction of the interarytenoid muscles approximates the arytenoid cartilages. These muscles are innervated by both recurrent laryngeal nerves and will remain functional in cases of unilateral vocal fold paralysis secondary to recurrent laryngeal nerve palsy. The result is some movement of the arytenoid cartilage on the affected side due to contraction of the bilaterally innervated interarytenoid muscles, often confused with early signs of recovery (**Fig. 2.9**).

◆ Laryngeal Surface Anatomy

The clinical examination of the larynx is typically from above with a view of the superior surface of the laryngeal structures. It is therefore the laryngeal surface anatomy that is most pertinent to the clinical examination of the larynx and the use of laryngeal imaging. The entry into the larynx is called the vestibule. The vestibule is defined by the fold of mucosa at the tip of the epiglottis, the superior aspect

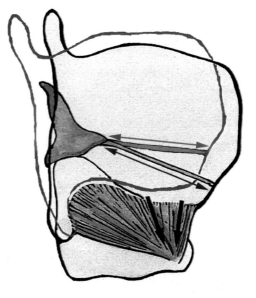

Fig. 2.11 Contraction of the cricothyroid muscle causes the thyroid cartilage to rotate forward and approximate the cricoid cartilage anteriorly. This movement increases the distance between the vocal processes of the arytenoid cartilages and the inner surface of the thyroid cartilage. As a result, the vocal fold elongates. The *purple arrow* depicts the relative length of the vocal fold before the cricothyroid muscle contracts and the *red arrow* depicts the increased length of the vocal fold with cricothyroid muscle contraction. (From Moore KL, Dalley AF. Clinically Oriented Anatomy, 5th ed. Baltimore: Lippincott Williams & Wilkins; 2006:1094.)

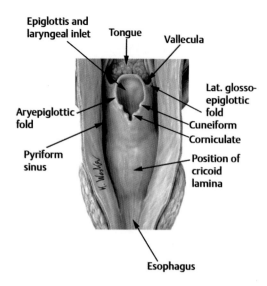

Fig. 2.12 Laryngeal surface anatomy: posterior view of laryngeal vestibule. (From THIEME Atlas of Anatomy, Neck and Internal Organs, © Thieme 2006. Illustration by Karl Wesker.)

of the aryepiglottic folds, and the top of the arytenoid cartilages (**Fig. 2.12**).

The Glottic Opening and the True Vocal Folds

The opening between the vocal folds during abduction is referred to as the *glottis* or the *glottic opening*. The margin of the glottic opening created by the edges of the vocal folds is called the *rima glottis*. The *membranous* portion of the vocal folds accounts for the anterior 52% of the margin of the rima glottis, and the *cartilaginous* portion of the vocal folds makes up the posterior 48% of the margin of the rima glottis (**Fig. 2.13**).[1] The rima glottis can only be adequately examined while the vocal folds are open, such as during quiet respiration. This also allows examination of the subglottic airway. It must be kept in mind that the undersurface of the vocal folds cannot be seen from a superior angle of view.

The membranous portion of the vocal folds is the portion of the vocal folds that vibrates during phonation and consists of the *thyroarytenoid* muscle and overlying *lamina propria* and epithelial covering. (Please see Chapter 3 for a more detailed discussion of the membranous vocal fold histology.) Healthy membranous vocal folds usually appear white in color and glistening with moisture. The membranous portion of the vocal folds inserts anteriorly in the midline into the *thyroid cartilage*. This area is referred to as the anterior commissure. Posteriorly, the membranous portion of the vocal folds inserts into the vocal process of the *arytenoid cartilage*. The cartilaginous portion of the vocal folds is created by the medial surface of the arytenoid cartilage and the overlying mucosa (**Figs. 2.14 and 2.15**). The interarytenoid portion of the rima glottis refers to the area between the arytenoid cartilages. The interarytenoid contours are the result of the interarytenoid muscles and overlying mucosa (**Fig. 2.13**).

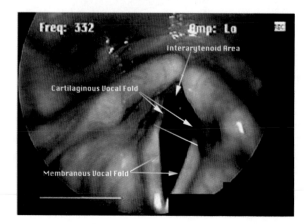

Fig. 2.13 Superior view of the larynx from imaging study. *White bar* over glottic opening defines the junction between the membranous portion of the vocal folds and the cartilaginous portion of the vocal folds.

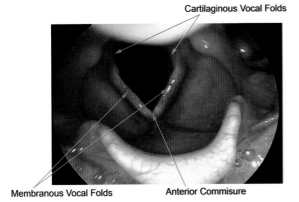

Cartilaginous Vocal Folds

Membranous Vocal Folds

Anterior Commisure

Fig. 2.14 Larynx viewed from above, vocal folds abducted.

The Quadrangular Membrane, the Ventricular Folds, and the Aryepiglottic Folds

The ventricular or "false" vocal folds and the aryepiglottic folds are the result of a sheet of connective tissue known as the quadrangular membrane. The quadrangular membrane is a rectangular sheet of connective tissue that attaches to the lateral margin of the epiglottis anteriorly and runs posteriorly to connect to the lateral margin of the arytenoid cartilage (**Figs. 2.15 to 2.17**). It is actually the inferior edge of the quadrangular membrane that creates the structure of the ventricular folds, and it is the superior edge of the quadrangular membrane that creates the superior margin of the aryepiglottic folds (**Fig. 2.16**). The laryngeal mucosa drapes over this connective tissue to create the folds. Within the superior margins of the aryepiglottic folds are located two small cartilages that act as batons, or stiffeners of the aryepiglottic folds. Those cartilages are the corniculate and cuneiform cartilages that sit at the apex of the arytenoids cartilages (**Figs. 2.12 and 2.18**).

The space between the superior surface of the true vocal folds and the ventricular fold is the ventricle. With a view from above, the contents of the ventricle cannot be evaluated as it is under the ventricular fold (**Figs. 2.16, 2.17, and 2.19**).

Right Aryepiglottic Fold

Vocal Process: Arytenoid Cartilages

Left Ventricular Fold

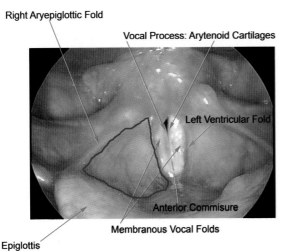

Anterior Commisure

Membranous Vocal Folds

Epiglottis

Fig. 2.15 Larynx viewed from above, vocal folds adducted. The location of the quadrangular membrane is outlined in purple.

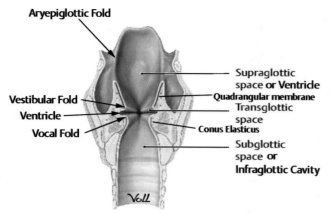

Aryepiglottic Fold

Vestibular Fold
Ventricle
Vocal Fold

Supraglottic
space or Ventricle
Quadrangular membrane
Transglottic
space
Conus Elasticus
Subglottic
space or
Infraglottic Cavity

Fig. 2.16 Laryngeal surface anatomy: coronal view. Note the conus elasticus and its role in shaping the vocal fold contour and the quadrangular membrane and its role in shaping the aryepiglottic fold and the ventricular fold. (From THIEME Atlas of Anatomy, Neck and Internal Organs, © Thieme 2006. Illustration by Markus Voll.)

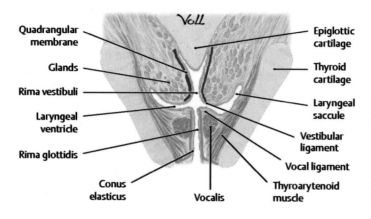

Quadrangular
membrane

Glands

Rima vestibuli

Laryngeal
ventricle

Rima glottidis

Conus
elasticus

Vocalis

Epiglottic
cartilage

Thyroid
cartilage

Laryngeal
saccule

Vestibular
ligament

Vocal ligament

Thyroarytenoid
muscle

Fig. 2.17 Histologic rendering of a coronal view. Quadrangular membrane is indicated in purple and conus elasticus in green. (From THIEME Atlas of Anatomy, Neck and Internal Organs, © Thieme 2006. Illustration by Markus Voll.)

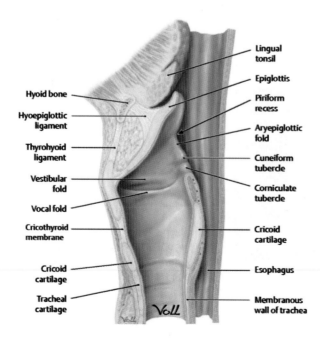

Hyoid bone

Hyoepiglottic
ligament

Thyrohyoid
ligament

Vestibular
fold

Vocal fold

Cricothyroid
membrane

Cricoid
cartilage

Tracheal
cartilage

Lingual
tonsil

Epiglottis

Piriform
recess

Aryepiglottic
fold

Cuneiform
tubercle

Corniculate
tubercle

Cricoid
cartilage

Esophagus

Membranous
wall of trachea

Fig. 2.18 Sagittal section of the larynx demonstrating the laryngeal surface anatomy. (From THIEME Atlas of Anatomy, Neck and Internal Organs, © Thieme 2006. Illustration by Markus Voll.)

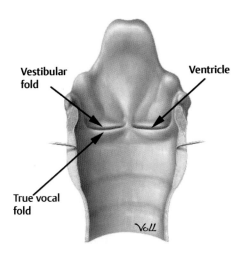

Labels on figure: Vestibular fold, Ventricle, True vocal fold, Voll

Fig. 2.19 Larynx opened from posterior midline to allow visualization of ventricular fold, ventricle, and vocal fold margin. (From THIEME Atlas of Anatomy, Neck and Internal Organs, © Thieme 2006. Illustration by Markus Voll.)

The Conus Elasticus and the Vocal Ligament

The true vocal folds contain connective tissue known as the vocal ligament. The ligament makes up the deep layer of the lamina propria and is involved in the attachment of the thyroarytenoid muscle to the connective tissue, that is, the lamina propria. The vocal ligament is the superior margin of another sheet of connective tissue known as the conus elasticus. The conus elasticus is attached to the inner surface of the cricoid cartilage and fans superiorly and medially to provide shape and contour to the undersurface of the vocal folds (**Figs. 2.6, 2.16, and 2.17**). It runs deep to the epithelial covering of the vocal fold and superficial to the deep musculature of the larynx.

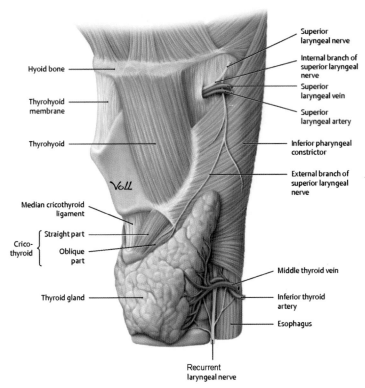

Labels: Hyoid bone, Thyrohyoid membrane, Thyrohyoid, Median cricothyroid ligament, Crico-thyroid { Straight part, Oblique part }, Thyroid gland, Superior laryngeal nerve, Internal branch of superior laryngeal nerve, Superior laryngeal vein, Superior laryngeal artery, Inferior pharyngeal constrictor, External branch of superior laryngeal nerve, Middle thyroid vein, Inferior thyroid artery, Esophagus, Recurrent laryngeal nerve, Voll

Fig. 2.20 Anterior-oblique view of the larynx demonstrating the course of the recurrent laryngeal nerve as it enters the larynx from the tracheo-esophageal groove. The external branch of the superior laryngeal nerve provides motor branches to the inferior laryngeal constrictor and the cricothyroid muscle. The internal branch of the superior laryngeal nerve enters the larynx via an opening in the thyrohyoid membrane. The blood supply to the larynx runs with the nerves. (From THIEME Atlas of Anatomy, Neck and Internal Organs, © Thieme 2006. Illustration by Markus Voll.)

◆ Innervation of the Larynx

The superior laryngeal nerve provides sensation to the laryngeal mucosa above the rima glottis. A motor branch of this nerve supplies the cricothyroid muscle. Recent anatomic studies indicate that branches of the motor part of the superior laryngeal nerve send fibers to the ipsilateral thyroarytenoid muscle in up to 47% of individuals.[2] This dual innervation of the thyroarytenoid muscle may account for the observation of persistent tone in the thyroarytenoid muscle despite no vocal fold movement in cases of recurrent laryngeal nerve injury. The nerve is a branch of the vagus nerve and enters the larynx via the thyrohyoid membrane (**Figs. 2.20 and 2.21**).

The recurrent laryngeal nerve (also a branch of the vagus nerve) provides motor branches to the rest of the intrinsic laryngeal muscles and sensory branches to the mucosa of the undersurface of the vocal fold and trachea. This nerve runs in the tracheoesophageal groove and enters the larynx from behind the cricothyroid joint (**Figs. 2.20 and 2.21**). The nerve then divides into an abductor branch that supplies the posterior thyroarytenoid muscle and an adductor branch that runs superiorly and anteriorly to supply the lateral cricoarytenoid muscle and terminates in the thyroarytenoid muscle.[3]

◆ Laryngeal Blood Supply

The blood supply to the larynx is from the superior laryngeal artery and inferior laryngeal artery, branches of the superior thyroid artery. The superior laryngeal artery travels with the superior laryngeal nerve and pierces

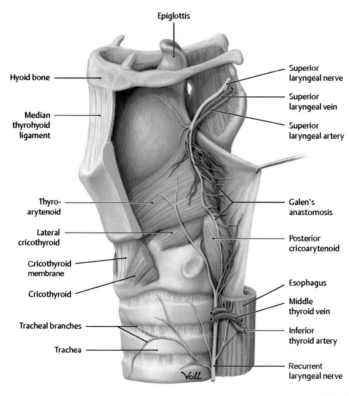

Epiglottis

Hyoid bone

Median thyrohyoid ligament

Thyro-arytenoid

Lateral cricothyroid

Cricothyroid membrane

Cricothyroid

Tracheal branches

Trachea

Superior laryngeal nerve

Superior laryngeal vein

Superior laryngeal artery

Galen's anastomosis

Posterior cricoarytenoid

Esophagus

Middle thyroid vein

Inferior thyroid artery

Recurrent laryngeal nerve

Fig. 2.21 Anterior-oblique view of the larynx with the thyroid cartilage removed demonstrating the course of the superior laryngeal nerve, vein, and artery and the recurrent laryngeal nerve along with the branches of the inferior thyroid artery and middle thyroid vein that supply the larynx. (From THIEME Atlas of Anatomy, Neck and Internal Organs, © Thieme 2006. Illustration by Markus Voll.)

the thyrohyoid membrane to enter the larynx. The inferior laryngeal artery runs with the external branch of the superior laryngeal nerve to supply the cricothyroid muscle (**Figs. 2.20 and 2.21**).

◆ Conclusion

Familiarity with basic laryngeal anatomy is critical for the interpretation of laryngeal imaging studies. Clinicians familiar with normal laryngeal anatomy are able to detect alterations in the anatomy and functioning of the larynx due to pathology.

References

1. Busuttil A, Davis BC, Maran AG. The soft tissue/cartilage relationship in the laryngeal glottis. J Laryngol Otol 1981;95:385–391
2. Mu L, Sanders I. The human cricothyroid muscle: three muscle bellies and their innervation patterns. J Voice 2009;23:21–28
3. Damrose EJ, Huang RY, Ye M, Berke GS, Sercarz JA. Surgical anatomy of the recurrent laryngeal nerve: implications for laryngeal reinnervation. Ann Otol Rhinol Laryngol 2003;112:434–438

3

Laryngeal Physiology

Murtaza T. Ghadiali and Gerald S. Berke

A thorough understanding of laryngeal physiology provides the foundation for the interpretation of laryngeal imaging in the evaluation of patients with laryngeal disorders. Once the clinician understands the interactions between the laryngeal structures and the pulmonary system that result in voice, it becomes clear that almost every case of laryngeal pathology interrupts the normal laryngeal physiology in a predictable way. Throughout the chapters in this book, authors will refer back to a discussion of the essential elements of normal laryngeal physiology to explain abnormalities of vibration or the impact of various pathologies on voice. This chapter describes the essential elements of normal laryngeal functioning and the unique histology of the larynx that allows the generation of the sound we all know as the human voice.

The human larynx is a highly specialized organ that provides many unique functions. Its primary function is as a gateway to the upper respiratory tract, and it plays an integral role in facilitating breathing, swallowing, and phonation. Laryngeal function and physiology relies on a sophisticated network of neural signaling, neuromuscular control, respiratory regulation, and vocal fold vibratory mechanics. A complete understanding of these complex interactions is still a distant goal of researchers, but much has been accomplished.

◆ Developmental Adaptations of the Larynx

The most primitive larynx (*Polypterus*, lungfish) serves as a sphincter to protect the lower airways from food or other foreign bodies.[1] Additionally, discrete muscular fibers provide active dilation of the glottic opening. With the need for additional ventilation in a terrestrial environment, active glottal dilation is enhanced by the acquisition of lateral cartilages that serve as a site for insertion of the dilator musculature. A cartilaginous ring arising between the glottis and the trachea on which these lateral cartilages sit adds further structural support and prevents collapse of this part of the respiratory system.[2] This phylogenetic development can be found in certain types of vertebrates such as reptiles. Phonation is a late adaptation, wherein the larynx functions like a flutter valve. This phenomenon is found only in mammals that have the appropriate respiratory machinery to power the vocal folds, including thoracoabdominal musculature. Among mammals, humans have developed the ability to create intricate sounds and spoken language using the glottis as a vibratory sound source to power the resonators of the pharynx, oral cavity, and nasopharynx.

The separation of the upper aerodigestive tract into channels for breathing and deglutition is a basic finding among all mammals. Furthermore, the larynx is in a relatively high position in close proximity to the posterior nasal cavity. This nasolaryngeal relationship provides a continuous airway from the nose to the lungs thus decreasing the risk of pulmonary compromise from swallowed food and permitting some species to smell approaching predators while grazing.[2] The human infant demonstrates a similar relationship with the close location of the epiglottis to the posterior soft palate. A common airway is formed that protects the newborn from aspiration. This relationship is lost after 6 months of age in humans, as the larynx descends in the neck.[3] At the base of the tongue, the epiglottis is uniquely shaped to direct food laterally to the pyriform sinuses and away from the midline glottis. A fold of tissue running between the epiglottis and the lateral cartilages (also termed the arytenoid cartilages), or the aryepiglottic folds, acts as a further barrier, directing food toward the lateral pharyngeal walls and away from the laryngeal opening or glottis. Thus, many of the central adaptations of the human larynx serve to facilitate its primary function of airway protection.

◆ Vocal Fold Histology

The vocal fold, or vocal cord, is a fold of tissue spanning the distance between the anterior aspect of the arytenoid cartilages and the inner surface of the front of the thyroid cartilage. This fold of tissue has a complex histologic organization that permits it to vibrate when air is passed across the tissue. To understand fully vocal fold vibratory functioning, it is important to describe the histologic complexity of the vocal fold (**Fig. 3.1**).

The vocal fold consists of five histologic layers: epithelium; superficial, intermediate, and deep layers of the lamina propria; and the thyroarytenoid muscle. The surface epithelium contains stratified squamous cells devoid of mucous glands, unlike the pseudo-stratified ciliated, columnar epithelium found in the remaining respiratory tract.[4] This modification allows the vocal fold to maintain shape and undulate freely over the underlying vocalis muscle.

A complex basement membrane zone connects the epithelium of the vocal fold to the superficial lamina propria (SLP).[5] The SLP is also known as Reinke's space and lies immediately deep to the surface epithelium. The basement membrane zone contains a delicate network of proteins and collagen fibers that

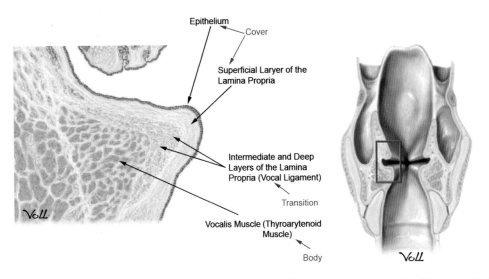

Epithelium
Cover
Superficial Laryer of the Lamina Propria
Intermediate and Deep Layers of the Lamina Propria (Vocal Ligament)
Transition
Vocalis Muscle (Thyroarytenoid Muscle)
Body

Fig. 3.1 Vocal fold histologic section demonstrating structural layers. (From THIEME Atlas of Anatomy, Neck and Internal Organs, © Thieme 2006. Illustration by Markus Voll.)

allow the epithelium to adhere to the gelatinous SLP.[6] The SLP layer contains loose fibrous tissue and a network of hyaluronic acid, mucopolysaccharides, decorin, and other extracellular matrix (ECM) components. The SLP contains very few fibroblasts and is primarily devoid of both elastic and collagen fibers. It provides little resistance to vibration and is very flexible, characteristics that are required for proper phonation to occur. Any change in the composition of the ECM can lead to a loss of vibratory function. In particular, alterations in levels of hyaluronan and fibronectin have been found in models of pathologic vocal fold lesions.[7] This has created significant interest in the development of novel therapeutic interventions for vocal fold scarring, including use of autologous fibroblasts and hyaluronan hydrogel.[7,8]

The intermediate layer of the lamina propria is similar to the SLP but contains higher amounts of collagen and mature elastin fibers arranged longitudinally. It is a highly hydrated structure, rich in fibrous and interstitial proteins as well as glycosaminoglycans and proteoglycans. The intermediate layer of the lamina propria also contains large quantities of hyaluronic acid that may act as a shock absorber.

The deep layer of the lamina propria is dense and contains the highest concentration of fibroblasts and collagen fibers. The properties of collagen limit its ability to stretch; therefore, the presence of this layer prohibits overextension of the vocal fold. The deep layer of the lamina propria is 1 to 2 mm thick. Together with the intermediate layer of the lamina propria, the deep layer forms the vocal ligament. The vocal ligament also forms the uppermost portion of the conus elasticus.

The deepest layer of the vocal fold consists of intrinsic laryngeal muscle, namely the thyroarytenoid or vocalis muscle.

A few histologic variations of clinical and physiologic importance exist at the anterior and posterior borders of the membranous vocal fold. Anteriorly, the intermediate layer of the lamina propria thickens to form an area called the anterior macula flava. This structure connects to the anterior commissure tendon, also known as Broyle's tendon, which provides a transition zone from the inner perichondrium of the thyroid cartilage.[9,10] Similarly, posteriorly, the intermediate layer of the

lamina propria of the vocal fold thickens again to form the posterior macula flava, which transitions into the arytenoid cartilage. These modifications are thought to facilitate a transition from the membranous vocal fold to the stiffer thyroid and arytenoid cartilage. In addition, they may serve to protect and cushion the vocal fold from damage during phonatory vibration and may contain stem cells with which to repopulate the vocal fold tissues.[9,10]

The biomechanics of fold vibration is intimately associated with the fold's layered structure. The five histologic layers of the vocal fold function as three different mechanical groups (**Fig. 3.2**). The epithelium and SLP make up the *cover* of the vocal fold; the intermediate and deep layers of the lamina propria make up the vocal ligament or the *transition*; and the thyroarytenoid muscle makes up the *body* of the vocal fold. The relationship between these three layers and the gradient of increasing stiffness provides the mechanics for the complex mucosal wave. Vibration of the vocal fold *cover* (epithelium and SLP) results in the rhythmic opening and closing of the folds, which is critical to the creation of the intermittent pulses of air that we perceive as sound. Stiffness in the cover will result in impairment of vibration and hoarseness. The special components (cells, proteins, matrix scaffolding) and organization of the lamina propria layers (superficial, intermediate, and deep) are all crucial in vocal fold vibration. Any changes to any of these components results in decreased pliability, thus altering

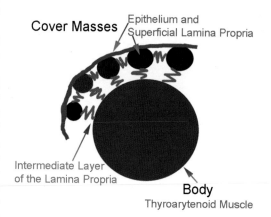

Fig. 3.2 Body-cover theory of vibration.

vocal fold vibration. It is important for surgeons to keep in mind that unintentional violation of the transition zone during surgical excision of superficial lesions of the vocal fold can lead to scarring of the epithelium to the deeper tissue layers and stiffness. On the other hand, decorin, found in the superficial layer of the lamina propria, reduces fibrosis and scarring after injury. Therefore, surgery and inflammation limited to the SLP is less likely to result in scar formation. The *body* (vocal ligament and vocalis muscle) of the vocal fold affects vocal fold tension and regulates the resistance to airflow.

◆ Laryngeal Respiratory Physiology

The larynx has an integral role in respiration, although its primary role in this regard remains a protective one. By closing during deglutition, it guards the lower airways from ingested or inhaled materials. The importance of the larynx as a valve that regulates airflow, both in inspiration and expiration, has been clearly established.[11] A variety of laryngeal receptors under central nervous system control also exists to regulate both protective and pathologic glottal reflexes. The glottal inlet generally opens with inspiration and closes reflexively during swallowing and in response to chemical or tactile stimulation.

The larynx regulates resistance to airflow in and out of the lungs and is protected from inspiratory collapse by the rigid cricoid cartilage, which forms a complete ring around the laryngeal airway.[11] The vocal folds form a laryngeal valve mechanism that regulates the transglottic pressure difference during both respiration and phonation.[12] Laryngeal and upper tracheal airflow is predominately turbulent as a result of the significant reduction in cross-sectional area at the level of the glottis.[13]

In the resting breathing state, contraction of the posterior cricoarytenoid (PCA) muscles results in abduction of the vocal folds during inspiration, providing a patent laryngeal airway.[14] The synchronous action of the cricothyroid muscles may contribute slightly to this dilatory function.[15] The vocal fold movement during inspiration is coordinated such that abduction occurs just before diaphragmatic contraction.

This provides a mechanical advantage by preventing airflow from occurring against a closed glottis.[11] The passive relaxation of the PCA muscles during expiration allows for adduction of the vocal folds, with the other adductory muscles such as the thyroarytenoid muscle providing some support and a small amount of positive end expiratory pressure slowing the rate of exhalation and preventing collapse of the distal bronchioles.

During hyperpneic and hyperthermic states of breathing, and as a result of underlying hypercapnia, the vocal folds abduct more widely during inspiration. This phenomenon continues into the expiratory phase and significantly reduces laryngeal resistance in addition to decreasing both the rate and duration of expiration.[16]

The larynx has an abundant network of afferent sensory innervation that facilitates feedback control of its protective mechanisms. The afferent fibers run primarily through the internal branch of the superior laryngeal nerve, although a few fibers are also transmitted via the recurrent laryngeal nerve.[17] Stimulation of sensory afferent receptors in the larynx can lead to sustained reflex adduction of the vocal folds. The underlying mechanism of a cough can be a result of similar laryngeal stimulation or coughing can be voluntary if mucus or foreign matter needs to be ejected from the lower airways. Coughs are initiated with a preparatory inspiratory phase where an increased inspiratory effort leads to exaggerated abduction of the vocal folds. This is followed by a compressive phase as the glottis tightly closes and intrapulmonary and subglottic pressure rises in response to expiratory muscle contraction. Finally, the cough is terminated with an abrupt opening of the vocal folds, allowing air to rush through at high velocities.[18,19]

The false vocal folds are also important during coughing, as they function as exit valves to prevent the egress of air from the trachea until sufficient subglottic pressure has been generated. In a closed position, they seal together tightly when pressure from the lower airway increases. The phenomenon of adducted false vocal folds is due to their unique shape and configuration and occurs independently of muscle tone.[2] Thus, expectorative functions of the larynx remain unimpaired even in bilateral laryngeal paralysis because passive closure of the false vocal folds is sufficient for effective cough production.

Several types of laryngeal receptors exist that control a variety of sensory and maladaptive reflexes. Mechanoreceptors include "pressure," "cold," and "drive" receptors.[20] Airflow receptors are activated by cooling of the laryngeal mucosa during inspiration. Other "drive" receptors respond to laryngeal movements or motion during breathing.[21] Laryngeal chemoreceptors are activated by various chemical and noxious stimuli, including liquids such as water. Intralaryngeal water can trigger an apnea reflex and is thought to play a role in the pathogenesis of sudden infant death syndrome.[22] Protective reflex glottal closure is usually replicated by direct electrical stimulation of the superior laryngeal nerve, but it can also be triggered by a variety of sensory stimuli. Afferent innervation of the laryngeal adductor reflex occurs via the internal branch of the superior laryngeal nerve and motor action from the recurrent laryngeal nerve branch of the vagus nerve. One example of a pathologic exaggeration of this reflex is laryngospasm. Laryngospasm leads to forceful and prolonged glottal closure that usually lasts long after the offending stimulus has ceased. Typical irritants that can induce laryngospasm include instrumental laryngeal manipulation during general anesthesia, airway foreign bodies, and laryngopharyngeal reflux.[19]

Laryngeal stimulation can also lead to the activation of a multitude of cardiovascular reflexes. These changes are usually found during intubation or extubation under general anesthesia or when the larynx is exposed to inhaled irritants.[23] Systemic hypertension and profound bradycardia have most commonly been described in previous studies.[24,25] The receptors for these reflexes have been characterized as polymodal and nociceptive although little is known about their morphology.

◆ Laryngeal Contribution to Swallowing

The mechanism of swallowing is controlled by the central nervous system and consists of both supratentorial and brain-stem components. The supratentorial component is found in the frontal cortex anterior to the sensorimotor cortex.[26] The brain-stem components are found in the dorsal aspect of the nucleus tractus solitarius in addition to the ventral aspect of the nucleus ambiguous.[27] Cortical and subcortical areas of the brain are integral for voluntary initiation of swallowing, whereas the brain stem is responsible for the involuntary stages of swallowing.[28]

Swallowing can be divided into three stages: oral, pharyngeal, and esophageal. The oral stage is controlled by voluntary neuromuscular function, whereas the pharyngeal and esophageal stages are involuntary. Intact laryngeal function is most crucial to the pharyngeal stage. During the pharyngeal stage, the larynx serves to primarily protect the airway while inspiration is necessarily inhibited.

At the initiation of the pharyngeal phase of swallowing, the larynx and the hyoid elevate and are pushed forward toward the tongue base. This movement enlarges the pharynx and creates a vacuum or negative pressure in the hypopharynx and larynx, thus allowing the food bolus to be pushed downward. This movement also contributes to the relaxation of the cricopharyngeus muscle. Next, and most importantly, the true and false vocal folds adduct, with closure beginning at the level of the true vocal folds and progressing up to the false vocal folds and then to the aryepiglottic folds. True vocal fold closure is the primary laryngopharyngeal protective mechanism that prevents aspiration during the pharyngeal swallowing stage. The epiglottis then descends over the superior portion of the larynx and protects the airway by diverting the ingested material toward and into the pyriform sinuses. If the ingested material is of a liquid consistency, then the epiglottis acts to slow the liquid movement through the pharynx, giving the vocal folds additional time to adduct and the larynx time to elevate.

The intricate nature of laryngeal movements and reflexes during the pharyngeal swallow stage can lead to significant aspiration and dysphagia when laryngopharyngeal sensation is compromised. This subject has been studied extensively in recent times, and new technology has emerged that allows for sensory testing during endoscopic examination of swallowing.[29] These studies have confirmed the importance of sensory feedback control during pharyngeal swallowing, although the mechanism has yet to be delineated completely.[30,31]

◆ Laryngeal Motion and Vibratory Physiology

Motor innervation to the intrinsic laryngeal musculature originates in the medullary nucleus ambiguus. The action of the intrinsic laryngeal muscles primarily determines vocal fold shape and movement. These muscles dictate the extent of abduction, adduction, length, mass, stiffness, and tension of the vocal folds (see Chapter 2, **Figs. 2.7, 2.9, and 2.10**). These six biomechanical parameters profoundly alter the vibratory characteristics of the vocal folds and thus the nature of the sound produced during vibration or phonation.

The chief adductory muscles include the thyroarytenoid, lateral cricoarytenoid (LCA), and interarytenoid. The LCA muscle originates from the lateral aspect of the cricoid cartilage and inserts onto the muscular process of the arytenoid. The thyroarytenoid muscle originates from the inner thyroid cartilage and inserts onto the muscular process of the arytenoid. The thyroarytenoid forms the body of the vocal folds and it also shortens, lowers, and thickens the vocal folds, in addition to altering the intrinsic stiffness of the folds during contraction. In this way, contraction of the thyroarytenoid muscle increases the resistance to airflow through the glottis. The LCA muscle is the stronger adductor, and its activity includes elongating and thinning the vocal fold, but it primarily functions to close the posterior portion of the folds.[32] Males require the posterior closure to generate enough subglottal pressure to set the folds into vibration. Conversely, women may not demonstrate complete posterior closure and do not need the extra subglottal pressure to phonate due to their less massive folds. The PCA muscle is the only abductory muscle. It originates at the posterior surface of the cricoid cartilage and inserts onto the muscular process of the arytenoid. Its action is accomplished by pulling the muscular process both posteriorly and inferiorly.

The PCA muscle also elevates, elongates, and thins the vocal fold and provides stabilization of the arytenoids allowing the other intrinsic muscles to function more efficiently. The cricothyroid muscle originates from the cricoid cartilage and has dual insertions into both anterior and posterior aspects of the thyroid cartilage lamina.[33] Contraction of the cricothyroid muscles increases vocal fold tension and length by increasing the distance between the posterior cricoid cartilage and the anterior commissure. This muscle is central to controlling and increasing vocal pitch by its ability to thin and simultaneously stretch the fold.

The normal vibratory-phonatory cycle is regulated by several principles that include adequate respiratory support, appropriate glottal closure, an intact vocal fold cover, and fine-tuned control of vocal fold length and tension.[9] The vibrating vocal folds convert the airflow and pressure energy generated by the lungs, the diaphragm, and the thoracoabdominal musculature into acoustic power. Many factors affect the production of sound at the glottal level, and these include subglottal pressure, glottal impedance, volume velocity of glottal airflow, and supraglottal pressure.[10]

Voice is achieved by a complex repeating cycle in which glottal opening and closing modulates the transglottic air-stream at anywhere from 50 to 1000 cycles per second. Despite many years of mathematical and tissue modeling studies on the nature of fold vibration, the essential factors permitting sustained vibration of the vocal folds is not yet understood. However, the series of events characterizing a vibratory cycle have been described. Each cycle begins with the subglottic pressure pushing against the undersurface of the closed vocal folds. The pressure from the lungs eventually overcomes the medial closing forces holding the folds together, also termed the phonatory threshold pressure, and pushes the vocal folds apart. The inferior-most part of the folds opens first, and the tissue is progressively compressed as an "air bubble" rises to the superior surface of the folds. This compression from inferior to superior is called a traveling wave. When the "bubble" or wave reaches the superior portion of the folds, they start to unzip, and pressurized air begins to escape from the folds as a jet. This jet can attain velocities of 50 or more meters per second. The vocal folds open first anteriorly.

At the superior portion of the folds, the tissue wave propagates out laterally. However, during this lateral wave propagation, the inferiormost portion of the folds now begins to move medially as a result of many factors, including a decrease in subglottic pressure, the recoiling force generated by the elasticity of the vocal folds, and a vacuum-like negative pressure phenomenon created by the Bernoulli effect.[9] The vocal folds contact again inferiorly, and this closure then progresses superiorly and anteriorly until the vocal folds close completely, leading to repetition of the cycle (**Figs. 3.3 and 3.4**). Studies of the medial surface of the vocal folds have confirmed significantly greater medial-lateral and vertical displacements than anterior-posterior displacement.[34] Sound is produced during fold oscillation by the inertial interaction of the pulsating jet against the air columns above and below the folds creating an air pressure wave that then interacts with the resonators of the vocal tract before exiting the lips. It is known that the maximum degree of air pressure modulation occurs at the moment of closure of the inferior vocal fold margin. In addition, the sound produced by the folds is complex in nature having both a fundamental frequency and associated harmonics decreasing at 12 dB per octave.

The simplest models of phonation are based on the principle that pitch depends on the frequency of vocal fold vibration, which is related to the vocal fold length, whereas loudness is the result of subglottic pressure and the amplitude of vibration of the vocal folds. Increases in subglottic pressure require greater resistance to airflow at the level of the glottis and greater air pressure generated by the lungs. Studies of vocal fold oscillation suggest, however, that the velocity and wavelength of the traveling wave controls the frequency of vibration.[35,36] As each traveling wave travels faster, the frequency of vibration increases and so does the pitch of the voice. Similarly, as the folds are thinned, the effective wavelength decreases, and the frequency of vibration increases along with the perceived pitch of the voice. Central neuromotor control of the intrinsic laryngeal muscles affects traveling wave characteristics. In other words, alteration in laryngeal muscle activity affects the phonatory sound quality. Thus, through central neuromuscular control, voice quality is altered.

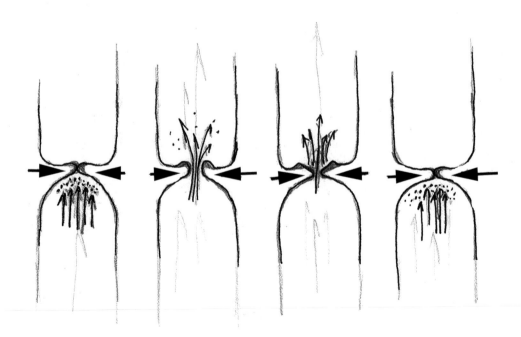

Fig. 3.3 Transglottic airflow and vocal fold vibratory cycle.

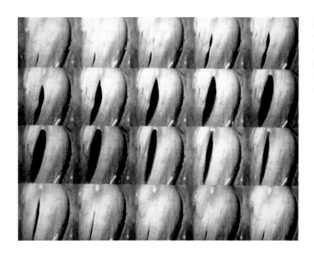

Fig. 3.4 Vocal folds viewed from above during one vibratory cycle. The anterior aspect of the vocal folds opens first with opening progressing posteriorly. The posterior aspect of the vocal folds closes first with closure progressing anteriorly.

The three main types of vibratory patterns that exist are modal, falsetto, and glottal fry. In the modal register, the vocal folds exhibit a normal vibratory topography as the mucosa vibrates independently of the muscle. In falsetto, glottal closure is incomplete, and only the uppermost free edges of the folds are involved in vibration, creating a high-pitched voice. Glottal fry is characterized by an excessively low-pitched voice with the vocal folds tightly approximated for a longer than normal duration during the vibratory cycle. These modes of phonation can be further characterized by the analysis of the open and closed phases of the vibratory cycle. The opening phase begins once the vocal fold margins are elevated and ends when the opening is maximal. A closing phase follows, which is finalized when the vocal fold margins are adjoining. The relationship between the two phases is based on the vocal pitch and intensity. During loud phonation, the closing phase is longer than the opening phase. The pitch also influences the closing phase, and the higher the pitch, the shorter the closing phase. The amplitude of displacement correlates positively with the intensity of phonation and negatively with the fundamental frequency and is decreased for breathy and pressed phonation modes.

Phonation would be incomplete without the modulation of the glottal output by the resonators in the chest, pharynx, and nasal cavities. These differing vocal tract configurations act as filters that modify glottal phonation to form the sound that is perceived as the human voice. Recent clinical research has led to the description of unique aerodynamic phenomena such as glottal and supraglottal vortical flow that may also significantly contribute to phonation.[37] Distortions in these rotational motions have been found in a variety of laryngeal pathologies, including disorders with asymmetric vocal fold tension.[38] In addition, the development of an ex vivo larynx model has the potential to facilitate the measurement of glottal variables in a neuromuscularly correct model.[39]

◆ Laryngeal Physiology and High-Speed Imaging

The advent of high-speed digital videoendoscopy has revolutionized laryngeal imaging. Digital video systems now exist with the ability to capture up to 10,000 high-resolution color images per second.[40,41] Stroboscopy is limited in its ability to provide information about individual vibratory cycles. High-speed imaging, on the other hand, has the potential to increase our understanding of vibratory physiology exponentially. The combination of laser technology with high-speed imaging systems has led to accurate measurements of vocal fold length, vibratory amplitude, glottal area, and vertical mucosal wave movements. Investigators are now using these systems to provide detailed visual playback of mucosal wave dynamics and vibratory symmetry.[41] The future of phonatory physiology is truly exciting and promising, as clinicians and researchers continue to uncover fascinating details about vocal fold vibration.

References

1. Negus VE. The Comparative Anatomy and Physiology of the Larynx. London, UK: Heinemann; 1949

2. Sasaki CT. Physiology of the larynx. In: English G, ed. Otolaryngology. Hagerstown, MD: Harper and Row; 1984

3. Sasaki CT, Levine PA, Laitman JT, Crelin ES Jr. Postnatal descent of the epiglottis in man: a preliminary report. Arch Otolaryngol 1977;103:169–171

4. Nassar VH, Bridger GP. Topography of the laryngeal mucous glands. Arch Otolaryngol 1971;94:490–498

5. Gray SD. Cellular physiology of the vocal folds. Otolaryngol Clin North Am 2000;33:679–698

6. Gray SD, Pignatari SS, Harding P. Morphologic ultrastructure of anchoring fibers in normal vocal fold basement membrane zone. J Voice 1994;8:48–52

7. Thibeault SL. Advances in our understanding of the Reinke space. Curr Opin Otolaryngol Head Neck Surg 2005;13:148–151

8. Chhetri DK, Head C, Revazova E, Hart S, Bhuta S, Berke GS. Lamina propria replacement therapy with cultured autologous fibroblasts for vocal fold scars. Otolaryngol Head Neck Surg 2004;131:864–870

9. Noordzij JP, Ossoff RH. Anatomy and physiology of the larynx. Otolaryngol Clin North Am 2006;39:1–10

10. Sataloff RT, Heman-Ackah YD, Hawkshaw MJ. Clinical anatomy and physiology of the voice. Otolaryngol Clin North Am 2007;40:909–929, v

11. Bartlett D Jr. Respiratory functions of the larynx. Physiol Rev 1989;69:33–57

12. Proctor DF. Breathing, Speech, and Song. Vienna, Austria: Springer-Verlag; 1980

13. Olson DE, Sudlow MF, Horsfield K, Filley GF. Convective patterns of flow during inspiration. Arch Intern Med 1973;131:51–57

14. Suzuki M, Kirchner JA. The posterior cricoarytenoid as an inspiratory muscle. Ann Otol Rhinol Laryngol 1969;78:849–864

15. Suzuki M, Kirchner JA, Murakami Y. The cricothyroid as a respiratory muscle. Its characteristics in bilateral recurrent laryngeal nerve paralysis. Ann Otol Rhinol Laryngol 1970;79:976–983

16. England SJ, Bartlett D Jr. Changes in respiratory movements of the human vocal cords during hyperpnea. J Appl Physiol 1982;52:780–785

17. Mathew OP, Sant'Ambrogio G, Fisher JT, Sant'Ambrogio FB. Respiratory afferent activity in the superior laryngeal nerves. Respir Physiol 1984;58:41–50

18. Macklem PT. Physiology of the cough. Ann Otol Rhinol Laryngol 1974;83:761–768

19. Nishino T, Tagaito Y, Isono S. Cough and other reflexes on irritation of airway mucosa in man. Pulm Pharmacol 1996;9:285–292

20. Mathew OP, Sant'Ambrogio G, Fisher JT, Sant'Ambrogio FB. Laryngeal pressure receptors. Respir Physiol 1984;57:113–122

21. Sant'Ambrogio G, Mathew OP, Fisher JT, Sant'Ambrogio FB. Laryngeal receptors responding to transmural pressure, airflow and local muscle activity. Respir Physiol 1983;54:317–330

22. Downing SE, Lee JC. Laryngeal chemosensitivity: a possible mechanism for sudden infant death. Pediatrics 1975;55:640–649

23. Nishino T, Kochi T, Ishii M. Differences in respiratory reflex responses from the larynx, trachea, and bronchi in anesthetized female subjects. Anesthesiology 1996;84:70–74

24. Tomori Z, Widdicombe JG. Muscular, bronchomotor and cardiovascular reflexes elicited by mechanical stimulation of the respiratory tract. J Physiol 1969; 200:25–49

25. Prys-Roberts C, Greene LT, Meloche R, Foëx P. Studies of anaesthesia in relation to hypertension. II. Haemodynamic consequences of induction and endotracheal intubation. Br J Anaesth 1971;43: 531–547

26. Jean A, Car A. Inputs to the swallowing medullary neurons from the peripheral afferent fibers and the swallowing cortical area. Brain Res 1979;178: 567–572

27. Jean A. Brainstem organization of the swallowing network. Brain Behav Evol 1984;25:109–116

28. Martin RE, Sessle BJ. The role of the cerebral cortex in swallowing. Dysphagia 1993;8:195–202

29. Aviv JE, Martin JH, Keen MS, Debell M, Blitzer A. Air pulse quantification of supraglottic and pharyngeal sensation: a new technique. Ann Otol Rhinol Laryngol 1993;102:777–780

30. Jafari S, Prince RA, Kim DY, Paydarfar D. Sensory regulation of swallowing and airway protection: a role for the internal superior laryngeal nerve in humans. J Physiol 2003;550(Pt 1):287–304

31. Setzen M, Cohen MA, Perlman PW, et al. The association between laryngopharyngeal sensory deficits, pharyngeal motor function, and the prevalence of aspiration with thin liquids. Otolaryngol Head Neck Surg 2003;128:99–102

32. Nasri S, Sercarz JA, Azizzadeh B, Kreiman J, Berke GS. Measurement of adductory force of individual laryngeal muscles in an in vivo canine model. Laryngoscope 1994;104:1213–1218

33. Hong KH, Ye M, Kim YM, Kevorkian KF, Kreiman J, Berke GS. Functional differences between the two bellies of the cricothyroid muscle. Otolaryngol Head Neck Surg 1998;118:714–722

34. Doellinger M, Berry DA, Berke GS. A quantitative study of the medial surface dynamics of an in vivo canine vocal fold during phonation. Laryngoscope 2005;115:1646–1654

35. Nasri S, Sercarz JA, Berke GS. Noninvasive measurement of traveling wave velocity in the canine larynx. Ann Otol Rhinol Laryngol 1994;103:758–766

36. Sloan SH, Berke GS, Gerratt BR, Kreiman J, Ye M. Determination of vocal fold mucosal wave velocity in an in vivo canine model. Laryngoscope 1993;103: 947–953

37. Khosla S, Muruguppan S, Gutmark E, Scherer R. Vortical flow field during phonation in an excised canine larynx model. Ann Otol Rhinol Laryngol 2007;116: 217–228

38. Khosla S, Murugappan S, Gutmark E. What can vortices tell us about vocal fold vibration and voice production. Curr Opin Otolaryngol Head Neck Surg 2008;16:183–187

39. Berke GS, Neubauer J, Berry DA, Ye M, Chhetri DK. Ex vivo perfused larynx model of phonation: preliminary study. Ann Otol Rhinol Laryngol 2007;116:866–870

40. Mehta DD, Hillman RE. Voice assessment: updates on perceptual, acoustic, aerodynamic, and endoscopic imaging methods. Curr Opin Otolaryngol Head Neck Surg 2008;16:211–215

41. Deliyski DD, Petrushev PP, Bonilha HS, Gerlach TT, Martin-Harris B, Hillman RE. Clinical implementation of laryngeal high-speed videoendoscopy: challenges and evolution. Folia Phoniatr Logop 2008;60:33–44

4

Indirect Laryngoscopy

Katherine A. Kendall

Prior to the introduction of flexible fiberoptic laryngoscopes in the mid-1980s, indirect laryngoscopy was the most important clinical tool for viewing the larynx and allowing the evaluation of laryngeal pathology. The technique involves placing a small mirror in the posterior pharynx and illuminating the larynx below with light reflected off of the mirror. Although indirect laryngoscopy is a "low-tech" method of laryngeal evaluation, facility with the technique requires significant practice, and most physicians have abandoned it in favor of the easily performed and well-tolerated flexible laryngoscopy. As a result, indirect laryngoscopy is rapidly becoming a lost art. Although the days of an otolaryngologist (let alone a primary care physician) wearing a head mirror may be numbered, indirect laryngoscopy is still commonly used as a screening tool for laryngeal pathology. Any complete review of laryngeal imaging must include a discussion of the indications, benefits, technical aspects, and the limitations of indirect laryngoscopy.

◆ Indications and Benefits

Indirect laryngoscopy is the simplest way to examine the hypopharynx and larynx because it does not require special equipment, other than a light source, a head mirror, and a dental mirror, to perform the examination. Indirect laryngoscopy is, therefore, also exceedingly cost effective because it does not require expensive equipment. It is indicated in any patient with symptoms referable to the throat such as dysphagia, globus sensation, and hoarseness. Indirect laryngoscopy is a good choice for the initial examination of the hypopharynx in all patients presenting to the otolaryngologist. It allows an evaluation of hypopharyngeal anatomy, mucosal color, and vocal fold movement. Indirect laryngoscopy uses incandescent light, which has the advantage of minimizing color distortion so that the assessment of tissue color is reliable.

◆ Technique

The light source used for indirect laryngoscopy is typically placed to the right of the patient's head and directed toward a head mirror worn by the examiner. The head mirror reflects the light onto the dental mirror held in the patient's mouth. (Alternatively, the examiner can wear a headlight and forego the external light source and head mirror.) A small hole in the center of the head mirror allows binocular vision as the examiner looks through the hole with the left eye (**Fig. 4.1**). The head mirror should be placed as close to the eye as possible (**Fig. 4.2**). The head mirror

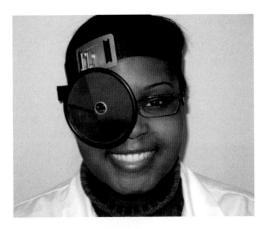

Fig. 4.1 Head-mirror position over the right eye. The examiner looks through the hole in the head mirror.

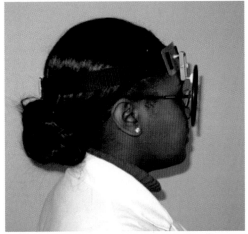

Fig. 4.2 Head-mirror position, close to the face.

is designed to focus the light at a convenient working distance. The position of the light source and the angle of the head mirror can be adjusted to focus the light onto the posterior pharynx properly.

Patient positioning for optimal indirect laryngoscopy is usually seated, with hips all the way to the back of the seat. The patient should be asked to lean forward, bending at the hips and lifting the chest and chin. A "sniffing" position with the jaw forward helps to position the tongue base anterior to the larynx (**Fig. 4.3**). Ideally, the head of the patient is above the head of the examiner. The examiner is seated in front of the patient with his or her knees to the right of the patient. Many patients will close their eyes during the examination, but it is helpful to have them keep their eyes open, looking upward. This prevents the patient from focusing solely on the sensation they are experiencing in the throat during the examination, precipitating a gag reflex.

Using tongue blades to hold the cheeks open, the posterior pharynx can be initially examined. This allows the examiner to make any minor adjustments of the light source and head mirror needed prior to beginning the indirect laryngoscopy. It also allows for an inspection of pharyngeal structures that will impact the ability to perform the examination such as size of tongue base, length of the soft palate, jaw opening, and so forth. It provides an opportunity to reassure the patient and prepare him or her for the indirect exam.

The size of the dental mirror chosen for the examination should be large enough to provide a good view of the larynx but should not be so large that it cannot be positioned in the pharynx and manipulated to allow examination of all of the hypopharyngeal structures. The mirror must be warmed to prevent fogging during the examination. Care must be taken to ensure that the mirror is not too hot. The patient is asked to protrude the tongue, which is then held out of the mouth by the examiner. A gauze sponge is used by the examiner to grasp the tongue with the left hand. It is important that the patient be instructed to relax the tongue as much as possible, allowing the examiner to pull the tongue forward. This will minimize discomfort for the patient and will also maximize the posterior pharyngeal opening through which the examination will be performed. The index finger of the left hand can be used to elevate the upper lip. The dental mirror is then placed against the soft palate and gently pushed up and back (**Fig. 4.4**). Sensation to the soft palate is provided by the trigeminal nerve, which is typically not involved in the gag reflex, so touching the soft palate with the mirror is generally well tolerated. On the other hand, the glossopharyngeal nerve, which provides sensation to the base of the tongue, is involved in the gag reflex, and thus touching the tongue base with the mirror should be avoided. Similarly, the pharyngeal walls, innervated by the vagus nerve, will stimulate a gag if touched.

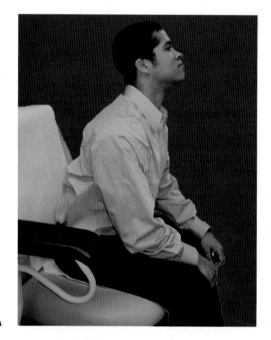

A

Back straight and slightly forward

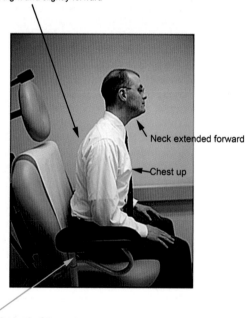

Neck extended forward

Chest up

B   Hips at the back of the seat

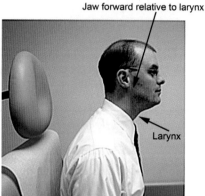

Jaw forward relative to larynx

Larynx

C

Fig. 4.3 (A) Optimal patient positioning for indirect laryngoscopy. Note head of the patient is positioned forward in a "sniffing" position. This moves the base of the tongue anterior to the larynx, improving a full view of the larynx. **(B)** Patient positioning during indirect laryngoscopy. The patient may need to bring his or her back off the backrest of the exam chair. **(C)** The anterior positioning of the head positions the jaw and tongue anterior to the larynx.

By angling the dental mirror back and forth, the larynx can often be viewed at this point in the examination. Asking the patient to say "EEEE" will also improve the ability to see the larynx. This maneuver elevates the larynx, depresses the tongue base, and brings the vocal folds together. It is important, however, to attempt to see the vocal folds while they are open, such as during respiration, as well, because lesions on the medial and undersurface of the vocal folds may be missed if the folds are only viewed during adduction.

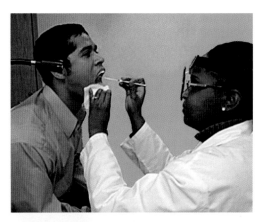

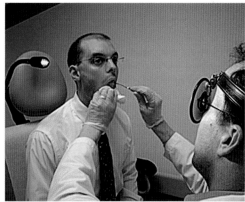

A

B

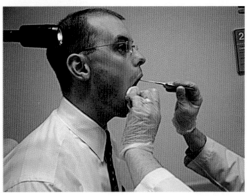

C

Fig. 4.4 (A) Indirect laryngoscopy: The patient is positioned above the examiner. Notice how the patient's mouth is at eye level for the examiner. **(B)** During indirect laryngoscopy, the light source is placed to the right of the patient's head, reflected off the examiner's head mirror and then reflected off the mirror placed in the oropharynx to illuminate the larynx. **(C)** Asking the patient to keep his or her eyes open during the examination helps the patient to tolerate the exam.

◆ Limitations

Ten percent of patients will not be able to tolerate the examination well enough to allow a complete evaluation of all of the hypopharyngeal structures.[1] A topical anesthetic applied to the posterior pharyngeal wall and tongue base can often aid in diminishing a strong gag reflex. Anatomic variations may also prevent a complete examination in up to 50% of patients.[2] The anterior commissure is an area that is often difficult to see, especially if the patient has a large tongue base or is unable to relax enough to allow the tongue base to be pulled forward. A very anterior larynx is usually easier to see if the patient is positioned well above the examiner, allowing angling of the mirror to see forward of the tongue base. Nevertheless, the ability to see the laryngeal structures may be fleeting during the examination, requiring the examiner to make judgments based on a very quick view of the anatomy. The examiner may be able to see the

larynx only during high-pitched phonation. This allows confirmation that the vocal folds are both moving but does not necessarily reflect conditions resulting in patient complaints. Subtle lesions are likely not to be detected, and vocal fold vibration cannot be seen with indirect laryngoscopy.

Because of the unnatural position of the patient during the examination and the restraining of the patient's tongue, only very simple vocalizing can be evaluated with indirect laryngoscopy. The technique does not allow assessment during connected speech. This means that functional abnormalities are likely to be missed with indirect laryngoscopy alone.

Furthermore, indirect laryngoscopy does not provide for documentation of the examination. Monnery et al. found a 29% error rate in documentation with indirect laryngoscopy when the examiner created a drawing of the larynx to record the examination. Most commonly the error involved placing an abnormality on the wrong side of the larynx.[1] Furthermore, descriptions or drawings of the larynx are too crude to allow detection of subtle changes in the findings on subsequent examinations. Because only one person can see the larynx during the examination, there is no possibility of simultaneous review of the findings by multiple individuals for the purposes of teaching, reviewing, or discussion.

In conclusion, indirect laryngoscopy is a long-established technique for laryngeal examination that is inexpensive and reliable in terms of tissue color assessment. It is limited by the technical skill required to achieve adequate examination, the patient's ability to cooperate with the examination, the inability to view vocal fold vibration, and the lack of documentation.

References

1. Monnery PM, Smith WK, Hinton AE. Laryngoscopy findings in outpatient notes: the accuracy of the recording of the side of the lesion. Clin Otolaryngol Allied Sci 2001;26:278–280
2. Barker M, Dort JC. Laryngeal examination: a comparison of mirror examination with a rigid lens system. J Otolaryngol 1991;20:100–103

5

Reliability in the Interpretation of Laryngeal Imaging

Claudio F. Milstein

> There are times when an experienced physician sees a visible lesion clearly and times when he does not. This is the baffling problem, apparently partly visual and partly psychologic. They constitute the still unexplained human equation in diagnostic procedures.
>
> —Henry Garland, MD, 1959

It came as a surprise to our group at the Cleveland Clinic that experts reading the same medical images frequently interpret them very differently. But in fact, early evidence for such varying interpretations goes back to 1947. At that time, Birkelo and colleagues reported that a study of the relative effectiveness of four methods of chest imaging for tuberculosis was inconclusive because the variation of opinion among observers was greater than the variety of techniques.[1] Until then, medical professionals had "naively assumed that what they perceive in images is a faithful representation of the images' information content, and have not been concerned with perception unless it fails," writes Harold Kundel.[2]

Our own work on this issue grew out of research conducted by an interdepartmental group at the Cleveland Clinic. This group was created through the frequent sharing of patients with throat-related gastroesophageal reflux disease (GERD) symptoms among the ear, nose, and throat, gastrointestinal, and surgery departments. Since the late 1980s, there has been increasing evidence that GERD causes laryngeal signs and symptoms secondary to tissue irritation. The goal of this group was to investigate the cause-and-effect relationship between GERD, laryngeal symptoms, and pathology, given that there was a lack of data and consensus on this topic among specialties. In several of the publications that came out of this group, we noted that one weakness was related to interobserver (agreement between raters) and intraobserver (how stable are the responses of the same observer at different time points) reliability.

For example, one of the studies investigated the prevalence of hypopharyngeal findings associated with GERD in normal volunteers.[3] A group of expert judges evaluated videolaryngoscopic examinations of 110 volunteer subjects and rated 10 hypopharyngeal structures based on signs of tissue irritation. Findings of edema, erythema, redundant tissue, surface irregularities, and other lesions under each structure were rated on a severity scale. We analyzed the interobserver and intraobserver variability data using a well-known statistical method, the Cohen's kappa coefficient, which establishes the strength of agreement between two independent evaluations. The significance of agreement is graded as a function of the calculated value. To appreciate the interpretations of kappa statistics more fully, the following value strength-of-agreement interpretations are provided: 0.00 to 0.20, slight; 0.21 to 0.40, fair; 0.41 to 0.60, moderate; 0.61 to 0.80, substantial; and 0.81 to 1.00, almost perfect. In this study, the agreement within and between raters was generally moderate at best, with several of the parameters rated resulting in poor agreement (e.g., erythema of the medial wall of the arytenoids, posterior cricoid-wall abnormalities, and presence of an interarytenoid bar).

A follow-up study involving the same sites of laryngeal irritation yielded similarly poor levels of agreement among our expert judges.[4] Thinking that we might have made errors of data entry, we evaluated the entire data set a second time. The results were the same. We did not seem to agree with each other very well.

This is unsettling. All raters in these studies are experts in this field with many years of experience. Individually, they evaluate those same signs of laryngeal irritation on a daily basis, and based on those observations, they make diagnoses and treatment plans. They have successful practices, and their patients get better. Yet, when their evaluations are compared with those of their colleagues, it becomes clear that they do not always agree on what they see.

◆ We Are Not Alone

Puzzled by these findings, we looked for answers in other fields, and we were surprised to find that we were not alone. It soon became clear that problems with perception and evaluation of medical images were pervasive across most specialties. The reality is that these problems affect not only raters' variability in research studies but also the ability of health professionals to diagnose patients accurately based on medical images.

For example, in a study of visual assessment of brain atrophy on magnetic resonance imaging (MRI), a team from The Netherlands asked four expert raters—three neurologists and one neuroradiologist—to rate medial-temporal lobe atrophy on MRI in 100 studies of elderly individuals. Complete agreement was limited to only 37% of the total sample (kappa = 0.44).[5]

When it comes to interpreting mammograms, it is well known that there is considerable variability among radiologists.[6] In one study, 10 radiologists interpreted mammograms showing clustered microcalcifications in 104 patients. They then made recommendations for biopsy or other follow-up measures. Analysis of their recommendations showed that the level of agreement was frighteningly low, about 13% (kappa = 0.19). This variability strongly highlights problems with diagnosis of breast neoplasms, which adversely affect clinical decision making. As a result, many women may be getting conflicting clinical advice when it comes to treatment of breast cancer.

Van de Steene and colleagues caution that variability in image interpretation plagues radiation therapy planning and evaluation for a variety of tumor sites, particularly in the assessment of lung cancer.[8]

Cardiology is similarly plagued by disagreements over medical image interpretation, and numerous studies show that kappa values for visual assessment are low. The most cited study in the stress echocardiography literature is probably Hoffmann et al.[9] In this study, experts from five experienced centers had greatly varying interpretations of 150 dobutamine stress echocardiograms obtained in patients undergoing coronary angiography. The number of studies evaluated as positive ranged from 38 to 102 (n = 150). Agreement on what constituted normal versus abnormal results was reached only in 73% of patients, for a mean kappa of 0.37. In other words, in 27% of cases, these expert cardiologists disagreed as to whether or not some patients were healthy or had heart disease! In another example, marked variability was found in the assessment of coronary stenosis severity and left ventricular function evaluation of coronary angiographies.[10] This study reported that agreement in the significance of a stenosis was found in only 13 of 20 coronary angiograms (65%) when read by four experienced coronary angiographers from the same institution. These data disturbingly suggest that a patient's diagnosis of "normal" versus "heart diseased" depends on which cardiologist reads the study.

Problems also exist in other specialty areas quite familiar to otolaryngologists. Evaluation of videofluoroscopic swallow studies has shown considerable variability in interpretation of certain parameters. In one study, nine independent observers from different international swallow centers rated 26 different parameters in 51 patients who had been referred for a modified barium swallow.[7] Kappa coefficients were as low as 0.01, 0.02, and 0.03 for parameters such as aspiration before swallow, penetration before swallow, and upper esophageal sphincter closing time, respectively. The authors concluded that modified barium swallow evaluations were highly reliable only in the case of aspiration, whereas reliability was poor for all other parameters of oropharyngeal swallow. To be sure, not all studies of evaluations of medical images show such low reliability scores. Nevertheless, in some areas, serious problems exist, and we have chosen to highlight those to point out a problem that needs to be addressed.

◆ Sources of Variability

The variability in interpretation of medical images affects the diagnostic accuracy of health professionals. In addition, it directly affects their clinical decisions and ability to recommend appropriate treatment. Given that this variability decreases clinical effectiveness, it should be recognized and improved whenever possible.

Variability may result from two sources: (1) the human element and how the visual input is processed, and (2) the instrumentation used to obtain, process, or display the image. The rapid technological advances in diagnostic imaging instrumentation—such as MRI, PET scans, virtual slide projectors, and other digital image acquisition devices used in all areas of medicine—also need to be considered, because of the potential to affect our perception. As Dr. Krupinsky, a researcher in the Departments of Radiology and Psychology at the University of Arizona, points out, "The emergence of new technologies raises important questions concerning optimization of the acquisition, storage, transfer and display of image, as well as text-based information, choice of appropriate

display media and format, optimization of image compression, and optimization of image processing and computer-aided detection (CAD) and diagnosis (CADx). It is only through systematic and objective evaluation of the entire imaging system—from hardware to human interpretation of images—that these questions can be answered."[11,12]

- ◆ **Human factors that affect diagnostic performance: observer variability**
  - ◇ Differences in reading criteria
  - ◇ Differences in thresholds or markers to classify results as positive or negative
  - ◇ Differences in level of expertise (expert vs novice)
  - ◇ Observer environment (time to evaluate an image, fatigue factor, etc.)
- ◆ **Technological factors that affect diagnostic performance: instrument variability**
  - ◇ Image quality (sharp or blurry)
  - ◇ Image processing and storage
  - ◇ Image display
  - ◇ Choice of instrumentation (eg, type of endoscope)
  - ◇ Technical efficacy (how accurately the images are obtained)

The following are examples of these factors that pertain to laryngology and how they can affect an evaluation:

- ◆ **Adjustments to the camera or display controls** can alter the overall color of the image. More redness in an image can indicate, or be interpreted as, a higher degree of erythema.
- ◆ **Endoscope position** (distance between the tip of the endoscope and the structure of interest, angle of vision, etc.) will change the size or view of the resulting image, potentially influencing diagnostic performance.

An important difference may result from the choice of endoscope and can affect diagnostic ability.[4] **Figures 5.1 and 5.2** show examples of images from the same patients obtained only minutes apart. The images on the left were taken with a flexible fiberscope, and the images on the right were obtained with a rigid endoscope. In both examples, the images on the left show a more edematous larynx, and furthermore, in **Fig. 5.2**, there is clear

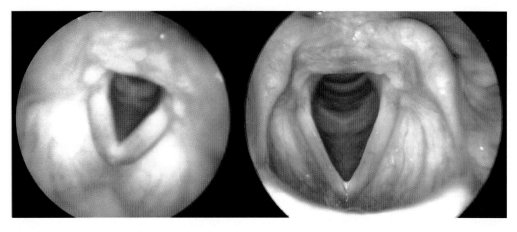

Fig. 5.1 Images taken from the same patient only minutes apart. with a flexible scope **(A)** and a rigid scope **(B).** In the image taken with a flexible scope, the larynx appears more edematous.

evidence of a bilateral pseudosulcus (subglottic edema) on the flexible fiberscope image, but the vocal folds appear less edematous, and pseudosulci are not evident when the same patient is evaluated with a rigid endoscope. These findings suggest that identification of laryngeal abnormalities depends not only on the examiner (intraobserver and interobserver variability) but also on the tools that are used. The choice of imaging technique (rigid versus flexible endoscopy) makes a difference in what we see and can therefore affect the accuracy and the objectivity of the laryngoscopic examination in certain settings.

◆ Research Interest and What Is Being Done

As noted above, research in this area began after World War II, when a study published in 1947 comparing methods for detecting tuberculosis in chest images found a high degree of interobserver and intraobserver variability. This study generated enough interest that eventually, the field of medical image perception was created. In the past 60 years, there has been significant progress in applying quantitative methods to the

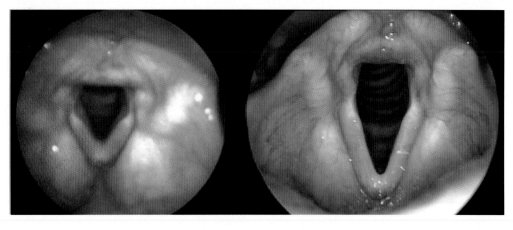

Fig. 5.2 Images taken from the same patient only minutes apart with a flexible scope **(A)** and a rigid scope **(B).** There is clear evidence of a bilateral pseudosulcus (subglottic edema) on the flexible fiberscope image, but the vocal folds appear less edematous and pseudosulci are not evident when the same patient is evaluated with a rigid endoscope.

assessment of visual diagnostic performance and to the evaluation of medical image quality in terms of task performance. The Far West Image Perception Conferences have been held biannually since 1985. These conferences have assembled an international group of radiologists, psychologists, physicists, engineers, and statisticians interested in the relationship of image perception and decision making, psychophysics, and diagnostic imaging.

In November 1994, the National Institutes of Health convened a meeting for developing a long-term plan for imaging research, which included, as a priority, issues of perception. The NIH generated five specific goals:

1. Develop psychophysical models for the detection of abnormalities in natural medical images.
2. Improve understanding of the mechanisms of perception as they apply to medical images.
3. Develop aids for enhancing perception by use of approaches that provide interactions between vision and display.
4. Study perceptually acceptable alternatives to sequential sections for viewing images from cross-sectional imaging examinations.
5. Perform methodological research aimed at improving the evaluation of medical imaging systems; alternatives to standard methods for measuring observer performance should be encouraged.

Then, in 1997, partly as a result of this meeting, the Medical Image Perception Society (MIPS) was established "to promote research and education in medical image perception, and provide a forum for the discussion of perceptual, psychophysical, and cognitive issues by radiologists and basic scientists." This society "seeks an improved understanding of the perceptual factors that underlie the creation and interpretation of medical images." The society's goals are:

1. The development of imaging systems to help optimize the interpretation of the visual diagnostic information.
2. Work on perception research that will
   a. identify the specific reasons for missed diagnoses and thus help train physicians and eliminate diagnostic errors; and
   b. clarify situations in which errors are a consequence of fundamentally ambiguous information rather than negligence.

Another group was created through collaboration between the U.S. Food and Drug Administration, the Center for Devices and Radiological Health, and the National Institute of Biomedical Imaging and Bioengineering, part of the National Institutes of Health. These agencies established the Laboratory for the Assessment of Medical Imaging Systems, run by Dr. Kyle Myers. The goal of LAMIS is to make safe and effective medical imaging products available to health care professionals in a rapid manner, as well as the development and evaluation of assessment methodologies for medical imaging systems.

Current projects cover the following areas:

- **Image acquisition**: Development of new digital imaging devices, with a broad range of performance characteristics.
- **Image display:** Displays are currently considered to be the weakest link of the imaging chain for many applications (eg, mammography), therefore development of measurement and analysis procedures to evaluate the performance of image display devices for digital diagnostic imaging systems are under way.
- **Computer-aided diagnosis:** Recent studies indicate that helical computed tomography may be an effective screening tool for lung cancer, and full-field digital mammography has been developed into a clinical tool. The primary goal of this project is to develop additional in-house CADx expertise.
- **Multivariate statistical assessment:** Development of study designs, objective measurements, and analytical methods for the laboratory and clinical assessment of medical imaging systems, systems for CADx used in medical imaging, and stand-alone image-based computerized diagnostic moda- lities such as high-dimensional DNA microarrays (DNA chips).[13,14]

Another academic group is the Vision and Image Understanding Laboratory at the University of California, Santa Barbara. This laboratory, run by Miguel Eckstein, "pursues computational modeling of behavioral, cognitive neuroscience and physiological data with the aim of elucidating the mechanisms and neural substrates mediating perception, attention, and learning." These investigators use acquired knowledge in conjunction with computer science and engineering tools to improve human performance in life critical decisions such as when doctors examine medical images for signs of tumors. The laboratory has done seminal work on improving detection of tumors on mammograms.

The University of Iowa's Department of Radiology also hosts an excellent group, headed by Kevin Berbaum. The Medical Image Perception Laboratory investigates the human component of image interpretation, studying the perceptual and intellectual aspects of how a physician interprets images, to be able to understand and correct the causes of interpretive failure.

Other researchers well known for their work in this area include Elizabeth Krupinsky at the Departments of Radiology and Psychology at the University of Arizona. Krupinski is the president of the Society for Perception of Medical Images, and her main interests are in medical image perception, assessment of observer performance, and human factors issues. Claudia Mello-Thoms at the University of Pittsburgh investigates image perception and image interpretation, as well as visual search, and modeling of the decision-making process involved in reading medical images.

◆ How to Improve Interpretation

Since the mid-1990s, and as computer technology and digital imaging systems have advanced, numerous groups have modeled human performance and proposed computer-aided detection and diagnosis algorithms. These have been applied to clinical settings and have helped improve the accuracy of diagnosis and interpretation. The use of CAD can have a dramatic impact on performance, as demonstrated in studies mentioned earlier in the chapter. When coronary angiograms were reevaluated with the aid of a computer-assisted quantitative program, the agreement in interpretation improved substantially, with an increase of kappa scores from 0.36 to 0.71.[9] Computer-aided

assistance also reduced variability and increased agreement among observers from 13 to 32% of the total cases (increasing kappa scores from 0.19 to 0.41) in the interpretation of mammograms showing microcalcifications.[6] However, problems remain. Even with computer assistance, clinicians continue to miss lesions, and new technologies frequently introduce new errors, showing that more work needs to be done.

To date, recommendations from these groups that can help improve accuracy include:

◆ Examine the image multiple times. Avoid diagnosis or rating upon first viewing.
◆ As image quality correlates with overall agreement on presence or absence of abnormalities, exclude poor-quality images.
◆ Optimize the image for the viewer.
◆ Optimize the display for the viewer.
◆ Be aware that there generally is higher agreement in extremes (normal or severe) but less agreement in more subtle findings.
◆ Additionally, the profession needs to act on certain issues. These include:
  ◇ The need to refine and unify reading criteria. Develop clear standards for classifying normal versus pathologic, and provide clear anchors for diagnostic or research tasks.
  ◇ The need to adapt methods for improving image interpretation from different fields to laryngology.

◆ Conclusion

The problems associated with the perception of medical images are of concern and undoubtedly account for errors in diagnostic interpretation that may result in poor patient care, lawsuits, and unnecessary health care spending. The problems are not restricted to the field of laryngology but are pervasive throughout most medical fields and likely inherent to any visual-perceptual task. The contributing factors to different interpretations are both human and technological. On the human side, differences in reading criteria, thresholds for classification, level of expertise, environment, and subjective conditions such as fatigue can alter interpretation. On the technological side, image quality, processing, storage, use of different instruments, displays, and the human-technological interface can all influence interpretation.

Fortunately, several groups are working creatively to mitigate this problem. As voice and larynx specialists, we routinely interpret medical images for diagnostic and research purposes. We can benefit from work done in other medical fields. By staying on top of research in this area, we can incorporate mitigating measures as they are developed and we can adapt innovations to our field to improve our ability to diagnose and treat our patients, providing them with the best possible care. Finally, understanding the widespread problem of interpretation of medical images should serve as a cautionary note against our overconfidence in the diagnosis and treatment of our patients.

References

1. Birkelo C, Chamberlain W, Phelps P. Tuberculosis case finding: a comparison of the effectiveness of various roentgenographic and photofluorographic methos. JAMA 1947;133:359–366
2. Kundel HL. History of research in medical image perception. J Am Coll Radiol 2006;3:402–408
3. Hicks DM, Ours TM, Abelson TI, Vaezi MF, Richter JE. The prevalence of hypopharynx findings associated with gastroesophageal reflux in normal volunteers. J Voice 2002;16:564–579
4. Milstein CF, Charbel S, Hicks DM, Abelson TI, Richter JE, Vaezi MF. Prevalence of laryngeal irritation signs associated with reflux in asymptomatic volunteers: impact of endoscopic technique (rigid vs. flexible laryngoscope). Laryngoscope 2005;115:2256–2261
5. Scheltens P, Launer LJ, Barkhof F, Weinstein HC, van Gool WA. Visual assessment of medial temporal lobe atrophy on magnetic resonance imaging: interobserver reliability. J Neurol 1995;242:557–560
6. Jiang Y, Nishikawa RM, Schmidt RA, Toledano AY, Doi K. Potential of computer-aided diagnosis to reduce variability in radiologists' interpretations of mammograms depicting microcalcifications. Radiology 2001; 220:787–794
7. Stoeckli SJ, Huisman TA, Seifert B, Martin-Harris BJ. Interrater reliability of videofluoroscopic swallow evaluation. Dysphagia 2003;18:53–57
8. Van de Steene J, Linthout N, de Mey J, et al. Definition of gross tumor volume in lung cancer: inter-observer variability. Radiother Oncol 2002;62:37–49
9. Hoffmann R, Lethen H, Marwick T, et al. Analysis of interinstitutional observer agreement in interpretation of dobutamine stress echocardiograms. J Am Coll Cardiol 1996;27:330–336
10. Zir LM, Miller SW, Dinsmore RE, Gilbert JP, Harthorne JW. Interobserver variability in coronary angiography. Circulation 1976;53:627–632
11. Krupinski EA, Jiang Y. Anniversary paper: evaluation of medical imaging systems. Med Phys 2008;35: 645–659
12. Krupinski EA. The importance of perception research in medical imaging. Radiat Med 2000;18:329–334
13. Department of Health and Human Services, U.S. Food and Drug Administration. About the Center for Devices and Radiological Health: Office of Science and Engineering Laboratories. Available at: http://www.fda.gov/cdrh/osel/programareas/medicalimaging.html. Accessed June 1, 2009
14. National Institute of Biomedical Imaging and Bioengineering. Research, NIBIB Intramural Labs. Laboratory for the Assessment of Medical Imaging Systems (LAMIS). Available at: http://www.nibib.nih.gov/-Research/Intramural/LAMIS. Accessed June 1, 2009

6

Normal Laryngeal Variability

Rebecca J. Leonard

There is ample evidence of variability in the "normal" larynx. Investigators using a broad array of investigative techniques directed toward either structure or function have contributed to this information base. Structural differences are reflected in size, shape, and, in particular, symmetry from right to left. For example, in a study of human cadaver larynges, Hirano et al. described asymmetry in all samples considered, regardless of age or gender.[1] Asymmetries were identified in the thyroid lamina, with the right tending to tilt laterally and the left medially. Further, the thyroid cartilage tended to shift right, against the cricoid cartilage. The right cricoarytenoid joint was typically located slightly more laterally, posteriorly, and inferiorly compared with the left joint.

Other authors have reported similar variability in the posterior larynx, as well as in the thyroid cartilage.[2] Reviewing computed tomography (CT) scans of the larynx, these investigators noted that the thyroid lamina in the majority of subjects was longer in the anteroposterior direction on the left side compared with the right. They related this finding to their observation that the most frequent pattern of corniculate cartilage crossover on vocal fold adduction involved the right crossing in front of or over the left. That is, the left aryepiglottic fold, positioned more posteriorly than the right due to the longer length of the left thyroid

lamina, is likely to remain posterior to the right on adduction. Differences in the shape of the thyroid lamina, possibly associated with aging, have also been described. Honjo et al. reported medial displacement of one false vocal fold in 10 elderly males.[3] CT scans of the underlying structures revealed a marked concavity of the thyroid ala on the same side as the false-fold protrusion.

In a study of 109 normal subjects, Lindestad et al. noted several types of asymmetries on vocal fold adduction assessed with rigid endoscopy.[4] The most common involved different placements of the corniculate or cuneiform cartilages, observed in 66% of individuals examined. Other asymmetries included one corniculate cartilage crossing over the other and differences in the angles of the aryepiglottic fold to the epiglottis. Of note, abduction asymmetries were rare in this group of normal individuals.

Such evidence of asymmetries in the paired structures of the larynx, though not uncommon in other bodily structures, is perhaps surprising in view of the coordination and symmetry required for normal vocal fold vibration and voice. As noted by Wang, evidence from human laryngeal embryologic development that the glottis and arytenoid cartilages are formed in adduction, not abduction, may offer one explanation for how vocal process approximation is achieved for normal vocalization.[5] Filho et al., examining characteristics of the vocal folds in 24 human cadavers, reported no significant within-subject differences in length, width, or thickness from right to left.[6] If the vocal folds demonstrate greater symmetry in size and shape than other laryngeal structures, this may further explain how normal vibratory behavior is achieved. If and how other compensatory mechanisms contribute to this process is not clear.

The longer length of the left recurrent laryngeal nerve, compared with the right, represents a particularly intriguing example of normal variability that has long been of interest to researchers and clinicians. The question raised is whether there are conduction time or other asymmetries that could account for coordination of bilateral laryngeal events, such as the opening and closing of the vocal folds. It has been suggested that, as the left recurrent nerve lengthens with the descent of the aortic arch, faster fibers may be preferentially retained in the right to left corticobulbar tract compared with the left to right corticobulbar tract.[7,8] Faster conduction times in the longer nerve would, of course, seem to provide a basis for the coordination observed in abduction and adduction and perhaps in other vocal fold behaviors.

Further evidence of variability, between individuals, but also across tasks and over time within the same individual, has been reported for voicing behaviors of the vocal folds. Electromyographic data reported by Poletto et al. have suggested that activation patterns of the cricothyroid and thyroarytenoid muscles on the same side demonstrated as high, or higher, correlations than activation patterns between the same muscles on opposite sides.[9] Digital high-speed laryngeal imaging of an individual speaker over a time period of 2 days revealed evidence of variability in opening and closing patterns as well as asymmetries between the right and left vocal folds that appeared related to voice usage, or vocal "loading."[10]

A stroboscopic examination of vibratory behavior provides additional evidence of normal variability across age and gender. For example, Bless and Hirano reported that closed phases of vibratory cycles tended to be longer and more complete in males than in females.[11] Children demonstrated a shorter closed phase than that of adult males, as well as larger posterior chinks. Older individuals were characterized as demonstrating lower amplitudes of vibratory displacement and greater asymmetry than that of their younger counterparts. Bonilha et al., using multiple imaging techniques, reported both left-right and anterior-posterior phase asymmetries in most of the 52 normal adult speakers examined. The findings were noted for both habitual and pressed phonation and were typically judged as mild.[12]

At some point, our expectation is that "normal" variability along the continuum of a laryngeal structure or behavior will become "abnormal." But even here, differentiation may not always be straightforward. For example, Elias et al., in stroboscopic examinations of professional singers with no vocal complaints, reported frequent observations of "abnormal" laryngeal findings, including evidence of reflux laryngitis, small benign lesions, varicosities, vibratory asymmetries, and weakness.[13] Complicating the matter further are frequent reports of poor reliability (or large variability) among examiners attempting to characterize the same vocal fold behavior, as well as the voice produced by the behavior.[14-17] What appears more or less normal to one observer or listener, for example, may seem less so to another, depending on many factors.

Several examples of normal variability in laryngeal structures and behaviors described here can be observed on routine clinical examination. In our experience, they are particularly well observed with rigid endoscopy, though variability is common to all imaging techniques discussed in this text. In the remainder of this chapter, examples of such observations, all based on rigid endoscopic examination, will be presented. For comparison, examples will range from very typical to less typical. The examples presented were considered within the range of "normal" by the laryngologists and clinicians who identified them. None of the observations presented was believed to be symptomatic in the individual in whom it was identified or to require intervention.

Perhaps one of the more striking examples of variability on endoscopic examination is the epiglottis. A typical presentation of this structure is illustrated in **Fig. 6.1A**, with less typical examples presented in **Fig. 6.1B–F**. It is apparent in the images that the concavity of the

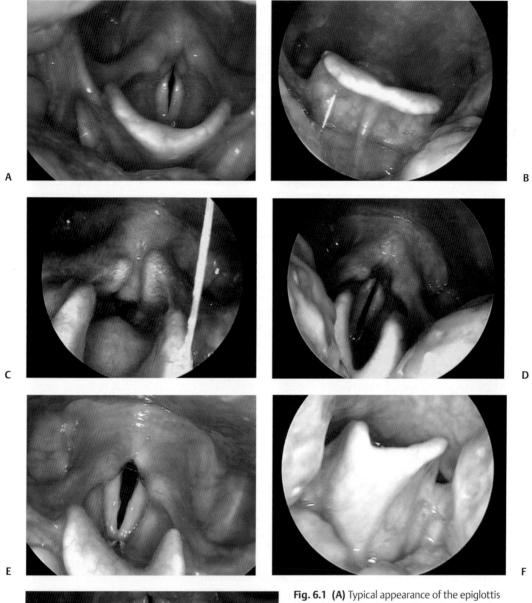

A

B

C

D

E

F

Fig. 6.1 **(A)** Typical appearance of the epiglottis from above during laryngeal imaging. **(B)** In this image, the epiglottis has less curvature as seen from the lingual surface of the structure. The vallecula is open and easily visualized in this example. **(C)** This is an example of an omega-shaped epiglottis. The rim is U-shaped, and the pediole is quite prominent. **(D)** Asymmetry of the epiglottis is within the range of normal variation. This example demonstrates an asymmetric and very curved epiglottis. **(E)** This epiglottis has a "normal" amount of curvature but is asymmetric, with an L-shape. **(F)** This lingual surface view of the epiglottis reveals the asymmetry in the shape of the epiglottic cartilage. **(G)** The pediole of the epiglottis is quite prominent in this example.

G

laryngeal surface of the epiglottis varies considerably, from an angle of 130 degrees in **Fig. 6.1A**, to 60 degrees or more in **Fig. 6.1D** and **E**. In **Fig. 6.1E**, the surface of the epiglottis appears in the shape of an "L," with one limb distinctly longer than the other.

Interestingly, Langmore has suggested that penetration of swallowed materials into the airway may be facilitated or hindered by epiglottic shape.[18] For example, an epiglottis that is relatively flat and lies against the base of the tongue at rest may obliterate the vallecular space and make it easier for bolus material to enter the laryngeal vestibule. We might also suspect that the somewhat omega-shaped epiglottis in **Fig. 6.1C** could facilitate airway protection, serving to divert bolus material around the larynx. Incidentally, an omega-shaped epiglottis in children has been associated with laryngomalacia, but it is not infrequently observed in adults on clinical exam. In **Fig. 6.1B**, the vallecular space is quite prominent, whereas in **Fig. 6.1D**, it is generally obscured. Some authors have associated a curled epiglottis that touches the tongue base at rest possibly with a globus sensation.[19] In **Fig. 6.1F**, both the position and angle of the cartilage make visualization with rigid endoscopy difficult. In **Fig. 6.1G**, the pediole of the epiglottis is quite prominent.

As previously discussed, the arytenoid cartilages, with the smaller corniculate and cuneiform cartilages composing their most superior portions, also vary substantially from left to right in many individuals. Examples are presented in **Fig. 6.2**. In **Fig. 6.2A**, the structures

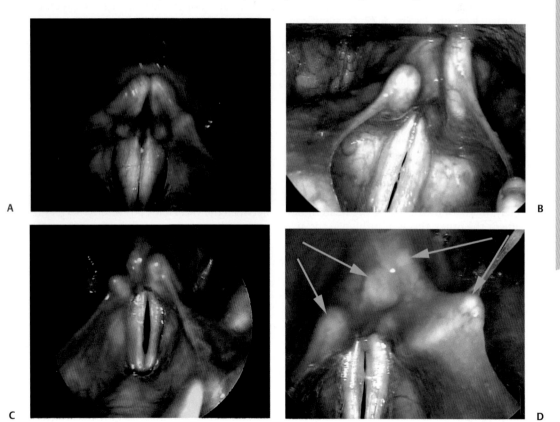

A

B

C

D

Fig. 6.2 **(A)** In this example, the arytenoid cartilages, with the smaller corniculate and cuneiform cartilages composing their most superior portions, appear quite symmetric in size, shape, and relative location.
(B) The arytenoid cartilages can be significantly asymmetric. This example shows the left side posterior to the right side. **(C)** Another example of arytenoid asymmetry with the left arytenoid posterior to the right arytenoid. **(D)** In this example, the arytenoid cartilages may be symmetric relative to each other, but the corniculate and cuneiform cartilages (*green arrows*) are asymmetric in their position giving an overall appearance of significant asymmetry.

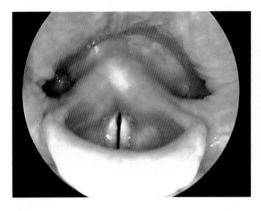

Fig. 6.3 The left pyriform recess appears larger in this example.

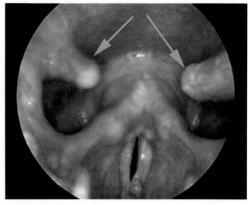

Fig. 6.4 The greater cornua of the hyoid bone project into the pharynx in this example (*green arrows*).

appear quite symmetric in size, shape, and relative location. In **Fig. 6.2B–D**, significant variability is apparent. Consistent with the findings of Lindestad et al., when asymmetry is present, it is more common for the left side to be located posterior relative to the right.[4] In all examples presented, arytenoid function was appropriate on abduction and adduction of the vocal folds.

Most typically in our experience, the pyriform sinuses appear approximately symmetrical and equal in size from side to side. Occasionally, however, one may seem to be smaller than the other, as in **Fig. 6.3**. Obviously, if a patient is turning the head to one side or the other, this will influence the size of the space. In elderly individuals, compared with younger individuals, the pyriform recesses may also appear to be deeper.

In **Fig. 6.3**, there is little evidence of the greater cornua of the hyoid bone present in the pharynx. This is in marked contrast with **Fig. 6.4**, in which these horns are unusually prominent.

Cysts, if not "normal," may nonetheless be benign and asymptomatic, not requiring intervention. Examples of vallecular or aryepiglottic cysts are presented in **Fig. 6.5**.

In **Fig. 6.6**, a slight notch in the uvula is apparent. This is not an uncommon observation, and is not indicative of a "bifid" uvula. In some individuals, the uvula is quite long and appears to separate only slightly from the tongue during production of "ee." If so,

examination of the larynx with a rigid endoscope or mirror may be difficult.

In **Fig. 6.7**, closure patterns commonly observed on rigid endoscopic examination are presented. All three examples are of normal speakers with no vocal complaints. In **Fig. 6.7A**, the vocal folds are adducted along the posterior vocal processes. Though typical, it can also be observed in individuals with some degree of glottic incompetence for voicing and may represent an adaptive response. In such cases, there will likely be evidence of thinness or bowing of the true vocal folds, as well. In **Fig. 6.7B**, a slight gap or chink is present between the vocal folds posteriorly. Secretions and mild erythema are also apparent on the vocal folds in this image. In **Fig. 6.7C**, there are slight gaps both anteriorly and posteriorly. The subjects in the figures were phonating at comfortable frequencies and intensities. Contact patterns can change depending on these variables, as well as with effort. See Chapter 15 for a more in-depth discussion of the variations in the normal glottic configuration.

The material presented here is not intended to be a comprehensive review of all aspects of normal laryngeal variability. Rather, the purpose is to introduce clinicians and, in particular, those who may be new to laryngeal imaging to the wide range of normal observations possible on *clinical* examination of the larynx. Further, based on studies representing a variety of investigational techniques, we have attempted to present evidence that offers

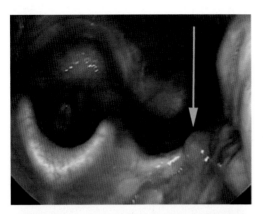

A

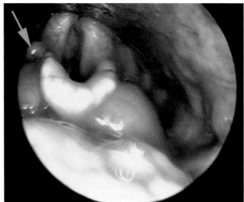

B

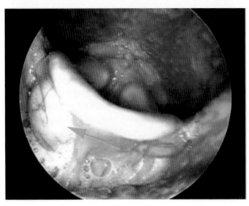

C

Fig. 6.5 (A) The green arrow points to a small vallecular cyst. **(B)** A small right aryepiglottic fold cyst is seen in this image (*green arrow*). **(C)** A right vallecular cyst can be seen on this image (*green arrow*).

explanations for, and speculation about, the examples of normal variability presented. Perhaps it is most important for clinicians to simply be aware that there is indeed a wide

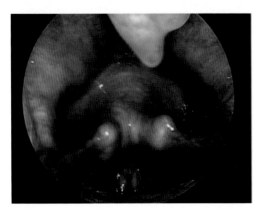

Fig. 6.6 A notch in the uvula is seen at the top of this image.

range of normal laryngeal and vocal presentation and to recognize when a deviation from normal is significant. Many contributors to this text have provided examples of normal and abnormal laryngeal function. Included here is a clip (**Video Clip 1**) of a normal subject engaging in a range of vocal tasks filmed with rigid endoscopy and stroboscopy. It will hopefully serve to illustrate, within a single subject, variability in laryngeal function associated with changes in frequency, intensity, and phonational mode. Changes in vibratory and mucosal displacements, length characteristics of the vocal folds, and involvement of other laryngeal structures are readily observed. The reader is encouraged to review this study, as well as others, and to perform as many examinations of normal laryngeal and vocal function as possible prior to engaging in the clinical assessment of patients with disordered voice.

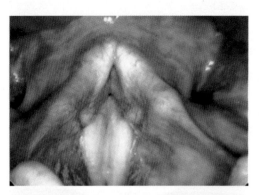

A

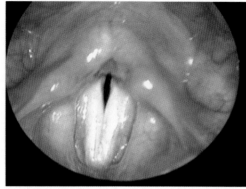

B

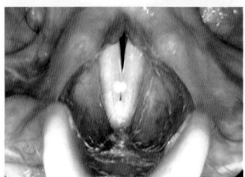

C

Fig. 6.7 (A) The vocal folds are adducted along the posterior vocal processes in this example. **(B)** In this example, a slight gap or chink is present between the vocal folds posteriorly. Secretions and mild erythema are also apparent on the vocal folds in this image. **(C)** This example demonstrates a case where there are slight gaps between the vocal folds both anteriorly and posteriorly.

References

1. Hirano M, Kurita S, Yukizane K, Hibi S. Asymmetry of the laryngeal framework: a morphologic study of cadaver larynges. Ann Otol Rhinol Laryngol 1989;98:135–140

2. Friedrich G, Kainz J, Schneider GH. [Impression of the thyroid cartilage lamina: differential diagnosis in hyperplasia of the ventricular fold]. Laryngol Rhinol Otol (Stuttg) 1988;67:232–239

3. Honjo I, Tanaka S, Tanabe M. Pathogenesis of protruded false vocal fold. Arch Otolaryngol 1985;111: 398–399

4. Lindestad PA, Hertegård S, Björck G. Laryngeal adduction asymmetries in normal speaking subjects. Logoped Phoniatr Vocol 2004;29:128–134

5. Wang RC. Three-dimensional analysis of cricoarytenoid joint motion. Laryngoscope 1998;108(4 Pt 2, Suppl 86)1–17

6. Filho JA, de Melo EC, Tsuji DH, de Giacomo Carneiro C, Sennes LU. Length of the human vocal folds: proposal of mathematical equations as a function of gender and body height. Ann Otol Rhinol Laryngol 2005;114: 390–392

7. Sims S, Yamashita T, Rhew K, Ludlow CL. An evaluation of the use of magnetic stimulation to measure laryngeal muscle response latencies in normal subjects. Otolaryngol Head Neck Surg 1996;114:761–767

8. Peters M. Cerebral asymmetry for speech and the asymmetry in path lengths for the right and left recurrent nerves. Brain Lang 1992;43:349–352

9. Poletto CJ, Verdun LP, Strominger R, Ludlow CL. Correspondence between laryngeal vocal fold movement and muscle activity during speech and nonspeech gestures. J Appl Physiol 2004;97:858–866

10. Doellinger M, Lohscheller J, McWhorter A, Kunduk M. Variability of normal vocal fold dynamics for different vocal loading in one healthy subject investigated by phonovibrograms. J Voice 2009;23:175–181

11. Bless D, Hirano M. Videostroboscopic Examination of the Larynx. San Diego, CA: Singular Publishing Group; 1993

12. Bonilha HS, Deliyski DD, Gerlach TT. Phase asymmetries in normophonic speakers: visual judgments and objective findings. Am J Speech Lang Pathol 2008;17: 367–376

13. Elias ME, Sataloff RT, Rosen DC, Heuer RJ, Spiegel JR. Normal strobovideolaryngoscopy: variability in healthy singers. J Voice 1997;11:104–107

14. Rosen CA. Stroboscopy as a research instrument: development of a perceptual evaluation tool. Laryngoscope 2005;115:423–428

15. Bassich CJ, Ludlow CL. The use of perceptual methods by new clinicians for assessing voice quality. J Speech Hear Disord 1986;51:125–133

16. De Bodt MS, Wuyts FL, Van de Heyning PH, Croux C. Test–retest study of the GRBAS scale: influence of

experience and professional background on perceptual rating of voice quality. J Voice 1997;11:74–80

17. Kreiman J, Gerratt BR, Kempster GB, Erman A, Berke GS. Perceptual evaluation of voice quality: review, tutorial, and a framework for future research. J Speech Hear Res 1993;36:21–40

18. Langmore S. Endoscopic Evaluation and Treatment of Swallowing Disorders. New York, NY: Thieme Medical Publishers; 2001

19. Agada FO, Coatesworth AP, Grace ARH. Retroverted epiglottis presenting as a variant of globus pharyngeus. J Laryngol Otol 2007;121:390–392

II

Flexible Laryngoscopy

7

Flexible Laryngoscopy

Yolanda D. Heman-Ackah

Flexible laryngoscopy is performed to gain a dynamic assessment of the larynx during phonation. It can serve as a useful adjunct to rigid and indirect laryngoscopy; as indirect methods of evaluating the larynx usually require protrusion of the tongue to facilitate adequate visualization of the larynx.[1,2] Flexible laryngoscopy, on the other hand, allows the examiner to evaluate the larynx in its normal anatomic position during various phonatory maneuvers and to gain a better understanding of the patient's vocal habits and vocal posturing during vocalization. Such an understanding can help with accurate diagnosis and in developing a treatment plan that addresses all aspects of the vocal mechanism contributing to voice complaints and vocal pathologies.

◆ Choice of Instrumentation

There are numerous options in instrumentation available currently for flexible laryngoscopy. These include systems that use a distal "chip-tip" camera versus a traditional camera positioned at the eyepiece of the laryngoscope. The chip-tip camera is a small camera positioned at the tip of the flexible laryngoscope. The advantage of the chip-tip laryngoscope is that the distal placement of

the camera allows a more magnified view of the larynx with better resolution than can be achieved with the placement of the camera at the eyepiece of the laryngoscope.[1,3–5] The light source chosen to be used with the flexible laryngoscope can be either a continuous halogen light or a stroboscopic light. Halogen light sources are often used for dynamic assessment of the supraglottic and glottic vocal tract during phonation and for anatomic evaluation of the larynx and its component structures. Stroboscopic light allows for the evaluation of the vibratory function of the vocal folds via flashing lights. The magnification and resolution achieved with currently available chip-tip flexible laryngoscopes for stroboscopic evaluation of the larynx is good, but more detail is usually appreciated with the greater magnification available with rigid endoscopes.[6,7] When portability is of benefit, flexible laryngoscopes with battery-operated light sources can be beneficial. In all cases, the ability to record the examination is invaluable not only in patient education but also in allowing the clinician the ability to take a sufficient amount of time to review subtle abnormalities of the larynx in great detail without the patient discomfort that often accompanies such attention in the absence of a video recording. Additionally, the ability to compare examinations over the course of time is a benefit of maintaining a video record.

◆ The Examination

The most valuable use of the flexible laryngoscope is in the evaluation of movement disorders of the larynx and in evaluation of supraglottic function during phonation.[2,8–10]

Anesthesia

The flexible laryngoscopic examination can be performed with or without topical anesthesia, and there are certain situations when either is appropriate.[11] Topical anesthesia in the larynx allows the clinician to position the laryngoscope within the laryngeal inlet, within several millimeters of the vocal folds without causing much patient discomfort, coughing, or choking. This can be particularly beneficial in patients with a significant amount of tongue base tension, in whom an adequate assessment of vocal fold mobility cannot be performed easily with the telescope positioned at or above the level of the tongue base. The use of topical anesthetics is also beneficial when stroboscopic evaluation of the larynx is performed with the flexible laryngoscope, as it allows a closer, more magnified view of lesions on the vocal fold and greater resolution for evaluation of the mucosal wave. When sensory deficits are suspected, the use of topical anesthetics can interfere with the ability to perform sensory testing, which usually is performed through a flexible laryngoscope that is designed to deliver calibrated puffs of air through an operating channel to laryngeal mucosa. However, in the absence of a need for sensory testing, topical anesthesia is usually recommended. Many clinicians use a nasal decongestant such as oxymetazoline hydrochloride or phenylephrine combined with a topical anesthetic in the nose such as Pontocaine (tetracaine) and a topical anesthetic in the mouth and laryngeal inlet such as Cetacaine. Because there is a slight risk of methemoglobinemia with use of local anesthetics, care must be taken not to use too much anesthetic and not to use anesthetic at all in those who are at risk of developing it.

Technique of Flexible Laryngoscopy

Positioning of the patient for flexible laryngoscopy is key for optimal examination results.[12] Ideally, the patient should be seated, with the head in the neutral position, eyes open, and face relaxed. A relaxed face allows for ease of passage of the laryngoscope into the nose. A small amount of lubricant on the tip of the scope will facilitate passage of the telescope through the nose with minimal patient discomfort, especially when sufficient amount of time has been allowed for nasal decongestion after application of oxymetazoline or phenylephrine. The scope should be passed along the floor of the nose, into the nasopharynx and then turned inferiorly for a view of the hypopharynx and, in particular, the larynx. Closure of the eyes during the examination results in posturing of the larynx that can easily be confused with supraglottic hyperfunction. For this reason, patients should be encouraged to keep their eyes open at all times during the examination. It can be extremely helpful to have a video monitor positioned behind the examiner for the patient to view during the examination. This provides excellent feedback to the patient and helps to reduce anxiety that can sometimes be provoked by the presence of the laryngoscope in the nose.

The flexible laryngoscope is passed through the nose, either beneath the inferior turbinate or between the inferior and middle turbinates in the nose. Care must be taken not to let the tip of the laryngoscope touch the turbinates or septum, as this will result in significant patient discomfort and/or pain. Once the laryngoscope reaches the back of the nose, it is flexed downwards, and the patient is instructed to breathe through the nose. In doing so, the patient will relax the soft palate, opening the posterior nasopharynx wide enough to allow the passage of the laryngoscope into the oropharynx and from there into the hypopharynx and laryngeal inlet.

At this point in the examination, it is best to use halogen light. It allows for evaluation of all of the anatomic structures of the upper aerodigestive tract, without distortion or shadows that can sometimes obscure the anatomy when stroboscopic light is used. A full evaluation of the nasal cavity, nasopharynx, eustachian tubes, soft palate, tonsils, base of tongue, vallecula, piriform sinuses, posterior oropharyngeal wall, posterior hypopharyngeal wall, and larynx should be performed during this portion of the examination. The telescope can be rotated from right to left in the back of the nasopharynx to visualize the eustachian tubes. Once in the hypopharynx, protrusion of the tongue will allow evaluation of the vallecula. Having the patient puff his or her cheeks with closed lips will distend the piriform sinuses. Evaluation of each of these structures for inflammatory, infectious, and neoplastic lesions should always be a routine component of the voice evaluation.

Assessment of Vocal Function

Once an anatomic survey has been completed, the examination can proceed to evaluation of vocal function. The first step in the examination is evaluation of quiet breathing. During normal respiration, the vocal folds should slightly abduct during inspiration and slightly adduct during expiration. When these movements are reversed, paradoxical vocal fold motions are said to exist. Such paradoxical movements can signify laryngeal hyperexcitability that could contribute to laryngeal spasms in response to environmental stimuli such as reflux or allergy. Other than these slight movements of the vocal folds with respiration, there should be no other spontaneous movements in the larynx during quiet breathing. The presence of involuntary, irregular, arrhythmic, jerky movements of the larynx implies laryngeal myoclonus. Rhythmic, involuntary twitches of the laryngeal muscles at rest imply a resting tremor. When similar involuntary, rhythmic twitches occur during phonation only, they are termed laryngeal intention tremors.[13]

After assessment of quiet breathing, an evaluation of the speaking voice is performed. Usually, the patient is asked to recite a familiar fact, such as his or her name and the date, to evaluate for evidence of supraglottic hyperfunction during speech. Ideally, the tongue base should be positioned anteriorly, away from the supraglottis; the vocal folds should meet in the midline with phonation, and the supraglottic muscles should be relaxed during phonation. With increased tongue base tension, the tongue will fall posteriorly and press against the epiglottis, narrowing the supraglottic inlet. When the false vocal folds and pharyngeal constrictors are overly recruited during phonation, there is squeezing of the false vocal fold mucosa in an anterior-posterior or lateral direction. In severe cases, the supraglottic mucosa may be squeezed circumferentially. Dysphonia plica ventricularis occurs when such squeezing results in approximation of the false vocal folds during phonation, so that the "voice" produced is a product of the false vocal folds vibrating against one another, rather than the true vocal folds doing so. Having the patient count from 1 to 10 helps to see whether any supraglottic hyperfunction observed during speech dissipates when the patient is performing a rote task or whether it remains the same. Hyperfunction that is present during thoughtful tasks and that disappears during a mundane task can signal task-specific hyperfunctional behavior. Having the patient raise the pitch of his or her voice to a Minnie Mouse–sounding caricature voice while counting to 10 should result in alleviation of much of the hyperfunction that is seen during normal counting. The inability to raise the pitch of the voice during this task may imply dysfunction of the superior laryngeal nerves. Strain in the voice that is present throughout speech implies supraglottic hyperfunction, which is also commonly referred to as muscle tension dysphonia. Strain that appears intermittently during speech can imply involuntary laryngeal spasms, such as can occur with reflux-induced laryngospasm, spasmodic dysphonia (also termed laryngeal dystonia), laryngeal myoclonus, laryngeal tremor, and some psychogenic laryngeal disorders.[9,12,13]

Occasionally, reflux-induced laryngospasm episodes are easily apparent during the examination. The examiner will see reflux material come up from the cricopharyngeal region and trickle onto the arytenoids and into the laryngeal inlet. At the moment that the refluxate touches the arytenoids or vocal folds, they will spasm, and a concomitant break in speech, characterized by sudden strain, is observed.

Spasmodic dysphonia is a focal dystonia of the larynx that can involve either the intrinsic adductor or abductor muscles of the larynx or both sets of muscles. Adductor spasmodic dysphonia is characterized by involuntary spasms of the adductor muscles of the larynx.

These spasms tend to occur during voiced sounds of speech. The best way to elicit adductor spasms is to have the patient count from 80 to 89. Usually, the /ay/ sound in "eighty" will cause an adductor spasm, and that sound will sound strained. This spasm will then make it difficult for the patient to produce the unvoiced sound of /ti/ that follows in the word *eighty*. Abductor spasmodic dysphonia is characterized by involuntary spasms of the abductor muscles in the larynx, and these tend to occur during unvoiced sounds of speech. It is easiest to elicit abductor spasms by having the patient count from 60 to 69. The sound /s/ that begins the word *sixty* is unvoiced and will cause an abductor spasm, making the rest of the word that follows sound breathy. Mixed spasmodic dysphonia is characterized by both adductor and abductor spasms. In all forms of spasmodic dysphonia, the spasms usually improve when the patient is asked to perform a phonatory task using a voice that is different from his or her usual and habitual communicative voice. Such tasks may include talking in a caricature voice like that of "Minnie Mouse" or singing.[9,12,13]

Laryngeal myoclonus will produce a "jerkiness" in speech that corresponds with the arrhythmic muscle spasms of myoclonus seen in the larynx. Similarly, laryngeal tremor produces a rhythmic roll in the voice that corresponds with tremorous movements of the laryngeal muscles. Psychogenic laryngeal disorders can be the most difficult to diagnose. They can present with muscle patterns and speech patterns that mimic physiologic laryngeal pathologies such as vocal fold paresis and supraglottic hyperfunction. However, with physiologic pathologies, the sound of the voice is the same regardless of the phonatory task. With psychogenic disorders, the patient does not normally associate phonatory tasks such as coughing or laughing with voice production, and when prompted to do so, the patient will produce a normal-sounding cough or laugh. In the case of paresis, the cough and laugh should be just as soft and breathy as the speaking voice. In trying to differentiate a psychogenic disorder from supraglottic hyperfunction, it is best to distract the patient and have him or her talk about something that is emotionally charged for him or her. Regardless of the emotional state,

true physiologic hyperfunction will always be present throughout all forms of speech. In a psychogenic disorder, feelings of anger, elation, or sadness will usually elicit, at least initially, a normal-sounding voice.

The next phonatory task specifically looks at superior laryngeal nerve function. It involves having the patient perform the glissando maneuver on the vowel /i/. In this task, the patient slides from the lowest pitch he or she can access to the highest pitch in his or her vocal range while phonating the vowel /i/, then sliding down from high to low. Ideally, both vocal folds should show a progressive and smooth increase in longitudinal tension (ie, the length of the vocal fold from the arytenoid to the anterior commissure should increase as pitch increases) as the patient goes from low to high and a reversal of this motion as he or she goes from high to low. The examiner is not only noting whether or not the vocal folds lengthen with voluntary increase in pitch but is also noting whether or not the lengthening of the vocal folds is symmetric and whether or not there is a tilting of the larynx as the pitch is increased. Asymmetric lengthening of the vocal folds with voluntary increase in pitch implies a relative weakness or paresis of the superior laryngeal nerve/cricothyroid muscle on the side that is foreshortened. Similarly, tilting of the larynx during voluntary increase in pitch implies a superior laryngeal nerve paresis on the side toward which the larynx tilts as the pitch is raised.[2,8–10,12–14]

The function of the abductor muscles of the larynx is evaluated by having the patient perform serial abductory laryngeal tasks. Having the patient sniff through the nose forcefully and quickly at least five times in rapid succession will assess the isolated function of the posterior cricoarytenoid muscles, the laryngeal abductors. Ideally, the vocal folds should abduct symmetrically during the sniffs. When assessing the degree of symmetry, the examiner is paying close attention to the extent to which the vocal folds open from the midline on each side, whether or not that excursion is the same or if one vocal fold appears to open slightly wider than does the other, and whether or not the quickness with which the vocal folds move is symmetric or if one vocal fold tends to move slightly more briskly than the other. Asymmetries in lateral excursion of the vocal folds or in the briskness of abduction of the vocal folds may imply dysfunction of the involved posterior cricoarytenoid muscle or the branch of the recurrent laryngeal nerve that innervates that muscle.

Having the patient whistle a tune, such as "Yankee Doodle," allows the examiner to evaluate the adductor and abductor functions of the larynx while at the same time eliminating the supraglottic hyperfunction that can accompany speech and that can obscure subtle abnormalities in vocal fold mobility. A tune with a quick beat will cause rapid adduction and abduction of the vocal folds, which is beneficial in assessing the rapidity of vocal fold motion. Attention is focused on symmetry of motion of the vocal folds, symmetry of both lateral and medial excursion of the vocal folds, and symmetry in briskness in movement of the vocal folds. Asymmetries in adduction may imply paresis or dysfunction in any of the adductory muscles of the larynx, including the thyroarytenoid, lateral cricoarytenoid, the interarytenoid, or the cricothyroid muscles. Asymmetries in abduction imply paresis or dysfunction of the posterior cricoarytenoid muscle. Asymmetries in adduction can also be elicited by having the patient alternate rapidly between the sounds /i/-/hi/-/i/-/hi/-/i/-/hi....[2,8–10,12–14]

The ability to coordinate the actions of the opposing muscle groups in the larynx is assessed by having the patient repetitively and quickly alternate between strong adductory and abductory movements. The task of repeatedly alternating between a forceful sniff and the sound /i/ is one of the best tasks for assessing coordination in the larynx. The inability to rapidly alternate between abduction and adduction implies laryngeal dysdiadokinesis. Any systemic neurologic disorder that can cause dysdiadokinesis in other muscle groups can also cause dysdiadokinesis in the larynx. These typically are signs of an extrapyramidal cause.[13] One of the most common causes in the larynx is laryngeal dystonia (spasmodic dysphonia). Parkinsonism is another. Laryngeal cogwheeling, seen as jerky movements of the adductor muscles as they attempt to go from the open position of the sniff to the closed position of the /i/, can also be elicited in this maneuver. Cogwheeling is a sign of laryngeal rigidity and can be seen in upper motor neuron disorders that cause spasticity as well as in Parkinsonism.[13,14]

Dysdiadokinesia can also be elicited by having the patient repeatedly say the sounds /pa/-/ta/-/ka/-/pa/-/ta/-/ka/-/pa/-/ta/-/ka/-/pa/-/ta/-/ka/-/pa/-/ta/-/ka/.... This task involves more rapid movement of the adductors and abductors and will elicit subtle abnormalities in coordination that may not be readily apparent in alternating between a sniff and the sound /i/. Additionally, the task /pa/-/ta/-/ka/-/pa/-/ta/-/ka/-/pa/-/ta/-/ka/-/pa/-/ta/-/ka/-/pa/-/ta/-/ka/... allows one to evaluate for rapidity of movement. The inability to say these sounds rapidly in succession implies laryngeal bradykinesia, which is often seen in basal ganglia disorders such as laryngeal dystonias and Parkinsonism.[13]

Whether or not the patient is a singer, it is always important to evaluate the singing voice as well as the speaking voice.[9,10,12] Usually, it is best to have the patient sing a tune with which he or she is very familiar, such as "Happy Birthday," or another similar tune in their native language if English is the second language. For instance, "La Cucaracha" is a song that most Spanish-speaking patients will know, and this can be used to evaluate the singing voice in this situation. Familiarity with a song that is commonly sung usually eliminates the desire for the patient to "perform" and allows for assessment of hyperfunction, breathing patterns, and vocal fold mobility during a task that the patient does not associate with normal speech. This can be particularly helpful again in patients with psychogenic voice disorders, as it is harder for the patient to manipulate the voice throughout the vocal range. During singing, inconsistencies in vocal fold mobility and longitudinal tension can be elicited that may be more difficult to ascertain during other phonatory maneuvers. Patients with spasmodic dysphonia will typically have a completely normal singing voice, regardless of the degree of severity of the dysphonia in the speaking voice. In patients who are singers, it is important to also have them sing a song or two from their normal repertoire to evaluate how they use their vocal mechanism during vocal performance. Oftentimes, laryngeal postures and habits are different during singing in professional and avocational singers than they are during speech, and it is important to make this distinction.

◆ Conclusion

Flexible laryngoscopy is an important tool in the evaluation of voice disorders and laryngeal pathology. It is most beneficial in diagnosing anatomic abnormalities throughout the upper aerodigestive tract and in evaluating vocal fold mobility and glottic and supraglottic postures during singing, speech, and other phonatory tasks. The flexible laryngoscope is a valuable tool in the diagnosis of neurologic abnormalities in the larynx, allowing for accurate assessment of mobility without artifact that can be induced from protruding the tongue, as is necessary with indirect methods of laryngeal examination. The ability to use stroboscopic light with the flexible laryngoscope makes it a useful tool in the evaluation of the vibratory function of the vocal folds as well, as is discussed in the chapters on videostroboscopy.

References

1. Sato K, Umeno H, Nakashima T. Stroboscopic observation of vocal fold vibration with the videoendoscope. Ann Otol Rhinol Laryngol 2003;112:965–970

2. Heman-Ackah YD, Batory M. Determining the etiology of mild vocal fold hypomobility. J Voice 2003; 17:579–588

3. Cleveland TF. Principles of stroboscopy. In: Ossoff RH, Shapshay SM, Woodson GE, et al., eds. The Larynx, 1st ed. Philadelphia, PA: Lippincott Williams & Wilkins; 2003:71–76

4. Boehme G, Gross M. Stroboscopy. London, UK: Whurr Publishers; 2005:18–106

5. Kaszuba SM, Garrett CG. Strobovideolaryngoscopy and laboratory voice evaluation. Otolaryngol Clin North Am 2007;40:991–1001, vi

6. Eller R, Ginsburg M, Lurie D, Heman-Ackah Y, Lyons K, Sataloff R. Flexible laryngoscopy: a comparison of fiber optic and distal chip technologies—part 2: laryngopharyngeal reflux. J Voice 2009;23:389–395

7. Eller R, Ginsburg M, Lurie D, Heman-Ackah Y, Lyons K, Sataloff R. Flexible laryngoscopy: a comparison of fiber optic and distal chip technologies. Part 1: vocal fold masses. J Voice 2008;22:746–750

8. Rubin AD, Sataloff RT. Vocal fold paresis and paralysis. Otolaryngol Clin North Am 2007;40:1109–1131, viii–ix

9. Rubin AD. Neurolaryngologic evaluation of the performer. Otolaryngol Clin North Am 2007;40: 971–989, vi

10. Rubin AD, Praneetvatakul V, Heman-Ackah Y, Moyer CA, Mandel S, Sataloff RT. Repetitive phonatory tasks for identifying vocal fold paresis. J Voice 2005;19: 679–686

11. Rubin AD, Shah A, Moyer CA, Johns MM. The effect of topical anesthesia on vocal fold motion. J Voice 2009; 23:128–131

12. Sataloff RT, Hawkshaw MJ, Divi V, Heman-Ackah YD. Physical examination of voice professionals. Otolaryngol Clin North Am 2007;40:953–969, v–vi

13. Merati AL, Heman-Ackah YD, Abaza M, Altman KW, Sulica L, Belamowicz S. Common movement disorders affecting the larynx: a report from the neurolaryngology committee of the AAO-HNS. Otolaryngol Head Neck Surg 2005;133:654–665

14. Altman KW, Schaefer SD, Yu GP, et al; Neurolaryngology Subcommittee of the American Academy of Otolaryngology-Head and Neck Surgery. The voice and laryngeal dysfunction in stroke: a report from the Neurolaryngology Subcommittee of the American Academy of Otolaryngology-Head and Neck Surgery. Otolaryngol Head Neck Surg 2007;136:873–881

8

Flexible Laryngoscopy in Speech-Language Pathology Evaluation

Rebecca J. Leonard

The term *phonoscopic* examination is used to describe the flexible endoscopic examination of dysphonic patients performed by the speech-language pathologist (or voice clinician). This term emphasizes the focus of the exam on understanding the relationship between laryngeal behaviors, including postures and gestures, and the voice. The term also clearly differentiates the assessment performed by the voice clinician, who is interested particularly in "vocal" pathology, from the diagnostic exam performed by an otolaryngologist, who is concerned about laryngeal or other pathology. The exam pairs laryngeal imaging with the voice evaluation traditionally performed by speech pathologists to both hear and see how the voice is produced.

The phonoscopic exam involves sampling laryngeal behavior and voice across a wide variety of tasks, including:

1. respiratory, vegetative, and phonatory;
2. the patient's available fundamental frequency range;
3. a range of intensities, from soft to loud, at different frequencies;
4. different phonatory modes (ie, whisper, falsetto);

5. different phonetic contexts (ie, single sounds, connected speech);
6. voicing for variable duration (as with sustained sound or repetition of voiced syllables).

If evidence of hyperfunctional and/or inappropriate behaviors is observed, efforts to modify them may be attempted. If the impression is that voice is produced more easily, or with improved quality, in certain contexts, these will be explored further. The process of identification and exploration is often referred to as "treatment probing."

The exam is performed with the patient seated in the usual position for a flexible endoscopic procedure, with back straight and torso angled forward. Depending on the protocols of the particular setting, a small amount of topical anesthesia may be applied to one or both nasal passages. In our own setting, typically only one nostril is anesthetized. If there is a question about mobility of one or the other vocal fold, viewing from both nostrils can be included. The exam may require 5 minutes or so and is usually well tolerated by the patient. The utility of the exam is dependent on several factors, including the patient's ability to cooperate, the experience of the clinician, and the quality of the imaging equipment being used.

A rigid endoscope with stroboscopy will permit laryngeal imaging during many of the tasks outlined here; for example, sustained sounds produced at different frequency and intensity levels and voice produced across phonatory modes. The inclusion of stroboscopy, with rigid or flexible endoscopy, also permits the assessment of vibratory and mucosal displacement details, including asymmetries in phase or amplitude that may imply subtle underlying pathology. The particular advantage of flexible endoscopy is the potential for evaluation of the larynx and voice during connected speech (or singing).

◆ Value

Assessment

Voice clinicians have long relied on the sound of voice in making judgments about a patient's dysphonia. Other perceptions, for example, the apparent effort associated with voice production and the relative difficulty of listeners in hearing and understanding what's been spoken, are also critical to this appraisal. More recently, a variety of acoustic and aerodynamic assessment tools have permitted greater insights into the nature of dysphonia in individual patients.[1] The increasing availability of normative data associated with these instruments and the emphasis on creating standardized approaches to their use have added further to our diagnostic and treatment repertoire. In particular, these measures help to distinguish clearly the disordered voice from normal voicing and allow objective comparisons of voice across time or treatments.

Over the past few years, many voice clinicians have been able to incorporate endoscopic imaging in the management of dysphonic patients. In our opinion, the use of imaging, and flexible endoscopy in particular, represents an enormous step forward in speech pathology practice. Quite simply, the advantage of not only listening to a voice but also observing simultaneously the structures that produce it is huge. Patients are typically referred to the voice clinician by an otolaryngologist who has performed a comprehensive examination of the head and neck, including the larynx. The physician's description of laryngeal pathology or voicing difficulty may be quite general, for example, "vocal nodules," "paralysis of left true vocal fold," or "functional dysphonia." This information, though important, says nothing about the patient's use of the larynx to produce voice. Yet, it is an understanding of how the patient uses his or her voice that, in our own experience, is required for the speech pathologist to develop the most efficient and effective treatment plan possible.

Vocal Pathology

Vocal pathology refers to a patient's inappropriate use of laryngeal structures to produce voice. In some cases, these behaviors may have produced laryngeal pathology. In other instances, they may be the result of laryngeal pathology or represent a response to some other stimulus. The provoking stimulus in these "adaptive dysphonias" (ie, edema, paresis, a lesion) may be clearly present on examination of the larynx. In other cases, the original pathology has resolved and laryngeal structures appear normal, but voice production continues to be abnormal. The onset of vocal pathology may also be associated with stress or psychopathology. Again, in response to some set of provoking stimuli, voice is produced in an atypical manner. Regardless of the origin of vocal pathology, however, the goal of the voice clinician is to redirect a patient's maladaptive behavior(s) to more appropriate behaviors; that is, ones more consistent with normal voice. If normal voice production is not a reasonable expectation, then voice produced in the most optimal manner possible (ie, best quality, least effort) is the goal. In both cases, the process is likely to require (1) relaxation of hyperfunctional postures; (2) elimination of inappropriate behaviors; (3) modification of both phonatory and vocal fold variables during voice production.

Our contention is that these goals can be much more directly, efficiently, and effectively completed if the clinician knows as much about the adaptive behavior as possible. In short, though the target of normal, or optimal, voice may be the same, the approach to achieving it will vary. Interestingly, whether a voice is "disordered" or not, at least from a listener's perspective, is largely determined by its sound; that is, how pleasant or unpleasant, strong or weak, audible or inaudible, it may be. But for the voice clinician, relying solely on the sound of voice to infer how it is being produced and developing a treatment plan consistent with this inference can be misleading, for several reasons.

First, in our experience, there is not a simple one-to-one correlation between laryngeal behavior and the voice perceived by this behavior. For example, voice generally characterized as "whisper" may be produced with the true vocal folds abducted, with both the false and true vocal folds adducted and constricted, or with the true vocal folds adducted but not vibrating, and, likely, in several other ways (**Fig. 8.1**). Relatively large changes in laryngeal behavior may sometimes produce only small or subtle changes in voice, whereas in other instances, small changes in behaviors or phonatory parameters (ie, frequency and airflow) produce large effects in voice. If the clinician is not both listening and observing, these relationships are not clear.

Another important benefit of the phonoscopic exam is realized when dysphonia is intermittent or variable. Inappropriate or hyperfunctional behaviors are sometimes "context-specific"; for example, occurring at the beginning or end of a breath group, when pulmonary support is compromised, or when fundamental frequency achieves a particular level. These kinds of behaviors are particularly common when patients are attempting to compensate for a laryngeal deficit, such as bowing, or glottic incompetence produced by the presence of a lesion. In other situations, for example, where scarring is present, voice quality may be better in selected contexts (ie, particular combination of frequency, intensity, and airflow) due to improved symmetry of vibration. Identification of such contexts can be quite useful to the voice clinician, providing insights into both laryngeal and vocal pathology. With imaging, specific behaviors can be associated with these contexts.

In some patients, there may also be a lag between the onset of a maladaptive behavior and its eventual manifestation in voice. Normal laryngeal behavior and voice may be apparent early in the production of a sustained sound and then be replaced with an increasing degree of false fold or supraglottic constriction; for example, when pulmonary support is compromised. The effect of the progressive hyperconstriction may not be apparent in voice initially but become more perceptible as increased effort or altered quality as pulmonary support is further compromised. If this effect can be further characterized, for example, by how many syllables can be produced before it is observed, or by where in a breath group it first appears, the information may be usefully incorporated into treatment planning. Examples of such context-specific behaviors are presented below (**Figs. 8.2, 8.3, 8.4**).

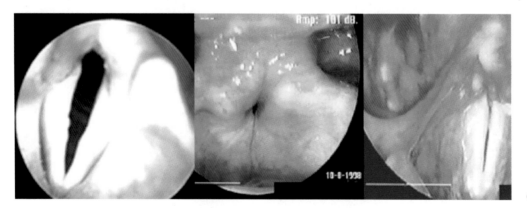

A,B

C

Fig. 8.1 Three different postures of the larynx, all of which produced voice characterized as "whisper," are illustrated. **(A)** The true folds are abducted. **(B)** The false folds are hyperadducted, obscuring the underlying true folds. **(C)** The true vocal folds are adducted but not vibrating.

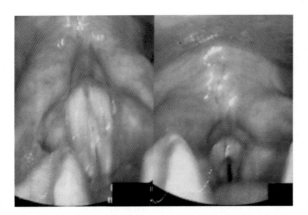

A   B

Fig. 8.2 (A) A patient complaining of vocal fatigue with singing reveals relatively better laryngeal behavior (and voice) at the onset of phonation. **(B)** Supraglottic constriction becomes apparent visually when sound is sustained beyond 7 seconds.

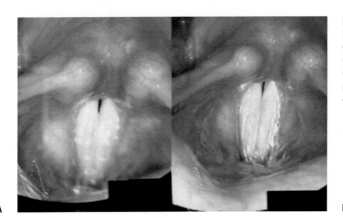

A   B

Fig. 8.3 In contrast with the illustration in **Fig. 8.2**, an individual with normal laryngeal and phonatory function is shown sustaining sound for 2 seconds **(A)** and 24 seconds later **(B)**. No evidence of excessive effort with increased duration is observed.

Laryngeal Pathology

As stated earlier, the intent of the phonoscopic exam is different from that of the diagnostic exam performed by an otolaryngologist. However, observation of the larynx over a wide range of voicing and other tasks may aid the diagnosis of tissue pathology, as well as vocal pathology. This is because laryngeal pathology, like vocal pathology, may be observed only intermittently or may be visualized more easily during certain laryngeal behaviors. A patient with bowing of the vocal folds may appear to have relatively normal vocal fold

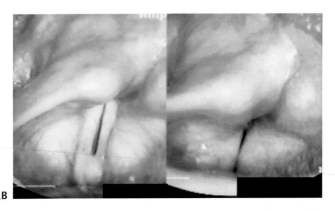

A,B

Fig. 8.4 (A) A patient with glottic insufficiency producing voice at soft intensity. **(B)** With even a small increase in loudness, evidence of false fold constriction and medialization become apparent. The inability of the true vocal folds to increase resistance with increased subglottal pressure (necessary to increasing vocal loudness) is likely related to the maladaptive behavior observed. The evidence of false fold behavior is readily observed visually but may not be apparent in voice until some time after its onset.

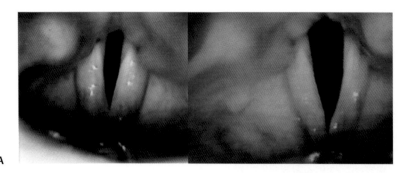

Fig. 8.5 The true folds remain partially abducted **(A)**, obscuring the lesion, which reflects greater abduction of the true folds **(B)**.

A

B

closure at higher fundamental frequencies but demonstrate significant glottic incompetence at lower frequencies. Because some larynges are difficult to observe at lower frequencies, due to a lowering of the larynx and shortening of the vocal folds, bowing of this type may be missed. Anterior commissure pathology may not be visualized unless the true vocal folds are widely abducted, and pathology that may be displaced below the vocal folds on voicing (ie, polyps, granulomatous lesions) may be more easily observed on voice produced on inspiration (**Figs. 8.5 and 8.6**). Infrequently, we have identified lesions that were not apparent until the patient was engaged in rigorous voice use for some period of time. This pathology (ie, ventricular cyst) appears to become pneumatized with such exercise and affects voice only in these circumstances. Careful questioning of the patient may prompt the clinician to simulate the situation implicated.

In other instances, the clinician may find that laryngeal pathology is masked by maladaptive laryngeal behaviors. This can be particularly true when voice production involves use of the false vocal folds or constriction of other supraglottic structures. Relaxation of these postures through treatment probing permits a more thorough evaluation of underlying structures and may lead to the identification of laryngeal pathology not previously recognized (**Fig. 8.7**). The possibility that voicing behaviors can mask laryngeal pathology also underscores the need for observing the larynx in nonphonatory tasks or in circumstances that permit thorough examination of laryngeal structures.

If laryngeal pathology related to voice use is present, it is important for the voice clinician to understand vocal and laryngeal practices likely to have produced the pathology, as well as practices that may have developed in response to the pathology. Secondary practices, in our experience, can often be dealt with relatively quickly to facilitate resolution of pathology. Behaviors likely to have produced the pathology initially, however, may be more long-standing and, consequently, more resistant to treatment. Careful interviewing of the patient will often be helpful in differentiating these issues.

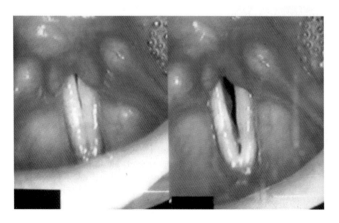

A,B

Fig. 8.6 (A) The vocal folds appear within normal limits. **(B)** Voice is produced on inspiration, and pathology on the inferior surfaces of the true vocal folds is apparent.

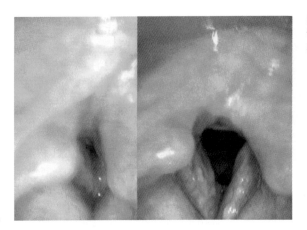

A   B

Fig. 8.7 Hyperconstriction of the false folds during voicing **(A)** obscures pathology apparent during respiration **(B)**.

Treatment

For patients who are voice therapy candidates, the use of endoscopy provides an excellent opportunity to engage in a process we refer to as "mapping vocal space." This process requires, first, identification of the patient's current vocal space; that is, the combination of phonatory and laryngeal behaviors where voice is being produced. Laryngeal and other behaviors that need to be changed in order for a patient to produce more appropriate voice are targeted for modification. Strategies for achieving these modifications, that is, for moving the patient into a more optimal vocal space, are then attempted. The goal will differ depending on the patient's current vocal capabilities. If laryngeal pathology is present, the goal is the elimination of inappropriate adaptive behaviors or the alteration of vocal fold contact patterns in a

way that facilitates resolution of pathology (**Figs. 8.8 and 8.9**). If maladaptive behaviors persist in the absence of observed laryngeal pathology, the goal is to restore optimal use of structures for voicing. Details of each patient's situation notwithstanding, the clinician's task is to elicit voice produced in the most appropriate manner possible (ie, best voice, no hyperfunction, no exacerbation of existing pathology, if present).

In our practice, the initial therapy objective is to identify voice produced as appropriately as possible on a single sound ("m" or "ee"). In some cases, a more normal target may be achieved, but at a frequency or intensity, for example, that is not ideal for a given patient. Continued modification of both laryngeal and phonatory variables may be required to produce sound that achieves both laryngeal and vocal appropriateness. Once (or if) produced,

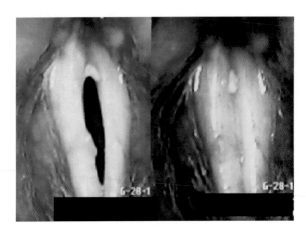

Fig. 8.8 Patient status after excision of resistant posterior granuloma reveals posterior contact pattern between the true folds. This pattern was typically observed on voicing tasks sampled.

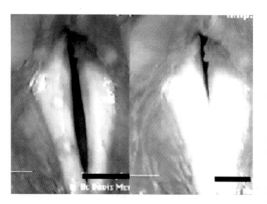

Fig. 8.9 Patient in **Fig. 8.8** after modification of contact pattern between folds. Note the small gap between vocal processes. The intent of modification was to reduce compression forces at the site of residual pathology.

the clinician then directs the patient in repeating the desired voice over several trials, again, on only one sound. Occasional rest breaks followed by another series of repetitions may be helpful in stabilizing the voice in this highly structured context. The clinician may counsel the patient to focus on a variety of available feedback sources during these attempts (ie, how it sounds, how it feels). When the patient is able to produce the voice readily and consistently, the vocal "space" in which the sound can be produced is expanded, for example, at different frequencies or intensities. For all phonatory parameters, including frequency, intensity, and airflow, which are perhaps the most frequently manipulated, there are normal ranges, low to high, soft to loud, less or more. The goal of mapping is to achieve normal or improved voice over a range of phonatory behaviors.

Once sound can be produced in this manner, the clinician expands the contexts in which the improved sound is produced; that is, on syllables, short utterances, and, ultimately, connected speech. The steps described here represent, in our opinion, a logical and often successful approach to voice therapy. With some patients, the progression from a target sound to its consistent use in connected speech may be quite brief, of the order of minutes. For other patients, progress may be significantly slower. When achieved, the clinician's next goal is consistent use of the improved voice in situations outside the clinic.

Laryngeal Imaging as a Feedback Tool

In our practice, treatment probing is most often performed without providing feedback from laryngeal imaging to the patient. Once our goals and the strategies for achieving them are defined, and when the target voice has been achieved in some contexts, feedback from imaging can prove extremely useful. For this purpose, the patient is seated as comfortably as possible in front of a monitor that permits easy visualization of the larynx. Ideally, the clinician can also view the monitor and be close enough to it to point out various features of the larynx. At this stage of treatment, it becomes important for the patient to understand mechanisms of normal voice production, as well as what has been inappropriate about his or her own use of the larynx to produce voice. By combining visual information with available feedback (ie, auditory and other sensory feedback), the clinician hopes to help the patient develop an ability to identify and self-correct any deviations from the target voice. If the patient can leave the treatment room with these skills, it bodes well for the success of therapy.

One example of the particular utility of imaging in treatment involves its use in patients with vocal process granuloma.[2] Patients appropriate for this approach have usually failed multiple medical and surgical treatments for vocal process granuloma. The relationship between patients' granuloma and laryngopharyngeal reflux should be documented on esophagram or by pH probe. The therapy program is usually offered to patients who demonstrate contact of the vocal processes at the site of pathology on voicing. Though such a pattern is thought to be within the range of normal variability, in the case of a vocal process granuloma it may be interfering with the desired resolution of vocal process pathology (**Fig. 8.8**).

The goal of the treatment is to produce voice without contact between the cartilaginous portion of the vocal folds, thus minimizing adductor forces at the site of pathology (**Fig. 8.9**). Treatment probing is first attempted to determine if such a pattern can be identified; that is, if voice can be produced with the patient maintaining a small gap between the vocal processes. The goal is first explained to the patient, and imaging equipment is positioned so that both patient and clinician can visualize contact patterns on a monitor. If achieved on a single sound, the pattern is then expanded across other phonatory contexts, as previously described. We found in a retrospective study of 10 patients who underwent therapy that 8 were able to achieve the treatment objective, and all 8 experienced resolution of pathology or a marked reduction in its extent. Six patients who did not undergo treatment, and the two who were unable to achieve the treatment objective, demonstrated minimal or no improvement, or worsening of their pathology, over the same period of time. This approach to treatment, while certainly not successful with all patients, has become a standard part of our protocol for patients with granuloma resistant to other treatments. A patient's candidacy for the treatment can typically be determined within the context of a single phonoscopic session, adding to its reasonable inclusion in the voice clinician's treatment repertoire.

◆ Flexible Endoscopy versus Phonoscopy

We previously reported results of a retrospective review undertaken in an attempt to assess objectively the value of the phonoscopic evaluation just discussed.[3] In particular, we were interested in a comparison of findings on a phonoscopic evaluation with results of flexible endoscopic exams performed on the same patients by referring physicians. Patients included in the review had undergone a laryngeal exam by the referring otolaryngologist prior to evaluation in our voice clinic. All patients underwent our typical voice clinic protocol, including case history/medical records review; a traditional voice evaluation from which maximum performance, habitual performance, perceptual and acoustic measures are obtained; a laryngeal function study that provides airflow data and estimates of glottal resistance and subglottal pressure; a pulmonary function screen; and phonoscopic evaluation with flexible and rigid endoscopy. For purposes of the study, no patient whose findings were dependent on stroboscopic exam (eg, asymmetry in vibration, mucosal stiffening, lesion differentiation) was included

for review. In addition, no patients with laryngeal or vocal tremor were included.

In 26 of 100 cases, our observations were consistent with those of the referring otolaryngologist. In 32 cases, we agreed with the referral diagnosis but found additional factor(s) related to pathology. In 12 of the 32 cases for whom additional pathology was identified, we agreed that the patient demonstrated a particular hyperfunctional behavior, but we believed it was a consequence of underlying pathology (eg, bowing, paralysis, lesion). The diagnosis on referral was of either the hyperfunctional behavior exhibited (eg, plicae ventricularis) or of a "functional" dysphonia, without evidence of any underlying laryngeal pathology. In the remaining cases, we agreed with the referral diagnosis but found additional pathology. Frequently, this was a smaller, for example, contrecoup lesion on the opposite vocal fold. However, in a few cases pathology distant from that noted on referral was identified. In 14 instances of pathology identified, our impression was that it may have been *context-specific*; that is, more easily identified on some voicing tasks than on others.

In 42 cases, our findings differed from those of the referring physician. The most frequent example in this category was of a lesion identified on phonoscopy that had not been noted in the referral. In contrast with lesions that were believed to be masked by hyperfunctional behaviors or postures, these lesions were not obscured from visualization by the behavior of overlying structures. In several instances, pathology noted on the phonoscopic exam was apparent primarily on particular vocal tasks; that is, context-specific. Interestingly, in seven of these cases, patients were diagnosed with "plicae ventricularis dysphonia" when, in fact, other hyperfunctional postures were responsible for the dysphonia. In one patient, for example, aberrant voice was produced by an arytenoid contacting the epiglottis. In another, the false folds were perhaps slightly medialized on voicing, but the major source of dysphonia was true vocal folds that were abducted and apparently quite tensed. Though these distinctions may seem subtle, and perhaps not that pertinent to the otolaryngologist, they are important to a voice clinician charged with modifying the aberrant behavior.

◆ Indications for Phonoscopic Examination

In our clinic, the phonoscopic examination described here is of particular value in the following situations:

1. *Patient is a candidate for voice therapy.* The phonoscopic exam will aid the voice clinician in understanding the relationship between laryngeal behavior and voice production. If inappropriate or hyperfunctional behaviors are a primary factor in the patient's dysphonia, identification and elaboration of these may be a key to the efficiency and effectiveness of voice therapy. If laryngeal pathology is present, the ability to probe laryngeal behaviors likely to produce optimal voice and minimize exacerbation of pathology is equally helpful. Visual feedback provided by endoscopy can also be a valuable tool in educating patients regarding how the larynx works, for voice or other purposes, and in directing their efforts to modify behavior consistent with treatment objectives.
2. *Patient's dysphonia is unexplained after non-phonoscopic laryngeal exam.* As described earlier, subtle laryngeal pathology is sometimes visualized more readily in particular contexts or circumstances not typically included on standard laryngoscopic exams. If there continues to be a question about the cause of a patient's dysphonia after this type of exam, the more task-oriented phonoscopic exam may prove quite useful.

If the referring otolaryngologist is aware that a speech-language pathologist who is working with a patient will be unable to perform an imaging study, the following information should be provided:

1. Details of benign pathology (ie, site, compressibility, evidence of acuteness vs chronicity).
2. Details of vocal "space" (ie, combination of frequency, intensity, airflow) where voice and laryngeal behavior appear improved.
3. Details of behaviors that appear to be maladaptive (ie, use of false folds during voicing, arytenoid-epiglottis approximation).

With respect to the latter, it is important to know that "maladaptive" behaviors may not necessarily be hyperfunctional. The illustration presented earlier of vocal folds that were adducted but not vibrating is one example of a behavior that, though inappropriate for normal voicing, did not appear to be associated with excessive effort.

◆ Limitations of Flexible Endoscopic Examination for Speech-Language Pathology

Traditional nasopharyngoscopes are composed of three components. These include a bundle of fiberoptic rods (typically around 3 to 3.5 mm in diameter) that transmit light to illuminate structures of interest, an external light source, and a video camera with lens attached to the viewing portion of the scope. The camera is attached to a monitor and, if desired, a recorder (video or digital) for storage of images. Recording the image through the fiberoptic bundle produces some pixelation of the image. In addition, the central portion of the image visualized appears larger than the image at the periphery. Newer versions of these scopes may accommodate an internal, battery-operated light source, making the entire system lighter and more portable.

Because of the scope's insertion through the left or right nostril, it may not be possible to center the scope tip exactly above the vocal folds on imaging. The image viewed, depending on its distance from the scope tip, may appear disproportionately large or small as a consequence or may appear to move more or less briskly/extensively. Casper et al. provided an example of two lines drawn in parallel that appeared to intersect at one end when viewed through the flexible nasopharyngoscope.[4] These limitations can typically be accounted for when they are understood and underscore the importance of experience with both normal and disordered anatomy and physiology in accurately interpreting the endoscopic exam.

Newer technology has produced flexible scopes that have a camera chip in the tip of the scope, minimizing several of the technical problems associated with older instruments. These videoscopes or "chip-in-the-tip" scopes produce high-resolution digital images of excellent quality. The diameter of these scopes may be somewhat larger than that of traditional scopes, though smaller versions are increasingly available. The powerful light sources and digital signal processing hardware associated with the videoscopes add weight to these systems, but the image resolution is excellent.

In our experience, stroboscopic imaging with a flexible endoscope, even a digital videoscope, does not typically provide the same quality of information regarding mucosal and vibratory displacements as stroboscopy with a rigid scope (in patients who can be visualized with rigid endoscopy). If a patient can be visualized well with rigid endoscopy, the large size and clear image possible are extremely useful to the voice clinician as well as the otolaryngologist.

◆ Flexible Endoscopy and the Speech-Language Pathologist: Training, Safety, Ethics

The use of flexible nasal endoscopy is often considered a "minimally invasive" procedure. Primary risks include a reaction to a topical anesthetic, a nose bleed, or other nasal injury, and a vasovagal response in a patient. In some states, laws pertaining to the scope of practice for speech-language pathologists have specifically allowed for the procedure if certain training requirements and setting restrictions are met. In California, for example, a licensed speech-language pathologist must first be successfully mentored in the use of the instrument by an otolaryngologist certified by the American Board of Otolaryngology. Settings in which flexible endoscopy can be performed are also restricted, with a primary requirement being the availability of documented emergency medical backup procedures, including a physician or other appropriate medical professionals. There is additional language specifying that the pathologist's use of an endoscope is not for the purpose of diagnosing pathology but, rather, for the elaboration and treatment of communication and swallowing impairment. It is incumbent on the voice clinician to know, and to be in compliance with, the pertinent state laws regarding the use of endoscopy by speech-language pathologists. These may differ from state to state and, unlike practice guidelines recommended by professional associations, are legally binding.

References

1. Leonard R, Dworkin J, Meleca R, Colton R, Leeper A, Till J. Assessment of the disordered voice: a roundtable discussion. J Med Speech-Lang Pathol 2002;10: 111–131
2. Leonard R, Kendall K. Effects of voice therapy on vocal process granuloma: a phonoscopic approach. Am J Otolaryngol 2005;26:101–107
3. Leonard R, Kendall K. Phonoscopy—a valuable tool for otolaryngologists and speech-language pathologists in the management of dysphonic patients. Laryngoscope 2001;111:1760–1766
4. Casper JK, Brewer DW, Colton RH. Variations in normal human laryngeal anatomy and physiology as viewed fiberscopically. J Voice 1987;1:180–185

9

Flexible Laryngoscopy for In-office Procedures

Seth H. Dailey

An aging U.S. population with higher general anesthetic risk profiles, new endoscopes with better imaging and features for office procedures, and digital recording systems have influenced a shift of upper airway procedures into the office from the operating room. Furthermore, the development of a new generation of vocal fold injectables and lasers with flexible fibers and other applications is transforming the range of opportunities for treatment of disorders of the larynx, pharynx, esophagus, and trachea.

◆ Background

Although access to the upper airway began in the office with the introduction of mirror laryngoscopy by Garcia in 1854, the movement of endoscopy to the operating room eventually evolved for better precision and improved imaging.[1] Specifically, the operating room setting provided direct, unimpeded access to the larynx, trachea, or esophagus, with better lighting and a minimum of patient movement.

In 1857, Czermak used artificial light sources and a tooth-held concave mirror to focus light into the larynx. Kirstein tirelessly promoted direct laryngoscopy in the office, which he described as "veritably a surgical method." "Autoscopy," as it was called, was performed with the patient in the sitting position and required an assistant to position and reassure the patient. Jackson formalized this surgical technique with his exhaustive teachings and original illustrations; he promoted the supine positioning of the patient, which heralded its evolution into an operating suite. The use of a suspension apparatus by Killian led to enhanced precision as the surgeon could employ two hands to operate.

The advent of reliable general anesthesia in the 1960s completed the triad of optimal conditions for laryngeal surgery in the operating room: direct visualization with suspension, stillness of the patient, and bimanual manipulation of tissues by the surgeon. The advances came at the expense of cardiovascular morbidity produced largely by anesthetic agents, a dilemma we still face today. The addition and popularization of microscopic laryngeal examination by Scalco, Jako, Kleinsasser, and others brought new precision through magnification.[2–4] Jako's addition of microinstruments with dimensions more appropriate to small-volume laryngeal pathology also aided in this regard, and they have not been substantially modified since their introduction in the 1960s.[5]

Despite the advantages of performing laryngeal surgery in the operating room, technological advances have also allowed better laryngeal visualization in the office setting. During the early 1970s, the advent of flexible fiberoptic technology and the reliable delivery of topical anesthetics such as lidocaine made awake examinations of the larynx, pharynx, trachea, and esophagus possible. Convenience, low cost, reasonable color, image veracity, and the breadth of applications soon influenced the practice of otolaryngologists, gastroenterologists, pulmonologists, and others. Rigid endoscopy of the larynx using angled telescopes transformed the field of laryngeal endoscopy in the office by allowing the consistent application of stroboscopic light. The color resolution and image resolution achieved with rigid endoscopes in the office were clearly superior to flexible fiberoptic technology, but the distance from the targeted lesion had limits; the endoscope could be angled in only so close to the larynx, limited by the tongue base.

We now live in what some have called the "Golden Age" of laryngology given the improvements in imaging, new office lasers, and vocal fold injectables. Arguably, the most influential component of the new technologies is the distal chip flexible endoscope. The most recent generation of scopes provides excellent lighting, proximal control of the distal tip, different sizes for various applications, image processing for video display, integration into photodocumentation units, and the critically important working channels. The features of upper airway endoscopes and their uses in office interventions are worth detailed discussion.

◆ Imaging Equipment and Access to the Upper Airway

A variety of visualizing and interventional tools are available to the surgeon for office-based procedures. Mirror laryngoscopy, though inexpensive and widely available, does not permit video archiving and is limited by patient tolerance. Mirror laryngoscopy does not permit effective visualization by a student. On the other hand, when flexible laryngoscopy is employed to examine the larynx, the endoscope is attached to a camera and a video monitor. By viewing the larynx on the video monitor, the surgeon enjoys a magnified view of the laryngopharynx, and multiple individuals can view the images simultaneously. After the examination, the images can be reviewed with the patient and family. Video archiving is also an available option when flexible laryngoscopy is employed. Archived images can be compared with subsequent examinations of the same patient, allowing a better evaluation of disease progression or response to treatment. Flexible transnasal endoscopy, using either fiberoptic or "distal chip" technology, permits excellent visualization of all segments of the upper airway.

More recently, transnasal esophagoscopes have allowed the surgeon to examine the esophagus while sparing the patient intravenous sedation. Recent reports confirm that diagnostic efficacy is comparable with that of the gold standard of larger endoscopes used by gastroenterologists.[6,7] A major advance in flexible technology is the advent of working channels within the endoscope itself. These channels permit the delivery of anesthetic agents, small biopsy forceps, laser fibers, and suction. Surgeons can therefore simultaneously visualize and operate on the esophagus or upper airway without the need of an operative assistant.

Telescopic rigid endoscopy, performed transorally, is generally employed for visualization of the laryngopharynx, with or without the addition of stroboscopy. If the patient holds his or her own tongue, the surgeon can perform bimanual tasks for simultaneous transoral visualization and placement of instruments for the delivery of therapeutic agents, as described by Ford.[8]

Delivery of treatment agents to the larynx, such as injectable bulking materials or steroids, can be achieved transorally, transnasally, or transcutaneously. The pathway of delivery is dependent upon equipment availability, patient tolerance, surgeon preference, and the availability and/or necessity of an operative assistant. Indirect surgery has been extensively reported on by Omori et al.[9] This technique employs transnasal visualization by an operative assistant using a flexible scope and transoral delivery of agents performed by the senior surgeon. Transoral delivery is often preferred as the delivery needle is directly viewed as it penetrates the vocal fold, ensuring accurate placement of the injection.[8]

Table 9.1 Factors for Selection: Inspection of and Surgery on the Laryngopharynx

Viewing Device	Operative Assistant Needed?	Pathway of Delivery Agent	Video Monitor/ Archiving Possible?	Biopsy Possible?	Laser Delivery Possible?
Mirror	No	Transoral	No	Yes	No
Flexible transnasal endoscope without channel	Yes	Transoral Transcutaneous	Yes	Yes	No
Flexible transnasal endoscope with channel	No	Transoral Transcutaneous Transnasal	Yes	Yes	Yes
Rigid transoral endoscope	No	Transoral	Yes	Yes	No

In patients with a gag reflex that cannot be controlled with topical anesthesia and coaching, a transnasal approach is available. A needle at the tip of a flexible cannula is passed through the working channel of a flexible endoscope for delivery of a glottic injectable.[10,11]

Transcutaneous delivery, with simultaneous flexible laryngoscopy allowing a superior view of the larynx, is performed through the cricothyroid membrane, the thyroid cartilage, or, as recently described by Getz et al., through the thyrohyoid membrane.[12–14] Transcutaneous delivery is a popular choice but may not allow the surgeon a direct view of the needle tip, which is below the vocal folds when using the cricothyroid membrane approach, potentially reducing precision.

Table 9.1 lists factors to consider in the selection of procedures to be performed in the office setting.

◆ Indications

Office-based laryngologic procedures involve visualization of the upper aerodigestive tract, specifically the glottic and supraglottic larynx, pharynx, subglottic larynx and trachea, and the esophagus. Indications for these procedures include diagnostic imaging and/or tissue manipulation. **Table 9.2** provides an overview of reported office-based procedures including the indications. Patients are selected for

Table 9.2 Applications of Office-Based Laryngologic Interventions

Region	Procedure	Indication
Glottis, supraglottis, and pharynx	Endoscopy	Anatomic visualization
	FEES	Dysphagia
	FEESST	Sensory testing of the laryngopharynx
	Cancer staging	Laryngopharyngeal cancer staging
	Mucosal injection (cidofovir)	Papillomatosis
	Mucosal injection (steroids)	Vocal fold nodules
		Reinke's edema
		Arytenoid granuloma

(Continued on page 82)

Table 9.2 (*Continued*)

Region	Procedure	Indication
	Muscle injection (Botox)	Spasmodic dysphonia
		Severe muscle tension dysphonia
		Arytenoid relocation
	Vocal fold augmentation	Vocal fold paralysis
		Vocal fold paresis
		Vocal fold scarring/sulcus
		Vocal fold atrophy
		Glottic insufficiency NOS
	Pulsed-dye laser	Papillomatosis
		Glottal dysplasia
		Arytenoid granuloma
	Mucosal biopsy	Suspicious lesion
	Scar lysis	Glottic web
	Vocal fold polyp excision	Vocal fold polyp
Subglottis and trachea	Diagnostic endoscopy	Suspected airway lesion
		Postprocedure evaluation
Esophagus	Transnasal esophagoscopy	Diagnostic imaging for reflux, globus, dysphagia
	Foreign body advancement	Smooth esophageal foreign body
	Tracheoesophageal prosthesis placement	Tracheoesophageal prosthesis placement

Abbreviations: FEES, flexible endoscopic evaluation of swallowing; FEESST, flexible endoscopic evaluation of swallowing with sensory testing; NOS, not otherwise specified.

office-based procedures for some of the following reasons:

1. surgeon preference to directly monitor vocal feedback;
2. surgeon preference to enhance efficiency;
3. patient preference to avoid general anesthesia;
4. patient desire to reduce cost if private-pay;
5. avoidance of general anesthesia if medically unsuitable;
6. poor laryngeal exposure under direct laryngoscopy;
7. refractory lesions previously treated under general anesthesia.[15,16]

◆ Contraindications

Contraindications to office-based procedures are determined by surgeon comfort, patient factors, and lesion type. If the surgeon does not possess sufficient experience with a particular technique or if there is a possible lack of necessary equipment, then microlaryngoscopy under general anesthesia should be selected.

A severe gag reflex that cannot be overcome with topical anesthesia and coaching or reduced jaw opening from trismus or temporomandibular joint disorders will likely preclude successful performance of office procedures.

Although bleeding diatheses from medications or systemic disease are cited as contraindications to office-based procedures, Bastian and Delsupehe report that none of 20 patients on aspirin, nonsteroidal anti-inflammatory agents, or warfarin had airway distress, although there was a longer interval required for spontaneous coagulation.[16]

The type of lesion may also dictate whether a surgeon opts for office management. For example, it is generally held that benign subepithelial pathology such as nodules, polyps, cysts, and Reinke's edema require a level of precision that office surgery does not afford.[15,17,18] However, Omori et al. have reported on the extensive use of indirect surgery for removal of vocal fold polyps using specially designed instruments.[9] Omori's group, while not excising nodules or Reinke's edema, has reported treatment using transoral steroid injection resulting in improved objective voice measures.[19,20] Tai et al. caution against the biopsy of overtly vascular lesions such as hemangioma.[18] If the full extent of a lesion cannot be establish by office examination, then direct inspection under general anesthesia is likely warranted. Additionally, given the delicate nature of the vocal fold and the relative imprecision of indirect surgery, Hogikyan and Pynnonen warn that biopsy of superficial lesions suspicious for malignancy may sacrifice normal tissue while not producing accurate information about the depth of lesion invasion.[15]

◆ Safety

Office-based procedures on the laryngopharynx and esophagus enjoy an excellent safety record. In 192 invasive procedures on the laryngopharynx performed mostly without intravenous sedation, Bastian and Delsupehe report no episodes of airway compromise, laryngospasm, cardiovascular event, undue bleeding, or unplanned hospitalizations.[16] Additional reports with more than 100 procedures on the laryngopharynx, including cancer biopsies, confirm no episodes of undue bleeding, aspiration, or laryngeal trauma. These reports describe a brief, self-limited period of production of blood-tinged secretions after many interventions.[9,18] Hogikyan and Pynnonen reported a case of excessive bleeding requiring temporary tracheotomy.[15] Tai et al. report a single case of airway compromise after Teflon injection that resolved after 1 week of medical therapy as an inpatient.[18]

Diagnostic evaluation of the laryngopharynx using flexible endoscopic evaluation of swallowing (FEES) with sensory testing has resulted in mild epistaxis in about 1% of cases.[21,22] A careful evaluation of safety by Cohen et al. also records no episodes of airway compromise or laryngospasm and no symptomatic events related to intraprocedural bradycardia or tachycardia.[22]

Use of the transnasal esophagoscope has been gaining in popularity, and a recent report by Postma et al. suggests an excellent safety record in 611 patients. None had epistaxis requiring packing, and only two had vasovagal episodes that were self-limited.[23]

One might expect to find an increased incidence of complications when evaluating the airway in the office setting. Reported series, however, do not support this assumption. In 37 transnasal examinations of the airway performed using only topical anesthesia, Hogikyan observed no airway distress or laryngospasm.[24] Even in the pediatric population and *without* specific topical anesthesia applied to the larynx and airway, there were no episodes of airway compromise or laryngospasm in 105 patients as reported by Lindstrom et al.[25]

◆ Uses

Bastian has elegantly reported on the specific use of the flexible endoscope for FEES testing.[26] The inclusion of colored dye into food products assists the endoscopic observer in an evaluation of the passage of different food consistencies through the pharynx. Aviv demonstrated the comparable efficacy of this modality in predicting aspiration pneumonia when compared with standard modified barium swallow.[27] Bastian et al. have employed FEES for cancer staging within the laryngopharynx.[28] Using variable-strength puffs of air to illicit the laryngeal adductor reflex, Aviv et al. have added sensory testing of the laryngopharynx to FEES. This addition allows the otolaryngologist to evaluate laryngeal sensation changes from aging, vocal fold paralysis, stroke, and reflux.[29–33]

In-office laryngeal tissue manipulations, including the injection of biologically active agents such as cidofovir for papilloma, have been reported.[34] Steroids have been successfully delivered into the glottis for treatment of vocal fold nodules, Reinke's edema, arytenoid granulomas, and contact ulcers.[9,15,16,18–20] Favorable results from these in-office procedures argue in support of their efficacy, although injections under general anesthesia have been the historic preference of surgeons for these pathologies. Transoral delivery of Botox for the treatment of spasmodic dysphonia has been championed by Ford and others to enhance precise delivery of the drug thereby reducing the required dosage.[35] Additional indications for laryngopharyngeal Botox injection include tremor, refractory muscle tension dysphonia, cricopharyngeal achalasia, and other neurologic disorders.

Injectable glottic bulking agents, once limited to Teflon, are multiple and can be used in the treatment of the diverse pathologies that produce glottic insufficiency.[36–40] These newer injectables offer favorable, short- to intermediate-term correction of glottic insufficiency. Patients should be counseled that the improvements in swallowing and voice, though substantial, will be temporary. Fortunately, reinjection is a viable option. Specifically, vocal fold paralysis, paresis, atrophy, scarring, and iatrogenic tissue loss (eg, cancer resection) can all be addressed with office-based glottic augmentation/medialization.

The successful application, in the office setting, of the 585-nm pulsed dye laser, delivered through a flexible endoscope, for treatment of various glottic pathologies has been reported. Use of the laser to vaporize tissue or coagulate vessels allows the reduction of small-volume refractory disease such as recurrent respiratory papillomatosis and dysplasia with keratosis (leukoplakia).[41]

Given the added safety concerns in the subglottis and trachea, aggressive interventions in these anatomic regions are generally reserved for the more controlled setting of the operating room. Pure visualization of these regions in the office, however, has proven effective and avoids repeated exposure to general anesthesia. Favorable safety records, even in children, argue for office-based airway evaluation in patients not at risk of imminent obstruction or rapidly evolving disease.

The in-office imaging of the esophagus is principally diagnostic in the evaluation of dysphagia, globus pharyngeus sensation, and esophageal reflux disease. In-office esophageal interventions make use of the internal side channel of the transnasal esophagoscope for delivery of small biopsy forceps and grasping instruments. In-office foreign body advancement into the stomach and assistance in the placement of tracheoesophageal prosthesis for postlaryngectomy voice restoration have been reported.[23]

◆ Conclusion

Advances in technology improving the resolution of flexible laryngeal imaging have resulted in a renewed interest in office-based laryngology procedures. The introduction of newer injectable bulking agents and flexible laser technology coupled with flexible imaging has already changed the treatment approach for many patients away from the operating room toward well-tolerated, quick, and effective treatments in the office. This trend is likely to continue, and the indications for office-based procedures will likely expand.

◆ Clinical Examples

Case Study 1

A 66-year-old man with a history of smoking was noted to have a suspicious supraglottic mass. Given the patient's reduced lung capacity and excellent office imaging of the mass, it was biopsied in clinic. For the biopsy, the patient sat in an examination chair opposite the surgeon (**Fig. 9.1**). After the application of topical anesthetic (atomized 4% lidocaine) to the posterior oral cavity, faucial pillars, and posterior pharyngeal wall, the patient held his own tongue so that the surgeon could use two hands—the left for holding the rigid endoscope (attached to a camera and video monitor) and the right for delivering three separate 1-mL aliquots of 4% lidocaine onto the larynx via an Abraham cannula (curved cannula seen in **Fig. 9.2**). The

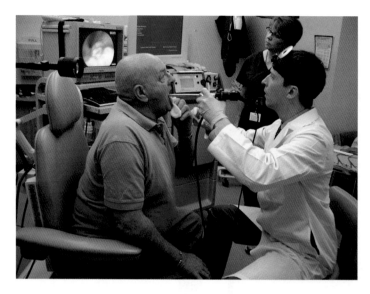

Fig. 9.1 The patient sits opposite the surgeon. The surgeon uses two hands while the patient holds his own tongue. The image on the video monitor is easy for the surgeon to see and allows for magnification and better precision.

right hand was then used to hold the transoral biopsy forceps and biopsy the area in question. This patient reported a 0 of 5 on the FACES pain scale when asked his pain level for the procedure (**Fig. 9.3**).

Case Study 2

A 25-year-old man with distal tracheal papillomatosis underwent a scheduled Revolix laser (AllMed Systems, Pleasanton, CA) treatment in the office. First, lidocaine/Afrin atomized spray was applied to each nasal cavity, and cottonoid

pledgets with the same solution were placed into each nasal cavity (**Fig. 9.4**). A distal chip endoscope with a working channel was introduced through the more patent nasal cavity and advanced toward the laryngopharynx. Three separate 1-mL aliquots of 4% lidocaine were introduced via a standard syringe at the level of the inferior supraglottis onto the vocal folds while the patient was phonating (**Fig. 9.5**). At the end of the phonatory gesture, the patient was instructed to breathe in deeply, at which time the lidocaine descended into the trachea allowing for dense tracheal mucosal anesthesia. The patient's cough reaction all but disappeared

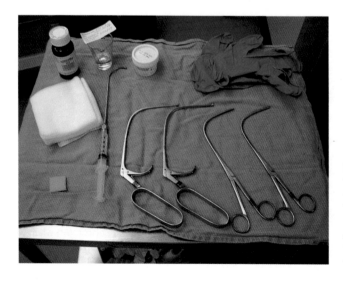

Fig. 9.2 A standard set of equipment for a transoral laryngeal biopsy. Pictured here are four curved biopsy forceps: two short and two long. Also present is the Abraham cannula attached to the plastic syringe; this is used to deliver lidocaine to the supraglottis and glottis.

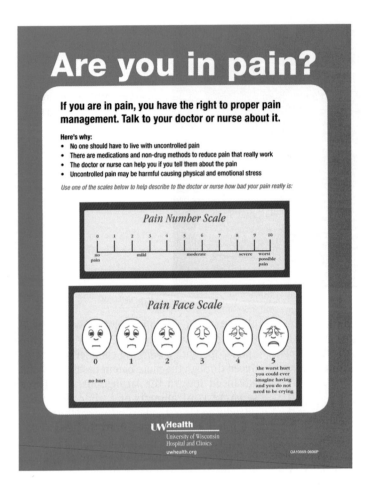

Fig. 9.3 This laminated placard is presented to the patient at the end of each procedure so that their pain scale can be assessed. Often, the patient is also asked where their pain was most intense (eg, the nose) and how to improve the experience if there were to be another procedure.

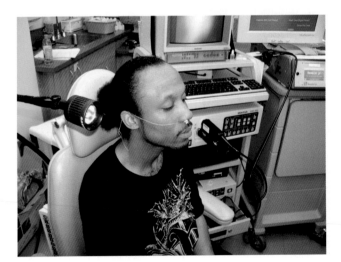

Fig. 9.4 The patient has had cottonoid pledgets moistened with a 50/50 mixture of 4% lidocaine and oxymetazoline placed into each nasal cavity to minimize discomfort when the flexible endoscope is passed through the more patent side.

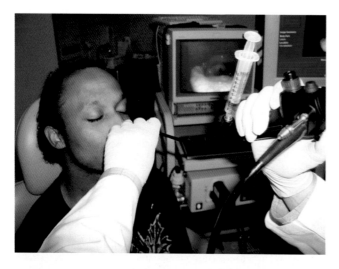

Fig. 9.5 One milliliter of 4% lidocaine is introduced into a syringe and the rest of the syringe filled with air. The syringe is then attached to the proximal port of the working channel via a Luer-Lok. When the endoscope is in position, the lidocaine is gently delivered onto the vocal folds as the patient initiates a prolonged phonatory gesture such as a sustained "ee."

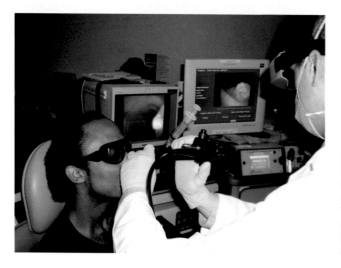

Fig. 9.6 The laser fiber has been introduced into the working channel of the endoscope until its tip exits the distal port of the working channel. The tracheal papilloma can be seen on the video monitor to the patient's left. Protective eyewear and masks are used during the procedure.

after the first application of the lidocaine. The flexible laser fiber was then delivered into the working channel of the endoscope that had been passed easily into the trachea (**Fig. 9.6**). The papilloma was then treated intralesionally and superficially with the laser to reduce it in size. This patient reported a 1 on the FACES pain scale.

References

1. Karmody CS. The history of laryngology. In: Fried MP, ed. The Larynx: A Multidisciplinary Approach, 2nd ed. St. Louis, MO: Mosby; 1996:3–11
2. Kleinsasser O. Mikrochirurgie im Kehlkopf. Arch Ohren Nasen Kehlkopfheilkd 1964;183:428–433
3. Kleinsasser O. Microlaryngoscopy and Endolaryngeal Microsurgery. Philadelphia, PA: W.B. Saunders; 1968
4. Scalco AN, Shipman WF, Tabb HG. Microscopic suspension laryngoscopy. Ann Otol Rhinol Laryngol 1960;69:1134–1138
5. Howard C, Jako GJ. General anesthesia for direct laryngoscopy and endolaryngeal microsurgery. Eye Ear Nose Throat Mon 1969;48:474–477
6. Thota PN, Zuccaro G Jr, Vargo JJ II, Conwell DL, Dumot JA, Xu M. A randomized prospective trial comparing unsedated esophagoscopy via transnasal and transoral routes using a 4-mm video endoscope with conventional endoscopy with sedation. Endoscopy 2005;37:559–565
7. Preiss C, Charton JP, Schumacher B, Neuhaus H. A randomized trial of unsedated transnasal small-caliber esophagogastroduodenoscopy (EGD) versus peroral small-caliber EGD versus conventional EGD. Endoscopy 2003;35:641–646

8. Ford CN, Roy N, Sandage M, Bless DM. Rigid endoscopy for monitoring indirect vocal fold injection. Laryngoscope 1998;108:1584–1586

9. Omori K, Shinohara K, Tsuji T, Kojima H. Videoendoscopic laryngeal surgery. Ann Otol Rhinol Laryngol 2000;109:149–155

10. Montgomery P, Sharma A, Qayyum A, Mierzwa K. Direct phonoplasty under local anaesthetic. J Laryngol Otol 2005;119:134–137

11. Trask DK, Shellenberger DL, Hoffman HT. Transnasal, endoscopic vocal fold augmentation. Laryngoscope 2005;115:2262–2265

12. Getz AE, Scharf J, Amin MR. Thyrohyoid approach to cidofovir injection: a case study. J Voice 2005;19:501–503

13. Berke GS, Gerratt B, Kreiman J, Jackson K. Treatment of Parkinson hypophonia with percutaneous collagen augmentation. Laryngoscope 1999;109:1295–1299

14. Ward PH, Hanson DG, Abemayor E. Transcutaneous Teflon injection of the paralyzed vocal cord: a new technique. Laryngoscope 1985;95:644–649

15. Hogikyan ND, Pynnonen M. Indirect laryngeal surgery in the clinical voice laboratory: the renewal of a lost art. Ear Nose Throat J 2000;79:350, 354, 357–358

16. Bastian RW, Delsupehe KG. Indirect larynx and pharynx surgery: a replacement for direct laryngoscopy. Laryngoscope 1996;106:1280–1286

17. Mahieu HF, Dikkers FG. Indirect microlaryngostroboscopic surgery. Arch Otolaryngol Head Neck Surg 1992;118:21–24

18. Tai SK, Chu PY, Chang SY. Transoral laryngeal surgery under flexible laryngovideostroboscopy. J Voice 1998;12:233–238

19. Tateya I, Omori K, Kojima H, Hirano S, Kaneko K, Ito J. Steroid injection to vocal nodules using fiberoptic laryngeal surgery under topical anesthesia. Eur Arch Otorhinolaryngol 2004;261:489–492

20. Tateya I, Omori K, Kojima H, Hirano S, Kaneko K, Ito J. Steroid injection for Reinke's edema using fiberoptic laryngeal surgery. Acta Otolaryngol 2003;123:417–420

21. Aviv JE, Murry T, Zschommler A, Cohen M, Gartner C. Flexible endoscopic evaluation of swallowing with sensory testing: patient characteristics and analysis of safety in 1,340 consecutive examinations. Ann Otol Rhinol Laryngol 2005;114:173–176

22. Cohen MA, Setzen M, Perlman PW, Ditkoff M, Mattucci KF, Guss J. The safety of flexible endoscopic evaluation of swallowing with sensory testing in an outpatient otolaryngology setting. Laryngoscope 2003;113:21–24

23. Postma GN, Cohen JT, Belafsky PC, et al. Transnasal esophagoscopy: revisited (over 700 consecutive cases). Laryngoscope 2005;115:321–323

24. Hogikyan ND. Transnasal endoscopic examination of the subglottis and trachea using topical anesthesia in the otolaryngology clinic. Laryngoscope 1999;109(7 Pt 1):1170–1173

25. Lindstrom DR III, Book DT, Conley SF, Flanary VA, Kerschner JE. Office-based lower airway endoscopy in pediatric patients. Arch Otolaryngol Head Neck Surg 2003;129:847–853

26. Bastian RW. The videoendoscopic swallowing study: an alternative and partner to the videofluoroscopic swallowing study. Dysphagia 1993;8:359–367

27. Aviv JE. Prospective, randomized outcome study of endoscopy versus modified barium swallow in patients with dysphagia. Laryngoscope 2000;110:563–574

28. Bastian RW, Collins SL, Kaniff T, Matz GJ. Indirect videolaryngoscopy versus direct endoscopy for larynx and pharynx cancer staging. Toward elimination of preliminary direct laryngoscopy. Ann Otol Rhinol Laryngol 1989;98:693–698

29. Aviv JE, Kim T, Sacco RL, et al. FEESST: a new bedside endoscopic test of the motor and sensory components of swallowing. Ann Otol Rhinol Laryngol 1998;107(5 Pt 1):378–387

30. Aviv JE. Effects of aging on sensitivity of the pharyngeal and supraglottic areas. Am J Med 1997;103:74S–76S

31. Aviv JE, Sacco RL, Mohr JP, et al. Laryngopharyngeal sensory testing with modified barium swallow as predictors of aspiration pneumonia after stroke. Laryngoscope 1997;107:1254–1260

32. Aviv JE, Liu H, Parides M, Kaplan ST, Close LG. Laryngopharyngeal sensory deficits in patients with laryngopharyngeal reflux and dysphagia. Ann Otol Rhinol Laryngol 2000;109:1000–1006

33. Tabaee A, Murry T, Zschommler A, Desloge RB. Flexible endoscopic evaluation of swallowing with sensory testing in patients with unilateral vocal fold immobility: incidence and pathophysiology of aspiration. Laryngoscope 2005;115:565–569

34. Shehab N, Sweet BV, Hogikyan ND. Cidofovir for the treatment of recurrent respiratory papillomatosis: a review of the literature. Pharmacotherapy 2005;25:977–989

35. Inagi K, Ford CN, Bless DM, Heisey D. Analysis of factors affecting botulinum toxin results in spasmodic dysphonia. J Voice 1996;10:306–313

36. McCulloch TM, Andrews BT, Hoffman HT, Graham SM, Karnell MP, Minnick C. Long-term follow-up of fat injection laryngoplasty for unilateral vocal cord paralysis. Laryngoscope 2002;112(7 Pt 1):1235–1238

37. Rosen CA, Thekdi AA. Vocal fold augmentation with injectable calcium hydroxylapatite: short-term results. J Voice 2004;18:387–391

38. Hertegård S, Hallén L, Laurent C, et al. Cross-linked hyaluronan versus collagen for injection treatment of glottal insufficiency: 2-year follow-up. Acta Otolaryngol 2004;124:1208–1214

39. Courey MS. Homologous collagen substances for vocal fold augmentation. Laryngoscope 2001;111:747–758

40. Chang HP, Chang SY. Autogenous fat intracordal injection as treatment for unilateral vocal palsy. Zhonghua Yi Xue Za Zhi (Taipei) 1996;58:114–120

41. Zeitels SM, Franco RA Jr, Dailey SH, Burns JA, Hillman RE, Anderson RR. Office-based treatment of glottal dysplasia and papillomatosis with the 585-nm pulsed dye laser and local anesthesia. Ann Otol Rhinol Laryngol 2004;113:265–276

III

Videostroboscopy

10

Introduction to Videostroboscopy

Katherine A. Kendall

Just like the beating of hummingbird wings, human vocal folds vibrate at a rate that is faster than can be perceived by the human eye. The evaluation of vocal fold anatomy, mucosal color, and gross movement can be performed while illuminating the vocal folds with a constant light source. But the evaluation of vocal fold vibration requires special imaging technology to "slow down" vibration for assessment. At this time, the most widely used technique for assessing the vibratory characteristics of the vocal folds is videostroboscopy, which has become an accepted and essential component of the comprehensive evaluation of voice disorders (**Video Clip 1**).

Oertel created the first stroboscope in 1895, but videostroboscopy did not become widely clinically available until the later part of the 20th century.[1] Chapter 1 in this text, on the history of laryngeal imaging, describes the development of laryngeal imaging techniques since Oertel's initial breakthrough. Much has been learned about vocal fold vibration as a result of the clinical use of videostroboscopy during the past several decades, and that knowledge can be applied to the evaluation of patients with voice disorders. Our ability to observe vocal fold vibration using videostroboscopy has also instigated further study of vocal fold histology and of how vocal fold structure affects vibratory physiology. The knowledge gained from those studies forms the basis for the contemporary clinical evaluation of patients with voice disorders.

◆ Indications

Videostroboscopy is indicated when a detailed visual analysis of vocal fold vibration is desired. It is usually performed in addition to an indirect or flexible examination of the larynx. Though videostroboscopy may be performed as part of a complete evaluation of a patient in whom the diagnosis is obvious, videostroboscopy is particularly indicated in any patient who complains of hoarseness but has an otherwise normal indirect or flexible laryngoscopic examination. If these examinations have ruled out an obvious abnormality of the anatomy, such as a mass or a lesion of the vocal fold, and have ruled out an obvious movement disorder, such as vocal fold paralysis, then a further evaluation of the vocal fold vibratory characteristics is warranted. In addition to providing information regarding vocal fold vibration, the image obtained with videostroboscopy is magnified, allowing a more detailed assessment of the vocal fold anatomy than is possible with indirect or flexible laryngoscopy. Video cameras can record a digital high-definition format with phenomenal image quality.[2] A detailed review of the recording, after the examination is completed, with slow motion or frame-by-frame analysis, allows for a comprehensive evaluation of the examination findings. As a result, videostroboscopy can often elucidate a vocal fold abnormality that was missed on indirect or flexible laryngoscopic examinations. Therefore, any patient with voice problems in whom the diagnosis is unclear is a candidate for videostroboscopy.

In addition to being an aid in the diagnosis of voice disorders, videostroboscopy is indicated to document vocal fold function prior to any treatment and to evaluate the outcomes of various interventions. The European Laryngological Society's Committee on Phoniatrics has proposed a basic protocol for the assessment of every patient with voice pathology that includes videostroboscopy. The European Laryngological Society cites videostroboscopy as being integral to the protocol because they believe that "Videostroboscopy is the main clinical tool for the etiological diagnosis of voice disorders." But the impetus behind the idea of using a protocol for the evaluation of every patient is that when the evaluation techniques are standardized across clinicians, the results of treatment can be compared between institutions.[3] Because videostroboscopy provides the benefit of documenting the examination findings, subsequent examinations can be compared, so that the results of treatment can be studied. Indeed, videostroboscopy has been used successfully to document the results of certain surgical interventions by demonstrating an improvement in the vocal fold vibratory characteristics after the treatment.[4,5] In addition, the results of videostroboscopy may be used during surgical planning. For example, videostroboscopy allows a detailed assessment of the degree of glottic closure, thus contributing to the planning of surgery in cases of vocal fold paralysis, along with an assessment of surgical results after treatment. Ford et al. took this concept one step further by using videostroboscopy during medialization procedures to determine when medialization was adequate as indicated by a return of the mucosal wave (indicating normal vibration) on the contralateral vocal fold.[6]

Videostroboscopy can be played back after completion of the examination so that patients can also view the examination during their evaluation, and the beneficial impact of patient education, with respect to the ultimate outcomes of treatment, should not be underestimated. Examination documentation and patient education have both become important indications for videostroboscopy.

◆ Examination

Videostroboscopy is performed with a rigid endoscope with a 70-degree or 90-degree angle of view. It is passed through the mouth, into the back of the pharynx, to visualize the larynx. A stethoscope on the patient's neck measures the frequency of vocal fold vibration and sets the frequency of strobe flashing to a frequency slightly off and several multiples slower than vocal fold vibration allowing images from sequential parts of the vibratory cycle to be recorded and viewed as a "virtual" slow-motion movie of vocal fold vibration. Recording rates are typically 30 frames per second. In addition to the "asynchronized" mode of stroboscopy described above, the strobe can be set to a "synchronized" mode wherein the strobe will flash at a frequency identical to the frequency of phonation. The "synchronized" mode records images from the same point in the vibratory cycle, and the resulting recording shows a "still" image of the larynx captured from the same point in the vibratory cycle (**Video Clip 2**). Chapter 11 describes the technical details of videostroboscopy and includes information about the equipment required to perform it.

Videostroboscopy allows evaluation of the following vibratory parameters:

◆ *Symmetry* of vibration refers to the movement of the right and left vocal folds relative to each other. The right and left folds normally vibrate as mirror images of one another. They begin to move laterally at the same time and at the same speed. They are displaced laterally to the same extent and reach maximal lateral displacement at the same time. They then begin to close together at the same time and at the same speed (**Video Clip 3**). Differences in the mechanical properties of the two vocal folds, however, will result in asymmetric movements. Symmetry of vibration is influenced by differences in the position, shape, mass, stiffness, elasticity, and tension of the vocal fold tissues.

- *Periodicity* of vibration refers to the relative length of the glottal cycle, and this should be stable from cycle to cycle. Use of the synchronized strobe setting can confirm that vibration is periodic (**Video Clip 2**). If the length of the vibratory cycle is stable from cycle to cycle, then a static image will persist with the strobe set to the synchronized mode. If changes in the length of the vibratory cycle are present, there will appear to be movement of the vibratory edge in the synchronized mode. Periodicity depends on the mechanical properties of the vocal folds and the expiratory force applied to them.
- *Phase closure* refers to the percentage of time that the vocal fold edges are open and/or closed during a single cycle of vibration. The phase characteristics are normally

influenced by the mode of phonation (falsetto, modal phonation, glottal fry) and the pitch and loudness of phonation (**Video Clip 4**) (**Fig. 10.1**).
- *Amplitude* of vibration refers to the amount of lateral movement of the vocal folds during vibration. Amplitude of vibration normally increases with increases in subglottic pressure, such as occurs during loud phonation. Amplitude of vibration also increases as the pitch or frequency of phonation decreases (**Video Clips 5 and 6**).
- *Glottic configuration* refers to the shape or contour of the glottic opening, if there is one, at the point of maximal closure during the vibratory cycle. Other terms for this characteristic include the "contour of the glottal margin" and the "vocal fold closure pattern." Chapters 14 and 17 cover the normal glottic configuration range and the differential diagnosis of abnormal glottic configurations, respectively.

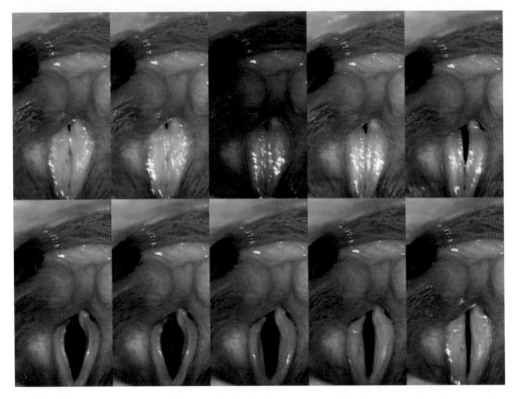

A

Fig. 10.1 (A) Montage function to evaluate phase characteristics. A normal open phase is 50%. *(Continued on page 94)*

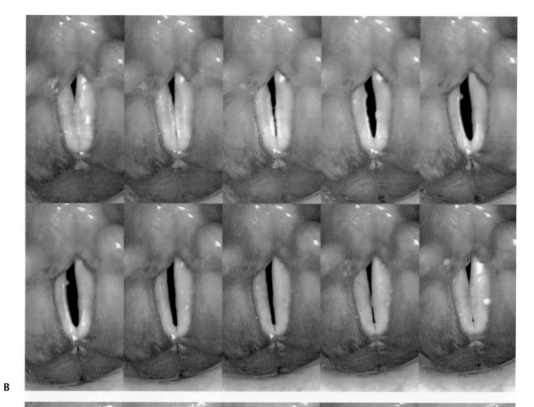

B

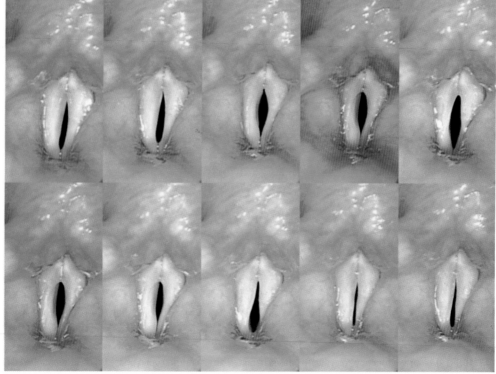

C

Fig. 10.1 (*Continued*) **(B)** Montage of a single cycle of vibration reveals a subtle predominance of the open phase. **(C)** A persistent glottic opening throughout the vibratory cycle is consistent with more significant presbyphonia.

- *Mucosal wave* refers to the movement of the superficial tissues over the vocal fold as the air moves through the glottis. The mucosal wave can be seen as a traveling wave in the superficial tissues over the top of the vocal fold surface from medial to lateral. Slow-motion or frame-by-frame analysis of the videostroboscopic recording is usually required for an adequate evaluation of the mucosal wave. The mucosal wave is interrupted with abnormalities of the vocal fold mucosal cover such as scarring, lesions, inflammation, and edema (**Video Clip 7**).

A detailed description of these vibratory parameters, including the range of normal findings, the impact of changes in loudness and pitch, and the expected findings in pathologic conditions of the larynx, is provided in later chapters of this book.

◆ Value of Videostroboscopy

The benefits of videostroboscopy in the evaluation of patients with voice symptoms have been well documented. Casiano et al. found that in patients with voice complaints and no abnormality identified on indirect laryngoscopy (previously diagnosed with a "functional voice disorder"), videostroboscopy resulted in a change of diagnosis in 44%. Furthermore, 20% of those patients diagnosed as having benign vocal fold lesions on indirect examination had a change in diagnosis after videostroboscopy. There was only a 3 to 5% rate of change in diagnosis in patients with malignant lesions of the vocal cords and neurologic disorders of the larynx, respectively, indicating that invasive vocal fold carcinoma and vocal fold paralysis are correctly identified on indirect laryngoscopy. In 70% of the cases where videostroboscopy resulted in a change of diagnosis, a previously unappreciated benign vocal fold lesion was found. In another 19%, vocal fold bowing that had not been appreciated on indirect examination was identified.[7] The benefits of videostroboscopy were confirmed by Sataloff et al, who reported that videostroboscopy, using a flexible laryngoscope, resulted in a change of diagnosis in 18% of patients and provided additional diagnostic information in 47% with changes in management based on these findings in 32%.[8]

Studies evaluating the accuracy of stroboscopy and the usefulness of specific stroboscopy parameters in the diagnosis of vocal fold pathology have illustrated the value of the technology. For example, stroboscopy in patients with bilateral vocal fold nodules typically demonstrates symmetric but reduced amplitudes of vibration, normal periodicity, an intact mucosal wave, and an hourglass glottic opening at maximal closure.[7] Dailey et al. found that in patients with vocal fold nodules, videostroboscopic findings correlated with surgical findings 100% of the time.[9] The accuracy of stroboscopy was also high in patients with vocal fold polyps who often present with asymmetric vibration and variable periodicity on videostroboscopy. With polyps, the mucosal wave may be present or absent and, due to the irregularity of the vocal fold margins, glottic closure is usually irregular and asymmetric.[10] In patients with polyps, stroboscopy findings have also been correlated with surgical findings in up to 100% of cases.[9] The situation is similar for vocal fold cysts. Typically unilateral, cysts cause asymmetric and aperiodic vibration. An hourglass glottic configuration results from protrusion of the medial vocal fold margin over the cyst, and the mucosal wave is frequently absent over the cyst.[9–11] Videostroboscopic results have been found to correlate with surgical findings 78 to 100% of the time in patients with cysts.[9,11]

◆ Limitations of Videostroboscopy

Although the extent of benign vocal fold lesions and their impact on surrounding vocal fold structures can be determined using videostroboscopy, superficially invasive cancer of the larynx cannot be distinguished from a benign process with videostroboscopy. If a reduced mucosal wave is identified in the area of a suspicious lesion, this may be the result of a superficial pathologic process such as epithelial atypia but could also be the result of an invasive malignancy involving deeper structures. It must be kept in mind that videostroboscopy is a two-dimensional representation of a three-dimensional process, and it is not a reliable way to diagnose cancer or to determine the depth of its invasion.[12]

Similarly, it is difficult to see the medial glottal surfaces using videostroboscopy, and lesions in this area may not be identified. Thus, the evaluation of cancers involving the medial vocal fold surface may be incomplete using videostroboscopy, and sulcus vocalis, a lesion of the medial surface of the vocal folds, can be difficult to diagnose on videostroboscopy. Although sulcus vocalis may present with an absent or decreased mucosal wave and a defect of glottic closure, videostroboscopy has been unable to identify sulcus vocalis in some studies and correlates with surgical findings in only 69% of cases in other studies. Similarly, mucosal bridges are frequently missed with stroboscopy.[8,9]

In addition to not being appropriate for the evaluation of all lesions, videostroboscopy cannot be used effectively in all patients. Videostroboscopy requires a stable phonation frequency to activate the strobe. In other words, patients must have periodic phonation for optimal recording of vocal fold vibration with videostroboscopy. Patients with severe hoarseness, however, may have aperiodic phonation or significant, rapid changes in phonation frequency that preclude videostroboscopy. Images obtained when the strobe is unable to track due to aperiodic voicing jump from one part of the vibratory cycle to the other, rather than display vocal fold motion in a smooth sequence. Additionally, several seconds of phonation are required to activate the strobe and record a sample of vibration that is adequate for analysis. In patients who cannot phonate for 3 to 5 seconds at a stable frequency, videostroboscopy may not be possible. This may occur in up to 34% of individuals.[7] Similarly, because significant aperiodicity occurs during the onset and offset of voicing, it is not possible to use videostroboscopy to evaluate vibration during those parts of phonation (**Video Clips 1, 8, and 9**).

Occasionally, an adequate or complete view of the larynx cannot be obtained with the rigid laryngoscope. Some patients may require topical anesthesia of the pharynx to tolerate the examination. Adequate examination may not be possible in up to 5% of patients due to anatomy or gag reflex.[7] In those patients, videostroboscopy can be performed with a flexible scope, but the image quality and magnification is usually not as good. Please refer to Chapter 13 on performing the examination for a full discussion of strategies for obtaining the optimal videostroboscopic examination.

Although the best image quality is obtained by using a rigid endoscope for videostroboscopy, a transoral rigid examination requires an abnormal head position with the patient's tongue out. Imaging is obtained during stable, periodic phonation and does not allow an analysis of what is happening during connected, articulatory speech production. As a result, functional dysphonias such as muscle tension dysphonia may be missed with videostroboscopy.

The analysis of the images recorded with videostroboscopy relies on visual perceptual judgments and is therefore susceptible to bias. Clinicians must avoid overdiagnosing or seeing pathology when none is present and also need to avoid missing pathology that is contributing to vocal symptoms. This may seem like a simple charge, but the task is complicated by the fact that vibratory features commonly associated with physiologic dysphonia are also frequently observed in the nondysphonic population and make it difficult to distinguish patients with physiologic dysphonia from nondysphonic subjects. Elias et al. discovered "abnormal findings" in 58% of healthy asymptomatic singers.[13] In other words, the finding of abnormal vibratory characteristics in any one patient may or may not be related to their vocal complaints.

Further complicating the issue is the fact that our ability to subjectively rate vibratory characteristics is not very reliable. Individual scrutiny of each vibratory parameter reveals that none of them have shown a high degree of intrarater reliability. Some studies have shown that reliability improves with experience, whereas others found inexperienced raters to be as reliable as the more experienced raters.[14,15] Looking at it another way, experience does not necessarily lead to greater reliability in rating videostroboscopic studies. Several factors, in addition to experience, have been shown to impact the way raters analyze videostroboscopic studies. Patient history has been demonstrated to influence severity ratings for the following parameters: vocal fold edge abnormalities, mucosal wave abnormalities, the identification of adynamic segments, and abnormalities of phase closure.[16]

Variations in nomenclature have also been identified and may be the source of some of the variability.[15] Overall, taking all the vibratory parameters together, the agreement in diagnosis based on videostroboscopic studies has been found to be as low as 62%.[15]

As long as videostroboscopy remains a subjective method of vocal fold vibration analysis, there are likely to be problems with reliable rating and interpretation of the findings. Unfortunately, given the situation, small changes in vibratory characteristics that could indicate initial stages of disease or a trend during treatment may escape undetected by the clinician observer. Currently, there exists no standard reference for calibrating videostroboscopic images and therefore allowing quantitative measurements and detection of small variations. Attempts to quantify vibratory properties have been undertaken using a two-point laser dot calibration for measurement of distances. This method of laser triangulation has been found to be very accurate. When used to measure glottal width and vocal fold length, laser triangulation has demonstrated less than 5% variability.[17]

Until commercially available videostroboscopy systems are equipped with a method of quantitative measurement, it is important that clinicians using stroboscopy be familiar with the limitations of the technology and the subjective characteristics of the analysis. Steps can be taken to minimize rater influence on image analysis including the development of a working knowledge of the layered structure of the vocal folds, the normal appearance of the vocal folds, and how the mechanical properties of the vocal folds vary with changes in frequency and intensity.

In addition, the results of stroboscopy studies are influenced by the examiner's instructions to the patient regarding the pitch and loudness of phonation during the examination. A standard protocol for every stroboscopy study should be developed. Using a protocol minimizes the variation of the study parameters secondary to the pitch and loudness of phonation and also allows for comparison of individual patients over time and the comparison of one patient with another. A standard protocol may include imaging during low-, normal-, and high-pitch phonation in addition to phonation in range of the patient's speaking or singing problem. Documentation of vocal intensity at each pitch range should be performed, and the protocol may include loud and soft phonation at various pitches. Soft high-pitched phonation may provide differentiation of benign vocal fold lesions such as bilateral vocal fold nodules versus a unilateral vocal fold lesion with a contralateral reactive lesion.[18]

◆ Interdisciplinary Communication and the Videostroboscopy Report

Both otolaryngologists and speech-language pathologists perform videostroboscopy, although it is common for the otolaryngologist to refer a patient to the speech-language pathologist for videostroboscopy. Both specialties use the results of the videostroboscopic examination to evaluate patients with voice disorders but may have a different perspective based on their approaches to treatment. A speech-language pathologist may be more interested in the functional voicing technique demonstrated by the patient, whereas the otolaryngologist may be more interested in the anatomic pathology. Of course, these elements of the examination are not mutually exclusive. Optimal patient management involves a team approach with both the physician and the speech-language pathologist involved in the evaluation and management of any given patient. It is therefore critical that these two specialties communicate well with respect to the results of videostroboscopy.

The ideal videostroboscopy report not only includes a description of the vibratory characteristics of the vocal folds observed during the examination but also includes an interpretation of those findings with regard to optimal management. It must be kept in mind that the referral of a patient for videostroboscopy is usually done because the referring clinician is interested in evaluating the patient for evidence of disease to make treatment decisions. Perhaps the patient has an unexplained dysphonia or is a professional voice user with subtle voice difficulties. Perhaps the referring clinician wishes to further distinguish between a functional versus organic dysphonia. In any case, the information obtained from videostroboscopy will be integrated into a treatment plan designed to improve or resolve the patient's voicing difficulties. It is important that the speech-language pathologist is able to determine if pathology exists that will respond to voice therapy, and it is important that the otolaryngologist is able to make plans for surgical treatment if that is needed. For example, when the evaluation of the vocal fold vibratory characteristics identifies stiffness, the examination interpretation must then help the clinician to determine if the stiffness is secondary to scarring or is due to hyperfunction.

Information gleaned from the videostroboscopic examination that is important for surgical planning often includes an evaluation of glottic competence. The glottic shape during maximal closure is important because defects in glottic competence may be amenable to surgical correction. In cases of unilateral vocal fold paralysis, for example, the position of the arytenoid cartilage is variable. In some patients, the arytenoid position is abducted, resulting in a significant posterior glottic opening during maximal vocal fold closure (**Fig. 10.2**). In other patients, the arytenoid cartilage is positioned in such a way that the posterior glottis is closed during voicing (**Fig. 10.3**). In the first case, an arytenoid adduction should be part of the surgical correction of the defect, and in the second case, arytenoid adduction is probably not necessary. The videostroboscopy report in a patient

with vocal fold paralysis should include information about the position of the arytenoid cartilages and the closure of the posterior part of the larynx during voicing.

A description of the glottic configuration is also important in cases of vocal fold bowing due to presbyphonia. Subtle cases of presbyphonia may not be visible during indirect laryngoscopy, and videostroboscopy may be required to document this condition. A small anterior gap at maximal vocal fold closure may be all that is identified during the videostroboscopic examination. Very early presbyphonia can also present as mild abnormalities in the phase characteristics: a predominately open phase during modal phonation. A montage function can be used to identify the open phase characteristics (**Fig. 10.1**). When abnormalities of phase are identified on videostroboscopy, the question then becomes: Would the patient respond to voice therapy or would bilateral vocal fold medialization be of benefit? Other phonatory measures, such as maximum phonation duration, may be required to answer this question and can be integrated into the videostroboscopy report.

Benign vocal fold pathology will also likely impact the glottic configuration. Nodules typically result in an hourglass glottic configuration, whereas polyps and cysts cause irregularities of the glottic shape. It is important to distinguish between these types of pathology because the treatment approach can

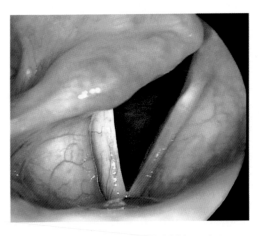

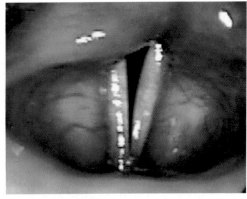

A

B

Fig. 10.2 (A) Unilateral right vocal fold paralysis with the vocal folds abducted. **(B)** When the vocal folds are adducted, there is a persistent posterior glottic gap identified. This patient would benefit from an arytenoid adduction as part of a vocal fold medialization procedure.

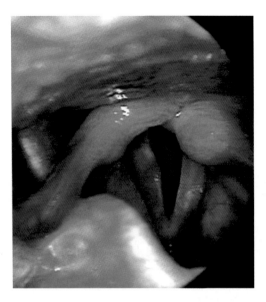

A

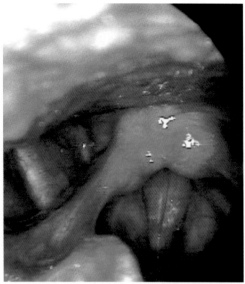

B

Fig. 10.3 (A) Unilateral left vocal fold paralysis with the vocal folds abducted. **(B)** During vocal fold closure for voicing, the posterior glottis is closed.

Arytenoid adduction is not likely to be necessary. An evaluation of phase characteristics would determine the potential benefit of vocal fold medialization.

be very different. The interpretation of the videostroboscopy report in such cases should include information about whether or not the lesions identified are responsible for the patient's voice complaints, and if so, will the lesions likely respond to voice therapy or is surgical correction required? If surgery is required, polyps ideally should be distinguished from cysts before surgery, as the surgical approach is different depending on the lesion. Nodules should be distinguished from a unilateral polyp or cyst with a contrecoup lesion (**Fig. 10.4**). An evaluation of vibratory symmetry as well as a description of the glottic configuration aid in making these distinctions and should be included in the interpretation of the results of videostroboscopy.

Ideally, clinicians who refer patients for videostroboscopy would communicate any specific clinical concerns to the stroboscopist before the examination to ensure that those concerns are addressed in the videostroboscopic examination and report. Performing the examination with a protocol can minimize the possibility that information critical to treatment decision-making will inadvertently be omitted from the examination. With respect to interpretation of the results of videostroboscopy, both

specialties must be cognizant of the other's point of view to maximize interdisciplinary communication for the patient's benefit.

◆ Conclusion

In summary, the use of videostroboscopy has greatly improved our diagnostic capabilities, has improved patient education, and has allowed for examination documentation. Like

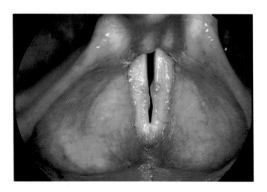

Fig. 10.4 Is this a left vocal fold polyp with a contrecoup lesion or bilateral polyps?

all medical testing methods, it has some limitations. A thorough understanding of both the utility and the limitations is required for optimal efficacy in use of the technology. Parts III, IV, and V of this book provide the reader with detailed information about the technology, performing the examination, and videostroboscopy study analysis.

References

1. Oertel MJ. Das Laryngo-stoboskop und die Larngosckopische Untersuchung. Arch Larngol Rhinol (Berl) 1895;3:1–6
2. Tsunoda A, Hatanaka A, Tsunoda R, Kishimoto S, Tsunoda K. A full digital, high definition video system (1080i) for laryngoscopy and stroboscopy. J Laryngol Otol 2008;122:78–81
3. Dejonckere PH, Bradley P, Clemente P, et al; Committee on Phoniatrics of the European Laryngological Society (ELS). A basic protocol for functional assessment of voice pathology, especially for investigating the efficacy of (phonosurgical) treatments and evaluating new assessment techniques. Guideline elaborated by the Committee on Phoniatrics of the European Laryngological Society (ELS). Eur Arch Otorhinolaryngol 2001;258:77–82
4. Chang HP, Chang SY. An alternative surgical procedure for the treatment of vocal fold retention cyst. Otolaryngol Head Neck Surg 2003;128:470–477
5. Finck C, Lefebvre P. Implantation of esterified hyaluronic acid in microdissected Reinke's space after vocal fold microsurgery: first clinical experiences. Laryngoscope 2005;115:1841–1847
6. Ford CN, Roy N, Sandage M, Bless DM. Rigid endoscopy for monitoring indirect vocal fold injection. Laryngoscope 1998;108:1584–1586
7. Casiano RR, Zaveri V, Lundy DS. Efficacy of videostroboscopy in the diagnosis of voice disorders. Otolaryngol Head Neck Surg 1992;107:95–100
8. Sataloff RT, Spiegel JR, Hawkshaw MJ. Strobovideolaryngoscopy: results and clinical value. Ann Otol Rhinol Laryngol 1991;100(9 Pt 1):725–727
9. Dailey SH, Spanou K, Zeitels SM. The evaluation of benign glottic lesions: rigid telescopic stroboscopy versus suspension microlaryngoscopy. J Voice 2007; 21:112–118
10. Kaszuba SM, Garrett CG. Strobovideolaryngoscopy and laboratory voice evaluation. Otolaryngol Clin North Am 2007;40:991–1001, vi
11. Hernando M, Cobeta I, Lara A, García F, Gamboa FJ. Vocal pathologies of difficult diagnosis. J Voice 2008;22:607–610
12. Colden D, Zeitels SM, Hillman RE, Jarboe J, Bunting G, Spanou K. Stroboscopic assessment of vocal fold keratosis and glottic cancer. Ann Otol Rhinol Laryngol 2001;110:293–298
13. Elias ME, Sataloff RT, Rosen DC, Heuer RJ, Spiegel JR. Normal strobovideolaryngoscopy: variability in healthy singers. J Voice 1997;11:104–107
14. Rosen CA. Stroboscopy as a research instrument: development of a perceptual evaluation tool. Laryngoscope 2005;115:423–428
15. Chau HN, Desai K, Georgalas C, Harries M. Variability in nomenclature of benign laryngeal pathology based on video laryngoscopy with and without stroboscopy. Clin Otolaryngol 2005;30:424–427
16. Teitler N. Examiner bias: influence of patient history on perceptual ratings of videostroboscopy. J Voice 1995;9:95–105
17. Popolo PS, Titze IR. Qualification of a quantitative laryngeal imaging system using videostroboscopy and videokymography. Ann Otol Rhinol Laryngol 2008;117:404–412
18. Rosen CA, Murry T. Diagnostic laryngeal endoscopy. Otolaryngol Clin North Am 2000;33:751–758

11

The Science of Stroboscopic Imaging

Robert E. Hillman and Daryush D. Mehta

During phonation, the vocal folds usually open and close over 100 times per second and vibrate at velocities approaching 1 meter per second, making it impossible to view this activity with the unaided eye.[1] Stroboscopy has become an essential component of the clinical voice evaluation because this approach enables the examiner to obtain a visual estimate of vocal fold vibratory function that can be recorded for later playback. This chapter explains the science that underlies stroboscopic imaging of vocal fold vibration and gives a description of the clinical systems that are currently used to perform stroboscopic examinations in the voice clinic.

◆ Overview of Stroboscopic Examination of Vocal Fold Vibration

In current practice, clinical stroboscopic examination involves using a video camera attached to a rigid (transoral) or flexible (transnasal) endoscope to observe (using a video monitor) and record images of the vocal folds. In the most common approach, illumination is provided by a strobe light that flashes at a rate that is synchronized with the patient's vocal fundamental frequency during sustained vowel production to produce what appears to be a slow-motion view of vocal fold vibration.[2]

Figure 11.1 shows the kind of simple schematic that is typically used to illustrate how stroboscopic examination of vocal fold vibration is accomplished.[3,4] The oscillating waveform along the top of **Fig. 11.1** represents the true pattern of glottal opening and closing that takes place as the vocal folds vibrate. The light bulbs indicate the instants when the flashes of the strobe light occur—at a slower rate than the vocal fold vibration frequency—timed to illuminate successive points (phases) in the repeating pattern of vibration from different vibratory cycles as time progresses. The lower waveform in **Fig. 11.1** represents the perceived composite stroboscopic (slow-motion) sequence, which is constructed by sequential presentation of the sampled images (represented by the arrows projecting from the upper waveform). This entire stroboscopic process is dependent on an adequately stable fundamental frequency, and the resulting sampled images form an averaged, down-sampled estimate of the true underlying tissue motion.

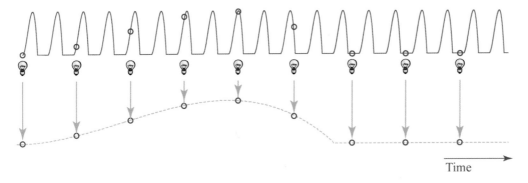

Fig. 11.1 A typical illustration of the stroboscopic sampling effect.

◆ Origins of Stroboscopy

In the early 1800s, it was discovered that the visual perception of motion could be evoked from viewing a discrete set of images.[5] Exploiting this phenomenon, several household toys of the day—the *phenakistiscope, zoetrope, daedaleum,* and *zoopraxiscope*—created striking visual illusions of motion by presenting successive images of a sampled event in rapid succession.[6] Regarded as the first application of stroboscopic principles, the *phenakistiscope* was invented by Plateau and independently conceived as Stampfer's *stroboscope* and Roget's *phantasmascope.* This device could make still images of objects, such as animals and dancers in different positions, appear to move by viewing the pictures through slits on a revolving disk. Motion was perceived because the periodic interruption of the viewer's line of sight occurred rapidly enough to produce a sequential sampling (strobing) of the individual pictures.

In the late 19th century, Oertel published the earliest application of stroboscopic principles for observing vocal fold vibrations.[7-9] Oertel used a revolving disk with equally spaced holes to mechanically shutter (strobe) a light source that was reflected by a laryngeal mirror to illuminate and observe the vocal folds. Provided subjects were able to adequately match their vocal pitches to the frequency of the rotating disk, the periodic flashes of the light produced a sequence of images that was perceived as a slow-motion representation of the vocal fold vibratory pattern.

◆ Visual Perceptions of Apparent Motion

Humans are able to perceive motion, even if no real motion exists, from the presentation of successive images if some temporal requirements of the human visual processing system are met. Wertheimer is credited with conducting seminal experiments that yielded temporal parameters necessary for the perception of apparent motion,[10-12] with refinements made by later investigators on more complex stimuli.[13] Wertheimer's experiments involved the successive presentation of two geometric figures separated by varying time intervals.[14] Although the specific time intervals necessary for evoking apparent motion varied depending on experimental conditions, general numeric boundaries were reported by Wertheimer based on his empirical data.

At presentation intervals shorter than 30 msec, the two figures were perceived to exist simultaneously. At intervals above 200 msec, the two figures were perceived to appear in succession. Two hundred msec, or 0.2 seconds, is often cited as the time an image persists on the retina after presentation, which has been erroneously linked to motion perception in much of the previous literature that has tried to explain how stroboscopy works for observing vocal fold vibration.[7,15,16] At intermediate interval durations, optimally around 60 msec, a single figure in motion was perceived. The 60-msec interval corresponds with a presentation frequency of ~17 images per second. These results define the optimal frequency

(17 Hz) at which a sequence of discrete images would be perceived to exhibit apparent, continuous motion. They also formed the basis for the frame rates at which motion pictures are filmed and played back, which has ended up at 25, 25, and 30 frames per second, respectively, for the phase alternating line (PAL), séquential couleur à mémoire (SECAM), and National Television System Committee (NTSC) standard analog video protocols.[17,18]

Common misconceptions that have been propagated in the laryngology literature involve the intertwining of *Talbot's law* with notions about the *persistence of vision* in attempting to explain how stroboscopy facilitates the examination of vocal fold vibration.[4,7,16,19,20] In actuality, Talbot's law states that "if a luminary of a certain brightness is exposed intermittently, the regular intermittences being too frequent for the eye to perceive, the resultant brightness is to the actual brightness as the time of exposure to the total time of observation."[12] In his experiments on estimating the intensity of light using time-based measurements, William Henry Fox Talbot rapidly rotated a white disk with a single black sector and noted that the perceived "obscuration" (Talbot's term for grayness) of the rotating disk was "proportional to the angle of the [black] sector."[21] Any point on the disk was intermittently illuminated (white) at periodic intervals, and the duration of illumination—the exposure time—was related to the grayness of the disk. This relationship became known as Talbot's law. Plateau further determined that this relationship was absolute (the Talbot-Plateau law); that is, the ratio between the apparent brightness of a rapidly rotating black-and-white disk and the brightness of an all-white disk is not only proportional to, but equal to, the ratio of the exposure time to the total time.[12,22] Talbot is mainly known for his seminal work in developing photographic chemical processes, particularly the calotype process that provided for the generation of multiple positive prints from a single negative.[23]

Subsequent experiments by others using painted disks and intermittently interrupted light sources have established that, under usual circumstances, the rate of strobed illumination (strobe frequency) should be greater than about 50 Hz to be perceived as *flicker free* (ie, having no perceived variation in light intensity or object illumination).[24–29] This frequency requirement is satisfied in laryngeal stroboscopy with the unaided eye, which employs strobe frequencies that are based on human fundamental frequencies well above 50 Hz. It follows that the visual perception of apparent motion (at frequencies above 17 Hz) is already created once the flicker-free threshold of 50 Hz is achieved. In addition, the idea that persistence of vision induces apparent motion in sequentially presented images has been shown to be a logical fallacy.[12,30]

◆ Principles of Stroboscopic Sampling

Once the requirements of the visual system are met to induce apparent motion, the task turns to selecting the images that will be displayed to create this motion. Stroboscopic sampling can be used to create the optical illusion of slowing down and better revealing (or even freezing) an underlying pattern of rapid motion, such as the vocal fold vibratory pattern. **Figure 11.2** illustrates a simple model of periodic motion to mimic the repeating vibratory pattern of the vocal folds. A circle is periodically rotated around its center and completes one revolution (360 degrees) in a given duration of time. For example, setting the fundamental frequency of rotation to 100 revolutions, or periods, per second would make each of the cycles (periods) 10 msec in duration. Each row in **Fig. 11.2** (from left to right) depicts one complete cycle of rotation, so with 10 rows, a total of 10 complete revolutions are displayed. Each column shows samples of the rotating circle taken at equal intervals of time, or phases, within each cycle. In this case, the samples are taken at 36-degree intervals, and each sampling interval is 1 msec in duration.

Stroboscopy can enable two views of periodic motion—it can appear to freeze the motion at a selected point (phase) in the repeating pattern or it can create an apparent slow-motion view of the repeating pattern (ie, display the entire period or cycle). The first view, freezing of the motion, is accomplished by matching the frequency of the strobe imaging to the fundamental frequency (repetition rate) of the motion. In **Fig. 11.2**, this principle is demonstrated by the blue squares sampling the circular motion once per revolution at the phase of 288 degrees. Freezing the motion at other phases can be accomplished by adding time delays to this

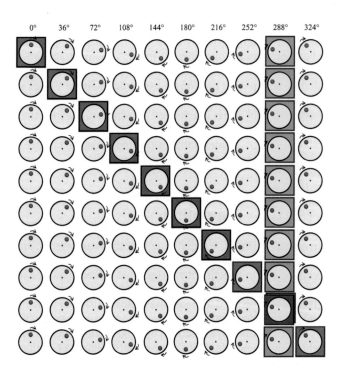

Fig. 11.2 The sampled motion of a revolving circle. See text for description.

stroboscopic sampling. For example, a delay of 1 msec would shift the sampling later in time by 36 degrees, resulting in a freezing of the motion at the 324-degree phase ([1 msec]/[10 msec] × 360 degrees = 36 degrees, and 36 degrees + 288 degrees = 324 degrees).

The second stroboscopic view creates an apparent slow-motion presentation of the underlying periodic movement by sampling successive phases of the movement across repeated cycles (the *strobe effect*). The method can be related to the beating that occurs between two auditory tones that are close in frequency, where the beat frequency is equal to the absolute difference between the frequencies of the two tones. By analogy, the number of cycles of slow-motion movement produced per second by the strobe effect is equal to the difference (*beat frequency*) between the fundamental frequency of the movement and the frequency at which the strobe images are being acquired (strobe frequency).[31] This phenomenon is illustrated by the red squares in **Fig. 11.2**, which shows a sequence of individual images being taken at successively later phases in each of the 10 repeated cycles of rotation.

Assuming a rotation period of 10 msec (ie, each cycle of vibration takes 10 msec to complete, producing a fundamental frequency of 100 Hz), the strobe effect requires sampling every 11 msec (ie, a 1-msec delay relative to the period) to progressively advance to the phase at which each subsequent image is taken. The strobe frequency must be lower (having a longer period) than the rotation frequency to sample successive phases of the cycle. If the strobe frequency were higher than the rotation frequency, the circle would appear to be rotating in reverse, a usually undesirable effect referred to as *time aliasing*. An 11-msec period corresponds with a strobe frequency of about 91 Hz (the reciprocal of 11 msec). The absolute difference between the strobe frequency (91 Hz) and the rotation frequency of the circles (100 Hz) is about 9 Hz, which is the *beat frequency*, or number of composite cycles actually presented per second. Thus, the actual rotation speed of 100 cycles per second would appear as 9 cycles per second during stroboscopy. The effective true sampling rate for this example, which would allow within-period sampling, would be 1000 Hz (calculated from 10 samples per period multiplied by the rotation frequency of 100 Hz).

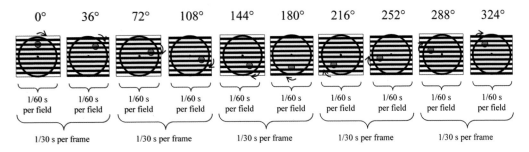

Fig. 11.3 An illustration of the effect of video interlacing on stroboscopic sampling.

◆ Stroboscopic Examination of Vocal Fold Vibration

Here it must be noted that there are two fundamentally different methods of stroboscopic examination of vocal fold vibration: real-time viewing by direct observation and real-time viewing and recording by video-based technologies. Up to this point, the principles of stroboscopy have assumed that the rapid motion of an object was to be viewed via direct observation with the eye. Consequently, as long as the strobe frequency is above 50 Hz, the conditions necessary for a flicker-free sequence of images and the perception of continuous, apparent motion will be satisfied. As already described, the earliest use of stroboscopy for direct observation of vocal fold vibration was accomplished using a laryngeal mirror and a shuttered light source.[9] As current clinical systems use video-based technology, it is necessary to have some understanding of how these systems integrate the video capture process with stroboscopic imaging.[2,32,33]

The video recording process often follows the NTSC standard that sets the capture rate at ~30 interlaced *frames* per second, with each frame comprising two *fields* that are captured at distinct times (actual frame and field rates are 30/1.001 Hz and 60/1.001 Hz, respectively).[17] Alternatively, the video capture process might follow one of two other international standards—PAL and SECAM—that also employ 2:1 interlacing but set the video frame and field rates at 25 Hz and 50 Hz, respectively.[18] A *field* consists of the set of either even-numbered or odd-numbered horizontal lines that are used to capture or encode the image. Thus, in the NTSC standard, every 1/60th of a second, half of the horizontal lines that comprise the image are captured and displayed on the monitor, and, in the subsequent 1/60th of a second, the other half of the horizontal lines that comprise the image are recorded and displayed. Therefore, a full image, or *frame*, is created every 1/30th of a second from the simultaneous display of two adjacent fields.

Figure 11.3 shows how the rotating motion (the moving red dot) in **Fig. 11.2** would be captured by the successive fields of the NTSC video capture process.

As with most digital camera technologies, a scene is captured by optically focusing light onto the image sensor of the camera, which then averages the scene information over the exposure time to create a static image. In the NTSC standard, the exposure time is maximized so that the camera sensor averages the scene information over the entire field duration (1/60th of a second). Any movement that occurs during the exposure time results in motion blur in the resulting field. To obtain nonblurred video recordings of stroboscopic images, the strobe light must be controlled so that it only flashes once (produces one strobed image) during the exposure time in each field. The video camera captures and plays back half the illuminated image every 1/60th of a second. The flicker due to the alternating pattern of horizontal lines is generally imperceptible because the field rate (60 Hz) exceeds the critical flicker frequency of 50 Hz. In addition, the perception of apparent motion is always achieved because the video rate (30 frames per second) is in the range at which discrete images are perceived as a continuous, moving sequence.

Thus, in a given system, the field and frame rates are fixed according to the NTSC, PAL, or

SECAM protocol. The rate of the strobe light, however, can be modified and controlled independently from the video capture rate. Early videostroboscopy systems by Atmos and by Brüel and Kjær set the strobe rate to a specified beat frequency to illuminate the vocal folds once per cycle.[33] A direct consequence of these strobe rates was that more than one strobe flash could occur during each video frame. For example, with the NTSC video field rate at ~60 Hz and a vocal fold vibratory frequency at 130 Hz, there could be two or three strobe flashes (once per vocal fold cycle) occurring during each video field. The captured vocal fold image within each video field would exhibit multiple-exposure artifacts, such as multiple edges and inconsistent field-to-field illumination, because the camera sensor would integrate spatial information across two or three illuminated images. Additional artifacts would be evident when viewing a composite (still) video frame combining two of the already degraded video field images. The degree of image degradation was directly linked to the fundamental frequency of vibration; that is, stroboscopic recordings of humans with higher fundamental frequencies suffered from increased artifacts.

◆ Current Clinical Stroboscopy Systems

To counteract the undesirable image degradation exhibited by earlier models, in 1992, Kay Elemetrics (now KayPENTAX) introduced the first laryngeal stroboscopy system that controlled the triggering of the strobe light so that it only flashed once per video field, thereby eliminating artifacts due to multiple exposures during each field. Modern clinical stroboscopy systems automatically derive an estimate of the patient's voice signal during phonation with a neck sensor (usually a contact microphone or electroglottograph) and use this signal as the basis for controlling the timings of the strobe light to produce high-quality stroboscopic images. Thus, the stability of the patient's voice is critical for generating an accurate slow-motion view of vocal function.

In current systems, the repetition rate of the slow-motion vocal fold vibratory pattern can be modified from 0.5 to 2 cycles per second.[2,32]

For example, with the slow-motion rate set to 1.5 cycles per second (the *fast* mode in the KayPENTAX system) and the (NTSC) video rate fixed at ~60 fields per second, it would take 40 fields (60/1.5), or 20 video frames, to capture one complete cycle of vibration. To emphasize, the number of images captured to represent one vocal fold cycle would be the same, regardless of the fundamental frequency of vocal fold vibration. The number of video fields per cycle defines the phase interval, in degrees, between successive strobe flashes in a complete 360-degree cycle. Thus for 40 fields per cycle, the phase interval would be 9 degrees (360 degrees/40). Consequently, the phase interval between each video frame would be 18 degrees. The voice signal from the neck sensor is used to trigger the flash of the strobe light at the appropriate phase interval for each successive video field. Once the strobe fires during a video field, the system waits for the next video field to start before triggering the strobe at the next desired phase in the voice signal. Some clinical stroboscopic examination systems provide a foot pedal for switching the recording/playback mode between slow-motion and freeze-frame modes of operation.[2] The freeze-frame mode is accomplished by setting the slow-motion rate to zero, which sets the phase interval parameter to 0 degrees. Instead of capturing successive phases within a vocal fold cycle, the same phase is obtained across vocal fold cycles for each video field.

There are two main types of videostroboscopic systems that differ in their methods used to capture stroboscopic images. The most common method is the use of a flashing strobe light as the illumination source, as in the KayPENTAX (Lincoln Park, NJ) Rhino-Laryngeal Stroboscope.[2] An alternative method makes use of a constant light source and performs stroboscopic sampling by electronic shuttering of the camera. An example of this type of system is the JEDMED (St Louis, MO) StroboCAM II.[32]

Modern clinical stroboscopic examination systems make use of some common components, including endoscopes and systems for image display and recording that are based on standard video protocols (as described earlier), in addition to specialized light sources and camera control technology.[2,32] Stroboscopy can be performed using any type of endoscope that transmits sufficient light to the camera sensor during the strobe process. For some time, this has been most easily accomplished with the standard transoral rigid endoscope (telescope) and, more recently, has been made possible with flexible transnasal *videoscopes* (containing a miniature-chip camera in the scope's tip) that attach to both the strobe light source and the camera to allow for illumination and imaging of vocal fold motion. Stroboscopy is also possible through older, flexible fiberoptic transnasal endoscopes, but the poorer image quality due to insufficient lighting compromises the utility of the strobe exam. The continued reliance on video-based technologies has resulted in the creation of the term *videostroboscopy* to describe clinical systems and the generated examinations. (Additional terms have been strung together to produce more expansive labels like *laryngovideostroboscopy*.) These days, most display and recording systems are essentially digitally based video systems.

◆ Example of Stroboscopic Sampling Using High-Speed Videoendoscopy as a Reference

This section uses reference images from high-speed videoendoscopy to provide a final comprehensive illustration of the principles that underlie the clinical use of stroboscopy to examine vocal fold vibratory function. Laryngeal high-speed videoendoscopy, with color video capture rates up to 10,000 frames per second, provides a much more accurate sampling of vocal fold tissue motion than that of stroboscopic imaging.[3] In addition, the digital cameras used for high-speed imaging capture the entire scene in each frame, in contrast with the video-based interlacing scheme inherent in clinical videostroboscopy.

Figure 11.4 shows the high-speed video data that were obtained from a subject without vocal pathology at a rate of 6250 frames per second (0.16 msec per frame) using state-of-the-art digital color camera technology.[3] Two transoral rigid endoscopes were simultaneously positioned to view the vocal folds while the subject produced a sustained vowel that approximated the /ae/ vowel. One endoscope

provided continuous illumination for capturing video images from the attached high-speed camera. The second endoscope was connected to the light source of a clinical stroboscopy system that delivered strobe flashes that were triggered off of the voice signal obtained from a neck-mounted contact microphone.[2] The fundamental frequency during the phonatory segment was estimated to be ~236 Hz (period = 4.23 msec), yielding 26.44 high-speed video frames per vocal fold vibratory cycle ([4.23 msec per period]/[0.16 msec per frame] = 26.44 frames per cycle).

A total of 477 frames (76.32 msec) from the high-speed recording of vowel phonation is shown in **Figure 11.4.** Each row consists of one period of vocal fold vibration, which mimics the organization of the schematic in **Figure 11.2** that was used to demonstrate stroboscopic sampling. Note that **Figure 11.4** compensates for a non-integer number of frames per period by alternating between displaying 26 frames in odd-numbered rows and 27 frames in even-numbered rows. The solid lines (yellow and orange) demarcate the number of high-speed images captured during the duration of NTSC video fields. Because one light source was continuously on, the brighter images in the figure indicate times when the stroboscopic light source was triggered to flash. The brighter images are meant to mimic the images that would have been captured with only a videostroboscopic system. This type of display gives a clear sense of how stroboscopy provides an undersampled and averaged estimate of the underlying temporal details in vocal fold tissue motion during phonation. Note that, as expected, the strobe light is triggered to flash only once during each video field and that three cycles are skipped between flashes.

In this example, the slow-motion rate of the strobe light was set to 1.5 Hz, resulting in the display of 1.5 periods of vibration per second (a common setting used on clinical strobe units). The strobe rate must be close to 60 Hz to provide exposure (exactly one strobe flash) for each video field. The strobe rate can be estimated by simply dividing the fundamental frequency (236 Hz) by the video field rate, in this example 236/60 ≈ 3.9, indicating that the strobe would flash approximately once every 4 cycles or periods of vocal fold vibration.

Phonation: f0 ≈ 236 Hz (period ≈ 4.23 milliseconds)
High-speed video: Frame rate = 6250 Hz (period = 0.16 milliseconds)
Displayed: 477 frames (76.32 milliseconds)

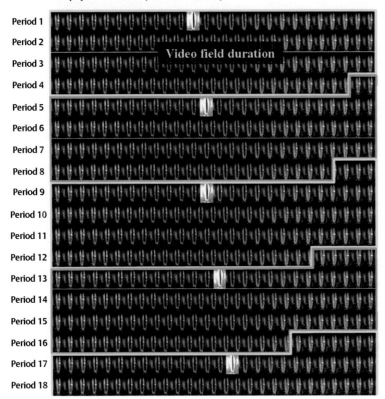

Fig. 11.4 The relationship between images acquired using stroboscopic sampling (brighter images) and high-speed video frames displaying true intracycle vocal fold motion.

◆ Further Reading

An illuminating account of the history of studies on flicker, apparent motion, and the propagation of the fallacy of persistence of vision can be found in an article by Galifret, "Visual Persistence and Cinema?"[12] Clear explanations of what happens when the strobe does not accurately track the phonatory pitch can be found in a chapter by Cranen and de Jong entitled "Laryngostroboscopy" in the book *Voice Quality Measurement.*[31]

◆ Video Examples

Stroboscopic recordings are an effective tool for assessing vocal fold vibratory patterns, facilitating real-time video and audio playback. Video clips on the DVD accompanying this book display stroboscopic video sequences created by the KayPENTAX Rhino-Laryngeal Stroboscope[2] and the Vision Research Phantom v7.3 color high-speed camera[3] (**Video Clips 10 to 14**).

References

1. Schuster M, Lohscheller J, Kummer P, Eysholdt U, Hoppe U. Laser projection in high-speed glottography for high-precision measurements of laryngeal dimensions and dynamics. Eur Arch Otorhinolaryngol 2005; 262:477–481

2. KayPENTAX. Instruction Manual: Stroboscopy Systems and Components. KayPENTAX, St Louis, MO; 2008

3. Deliyski DD, Petrushev PP, Bonilha HS, Gerlach TT, Martin-Harris B, Hillman RE. Clinical implementation of laryngeal high-speed videoendoscopy: challenges and evolution. Folia Phoniatr Logop 2008;60:33–44

4. Patel R, Dailey S, Bless D. Comparison of high-speed digital imaging with stroboscopy for laryngeal imaging

of glottal disorders. Ann Otol Rhinol Laryngol 2008; 117:413–424

5. Roget PM. Explanation of an optical deception in the appearance of the spokes of a wheel seen through vertical apertures. Philos Trans R Soc Lond 1825; 115:131–140

6. Wade NJ. Philosophical instruments and toys: optical devices extending the art of seeing. J Hist Neurosci 2004;13:102–124

7. Wendler J. Stroboscopy. J Voice 1992;6:149–154

8. Zeitels SM. Premalignant epithelium and microinvasive cancer of the vocal fold: the evolution of phonomicrosurgical management. Laryngoscope 1995; 105:1–51

9. Oertel M. Das Laryngo-stroboskop und die laryngostroboskopische Untersuchung. Arch Laryng Rhinol. 1895;3:1–16

10. Wertheimer M. Experimentelle Studien über das Sehen von Bewegung. Z Psychol Z Angew Psychol 1912;61: 161–265

11. Sekuler R. Motion perception: a modern view of Wertheimer's 1912 monograph. Perception 1996;25: 1243–1258

12. Galifret Y. Visual persistence and cinema? C R Biol 2006;329:369–385

13. Burr DC, Ross J, Morrone MC. Smooth and sampled motion. Vision Res 1986;26:643–652

14. Wertheimer M, Experimental studies on the seeing of motion. In: Shipley T, ed. Classics in Psychology. New York: Philosophical Library; 1912:1032–1089.

15. Ferry ES. Persistence of vision. Am J Sci 1892;44: 192–207

16. Yanagisawa E, Yanagisawa K. Stroboscopic videolaryngoscopy: a comparison of fiberscopic and telescopic documentation. Ann Otol Rhinol Laryngol 1993;102:255–265

17. The Society of Motion Picture and Television Engineers. SMPTE 170M-2004; Television–Composite Analog Video Signal–NTSC for Studio Applications (Revision of SMPTE 170M-1999). SMPTE; 2004

18. International Telecommunication Union. Characteristics of Composite Video Signals for Conventional Analogue Television Systems (Recommendation ITU-R BT.1700). ITU; 2005

19. von Leden H. The electronic synchron-stroboscope: its value for the practicing laryngologist. Ann Otol Rhinol Laryngol 1961;70:881–893

20. Colton RH, Casper JK, Leonard RJ. Understanding Voice Problems: A Physiological Perspective for Diagnosis and Treatment. Baltimore, MD: Lippincott Williams & Wilkins; 2006

21. Talbot HF. Experiments on light. Philos Mag Ser 3 1834; 5:321–334

22. Plateau J. Sur un principe de photométrie. Mém Acad R Belg 1835;2:52–59

23. Keller K, Kampfer H, Matijec R, et al. Photography. In: Ullman's Encyclopedia of Industrial Chemistry. New York, NY: Wiley-VCH; 2005

24. Porter TC. Contributions to the study of 'flicker.' Proc R Soc Lond 1898;63:347–356

25. Porter TC. Contributions to the study of flicker. Paper II. Proc R Soc Lond 1902;70:313–329

26. Porter TC. Contributions to the study of flicker. Paper III. Proc R Soc Lond Ser A 1912;86:495–513

27. Hecht S, Verrijp CD. Intermittent stimulation by light: III. The relation between intensity and critical fusion frequency for different retinal locations. J Gen Physiol 1933;17:251–268

28. Hecht S, Verrijp CD. The influence of intensity, color and retinal location on the fusion frequency of intermittent illumination. Proc Natl Acad Sci U S A 1933; 19:522–535

29. Hecht S, Shlaer S, Verriijp CD. Intermittent stimulation by light: II. The measurement of critical fusion frequency for the human eye. J Gen Physiol 1933; 17: 237–249

30. Anderson J, Anderson B. The myth of persistence of vision revisited. J Film Video 1993;45:3–12

31. Cranen B, de Jong F. Laryngostroboscopy. In: Kent RD, Ball MJ, eds. Voice Quality Measurement. San Diego, CA: Singular Publishing Group; 2000:257–267

32. JEDMED. StroboCAM II. St. Louis, MO: JEDMED; 2008

33. Nagashima H, Tuda K, Marui M. Larynx stroboscope for photography. US Patent No. 4,232,685;1980

12

Performing Videostroboscopy

Joseph C. Stemple and Lisa B. Fry

Laryngeal videostroboscopy has become the gold standard for the evaluation of laryngeal structure and function during voicing. The well-performed exam can offer a wealth of diagnostic as well as therapeutic information. This chapter will describe methods for achieving a successful and informative stroboscopic examination.

Those new to laryngeal visualization are referred to the American Speech-Language-Hearing Association's "Training Guidelines for Laryngeal Videoendoscopy/Stroboscopy" for a thorough review of the competencies and skills required for this procedure.[1] The document clearly outlines key competency areas (eg, anatomy, physiology, pathophysiology, equipment management, etc.) and serves as a comprehensive knowledge and skill checklist for clinicians and for those charged with their supervision.

Finally, it should be stated up front that laryngeal videostroboscopy can be performed with either rigid or flexible scopes. This chapter will focus on completing the stroboscopic exam using the rigid scope. Many of the principles discussed in the pages that follow apply to use of flexible scopes as well and should, therefore, be considered applicable to those exams. When appropriate, the authors have provided additional comments regarding the use of the flexible scope.

◆ Preparing the Clinician

The successful stroboscopic examination begins with the clinician's preparation. Skill in performing and interpreting stroboscopy comes only after hours of study and practice with willing volunteers. Once clinicians have reached an appropriate level of proficiency and confidence with the exam procedures, they bring a sense of comfort into the setting and set the stage for a successful exam.

Many experienced clinicians establish and follow a basic routine for arranging the room, setting up the equipment, positioning the patient, and placing their protective gear. Clinicians can set the tone for the exam by going through their preparation routine in a relaxed manner, maintaining light conversation with the patient.

At the start of the exam, the clinician's physical demeanor plays a significant role in either reassuring the patient or contributing to the patient's concerns. Consequently, the clinician should approach the patient in a slow, casual manner. Steady eye contact with the patient during this time conveys a sense of confidence and familiarity with the procedure and allays fears. During the exam, a relaxed posture with "soft hands" and "soft shoulders" will help to keep the patient calm as well.

◆ Preparing the Patient

Preparing the patient for the stroboscopic evaluation has as much to do with the success of the procedure as does scoping technique. Most patients have at least some level of anxiety about undergoing any medical procedure. Most of the patients seen for the stroboscopic procedure have had a previous mirror examination, which may or may not have been pleasant. The idea of a more extensive examination may be frightening. When a patient is anxious, his or her entire body is stiff, including the neck, jaw, and tongue. This stiffness contributes to a difficult examination. Consequently, relieving anxiety from the start should be a goal of the examiner.

Scheduling the Examination

Patients are scheduled for stroboscopic examinations several different ways. The exam may simply be a part of the routine otolaryngology examination or a later referral to the speech-language pathologist as a part of the diagnostic voice evaluation. When the examination is being scheduled for a later time, the scheduler actually becomes an important part of preparing the patient and reducing anxiety. Schedulers should be trained to describe the procedure to the patient, assuring them that the scope is merely placed in the mouth and will not be inserted deep in the throat. Patients are often given inaccurate information about examinations by friends and family—information that has no basis in truth. They often ask the schedulers if someone needs to accompany them; if they are permitted to eat; if there is recovery time; and so on. The scheduler can be extremely helpful in sharing accurate information and reassuring the patient.

Greeting the Patient

The examiner should make it a point to greet patients in the waiting room prior to a stroboscopic examination. This greeting gives the examiner the opportunity to shake the patient's hand and gauge the level of anxiety. If a patient's hand is cold and damp and his or her demeanor suggests anxiety, the clinician should begin discussing the examination with the patient as the clinician and patient walk to the exam room. The clinician may ask the patient what he or she knows about the test and immediately clear any misconceptions the patient might have. This 1- or 2-minute conversation along with the clinician's relaxed, friendly demeanor and obvious concern for the patient's feelings and well-being can make a significant difference in the quality of the examination.

Explaining the Procedure

There is no greater fear than fear of the unknown. Have you ever had a medical procedure where the technician, therapist, or physician is moving about the room, preparing instruments, handling supplies, putting on gloves, and so forth, while you wonder what it is all about? What are they doing? Are they going to use that with me? As medical professionals, otolaryngologists and speech-language pathologists are familiar with this environment and comfortably move about their instruments doing the routine "dance" of the day. However, for the majority of patients, the examination area is a scary, foreign environment. Because the goal is to reduce anxiety even before beginning the examination, it is very helpful for clinicians to talk the patient through every step of the procedure.

Once in the examination room, ask the patient to sit in the examination chair. While raising the level of the chair to the appropriate height, explain to the patient that raising the chair to eye level enables you to better see in the patient's mouth. At that point, show the patient the scope. Never point the scope right at the patient as this is a somewhat threatening posture; rather hold it parallel to your body. Explain to the patient that you will be placing the scope in his or her mouth and not down the throat. Tell the patient that you will be holding his or her tongue with a gauze pad, just to keep it out of the way, and that he or she will be saying "e-e-e-e" during the exam. Explain the purpose of the neck microphone and then turn the strobe light on to demonstrate the sound and the flashing light, so that

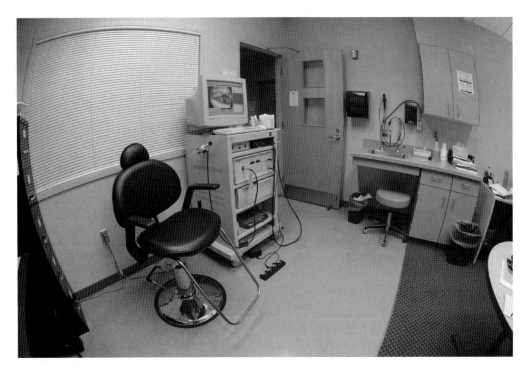

Fig. 12.1 View of the examination room set up to perform videostroboscopy.

the patient will be familiar with this during the actual exam. Place the scope back in the holder and wash and glove your hands. When the patient sees you hand washing, it provides a subtle comfort as to the sterility of the procedure. Some patients have even been known to inquire about how the scope is cleaned between examinations. By taking steps to demonstrate care and cleanliness throughout the preparation process, concerns such as this may be allayed and patient confidence increased. Once the above steps have been completed, tell the patient that you are ready to begin the examination.

◆ Preparing the Room

The room and equipment should be arranged in a manner that is convenient for the clinician yet not intimidating for the patient. Personal protective equipment, gauze, cleaning supplies, warming devices/solutions, topical anesthesia, and so forth, should be housed in close proximity to the strobe unit and should be arranged so that each can be accessed easily as the clinician works through his or her routine.

These authors recommend that the clinician arrange the room so that the sink and all needed supplies are located on a single side of the strobe unit, away from the patient. By doing so, you can prepare yourself and the equipment for the study without needlessly passing the scope, cords, or other supplies over or in front of the patient (**Fig. 12.1**).

Finally, management of lighting can be quite important during an exam. Dimming bright overhead lights and/or closing window blinds help to reduce glare on the screen and permit improved viewing throughout the exam.

◆ Examining the Patient

At this point, all of the pre-examination issues that will help ensure a successful stroboscopic study have been addressed. It is now time to do the study. A key to success for many clinicians is the development of a systematic routine for completing the exam. One might equate this to choreographing a dance. If clinicians develop and follow the same routine for each examination, all will go smoothly. When developing the routine, clinicians will need to consider and work through a variety of exam scenarios, eventually choosing the format that is best for them. For example, clinicians may ask: will I stand in front or slightly to the side of the patient? How will I turn toward the sink if I am warming the scope with warm water? Will the cords and wires easily reach? Where will I place the gauze and the waste receptacle for easy access? When do I tell the patient how to position himself or herself? Will I turn the light source on before or after I place the scope in the mouth, and will the patient begin saying the "e-e-e-e" before I actually see the folds? Choreographing and practicing this dance routine with many practice subjects prior to actual patient examination will serve clinicians well. The following are examination tips that clinicians might find useful with the majority of patients.

Positioning the Patient

Because patients vary anatomically, positioning all patients for a rigid scope exam in a single, standard posture is not possible. However, for the majority of patients, sitting up straight with the neck extended forward is often the position of choice. When the neck is extended forward, the pharynx is lengthened giving better unimpeded access to the 70-degree angle scope. At the onset of the examination, the patient should be instructed to sit up straight with the chin forward, mouth open, and tongue out.

Tongue Issues

Having taught many people over the years how to do stroboscopic examinations and having served as practice subjects, the authors are very sensitive to tongue issues. The manner in which the tongue is handled has a major impact on the success or failure of the examination. The importance of relaxed eyes, arms, shoulders, and hands of the examiner to a successful examination has been previously stated. The clinician's handling of the tongue is an extension of that discussion. Much can be learned in this area by considering how one is trained in riding horses. An important concept taught in riding lessons is that if the rider's hands are "heavy" or tight on the reins, the horse will respond in the same manner and be heavy against the rider's hands. The rider and horse will be fighting each other for control. The same holds true for clinician handling of the tongue in a stroboscopic examination.

If the clinician squeezes the tongue with his or her fingers, it will be painful, and the patient will pull back. If the clinician pulls the tongue too far forward, the same response will occur. This concept can be easily tested out with a colleague. After your colleague has washed and gloved his or her hands, assume the posture for the examination. Open your mouth and protrude your tongue. Ask your colleague to both pinch your tongue and pull it forward. You will see that your automatic response is to brace the back of your tongue in a protective manner which stiffens and decreases the diameter of your pharynx and makes the epiglottis less flexible thus less able to tilt forward. The examination is therefore unpleasant, and the view is often less than adequate. By working cooperatively with clients and allowing clients a degree of control over tongue position, improved tongue posture can be achieved, and improved viewing will result. Clinicians working in this manner may avoid situations such as that reported by a recent patient who was asked what the doctor saw when he looked at her vocal folds with the mirror. Her response was both humorous and telling. She said, "You're not going to do that are you? Why, it felt like he ripped out my tongue, threw it on the floor, and stomped on it!"

We would suggest that the examiner hold the tongue with the nondominant hand with the index and middle fingers on top and the thumb below. Ask the patient to stick out the tongue. Once holding the tongue in the above manner, say to the patient, ". . . now, let the tongue go back in your mouth." This request accomplishes two things. First, some patients protrude their tongues with extreme stiffness, and this request will encourage them to relax. Second, it reminds the examiner that he or she is simply controlling the tongue and not pulling it forward, thus permitting it to assume a more natural posture. Some endoscopists might suggest that pulling the tongue forward with the thumb on the top aids in viewing the vocal folds by forcing the epiglottis to tilt forward. However, others (including the authors) may argue that permitting the tongue to reside in a more natural position in the mouth and only controlling the tip will permit the patient to produce the "e-e-e-e" in a more natural manner that not only tilts the epiglottis but also permits a more natural vibration of the vocal folds.

Positioning the two fingers on the top of the tongue also permits the examiner to use the fingers as a fulcrum for the scope. Without this fulcrum, the scope is permitted to float in the mouth often hitting teeth and other oral structures. The fulcrum steadies the clinician's scoping hand and permits the subtle movements necessary to attain the desired view (**Fig. 12.2**).

The "eeee" Sound

Successful rigid scope exams require that the tongue base and epiglottis be moved out of the viewing area. Consequently, patients are instructed to produce the front vowel /i/. This task is quite challenging for some patients and may require additional guidance from the clinician. This author is in the habit of saying to patients during the examination, "more eeee-like." It is true that the /i/ will encourage the tilt of the epiglottis better than any other vowel. However, in the unnatural environment of someone holding a patient's tongue while a scope is placed in his or her mouth, some individuals need to be encouraged to produce

the sound as close to the /i/ as possible. Sometimes patients struggle so hard to produce the /i/ that they actually create excessive and unwanted tension in the oral and pharyngeal regions. If this is the case, remove the scope and have the patient practice the desired sound with a protruded tongue. This coaching can often make the difference between an adequate and an inadequate exam.

Breathing

Sometimes it is necessary to instruct the patient in how to breathe during the examination. Occasionally, patients attempt to breathe through their noses while being scoped, a posture that invites the tongue to block the oral cavity and impede the view of the scope. If this behavior continues, clinicians may place a nose clip to occlude the nares and force the patient to breathe through the mouth.

The "No-Fault" Gag

A good rule of thumb when performing stroboscopy is to never bring up the subject of a gag unless the patient does. The mere suggestion of gag often causes a gag. If a patient says, "is that going to make me gag" or "I gag when I brush my teeth," it is important to remind them that the scope is only going in the mouth, not down the throat. Notice when a patient does gag that the response is typically to apologize profusely. The more patients gag, the more they worry about the gag and compromise the exam

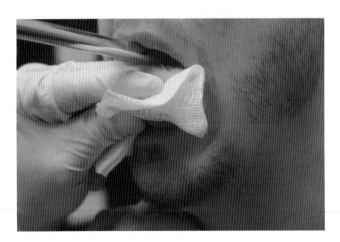

Fig. 12.2 The tongue is held between two fingers and the scope is steadied during the exam.

even further. At this point, to relieve the patient, it can be helpful to introduce the "no-fault gag." Explain to the patient that everyone has a gag reflex and, in fact, you worry if a patient does not show at least some sign of gagging during the exam. Consequently, their gagging is something that is natural and not something that they can be expected to control. This explanation often relieves them and reduces the intensity of their gagging behavior. If the protocols have been established for use of topical anesthesia in your facility, even a small touch of spray at this point may be all that is needed to control the reflex.

Other suggestions for reducing the gag reflex involve distraction. Never permit the patient to close his or her eyes during the examination. When the eyes are closed, the patient is able to concentrate more on the sensation of the scope in the mouth. Tell patients as the scope is entering the mouth to look up and instruct them to open their eyes if they close. It can also be helpful to have a second monitor in the room within the view of the patient so that the patient can see the exam, which will also distract them from being a part of the exam. Finally, asking the patient to pant like a dog in between saying /i/ may prove helpful. Realistically, some individuals possess significant gag responses. These patients will continue to exhibit that response no matter what the examiner tries. If a rigid scope examination is required, demonstrate patience and take the time to get the best examination possible.

◆ The Exam Protocol

Camera Setup

Just prior to initiating the exam, the clinician must attach the rigid scope to the unit's camera. Care should be taken to ensure that the scope is aligned properly on the camera base, allowing a straight, midline view. When the angle of alignment between the camera and scope is off, even by a slight degree, visual artifacts may taint the image observed by the clinician. Improperly positioned cameras can lead to erroneous conclusions regarding vocal fold symmetry and motion. Once attached, camera alignment can be confirmed by holding the scope over a reference point (eg, unit's keyboard, piece of typed text). If the text appears off midline or rotated, the scope's attachment to the camera should be readjusted slightly and reevaluated for its alignment.

After alignment is confirmed, the camera should be white-balanced. This step takes only a moment to complete and ensures that the coloration of the larynx is correctly represented on the recording. Though clinicians have a variety of ways of white balancing, many place the scope 2 inches to 3 inches from a white sheet of paper with black text, turn on the light source, and follow the unit's instructions to balance. (Step-by-step instructions for white balancing differ across systems and are generally provided with the camera unit's instruction manual.) Other clinicians confirm the balance and test the coloration by making a slightly opened fist with the non-scoping hand and placing the scope over the fist, as if to peer into the tube formed by the fingers. If properly balanced, the coloration of the skin should be true-to-life, and the lower aspects of the "tube" should be properly illuminated. Some cameras automatically white-balance, precluding the need for this step.

Scope Warming/Defogging

Placing a room-temperature scope into a patient's warm oral cavity generally results in fogging of the lens. When this occurs, views of the larynx are severely limited. Consequently, it is important that the scope be warmed prior to its insertion into the mouth. A variety of methods are currently used for this purpose. Commercially available defogging agents and warming beads are frequently used. These authors prefer to gently warm the scope by holding it under warm running water for a few seconds or by immersing it into a cup of warm water. This method effectively prepares the scope without exposing it to potentially harmful chemicals or rough surfaces and without the requirement of additional supply costs.

Scope Insertion

Proper insertion of the scope sets the foundation for a good examination. Though many different methods of holding and inserting the scope are available, several basic principles of

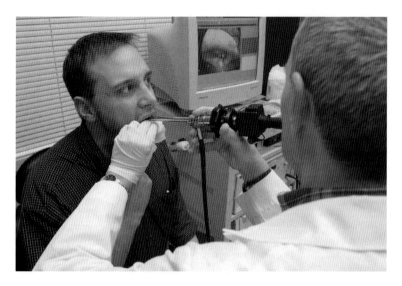

Fig. 12.3 View of patient and examiner during videostroboscopy.

scope management are quite helpful. As previously mentioned, the clinician's hand often has a way of drifting with his or her body's movements. It is therefore helpful to use the nonscoping hand not only to anchor the tongue but also to create a fulcrum on which the scope can tilt, slide, or rotate. Such a posture keeps the scope more steady in the mouth and allows the clinician to make small adjustments in the scope's position that are not bothersome to the patient. Once the clinician has established his or her hand position, the scope can be slowly advanced into the mouth, sliding along the fulcrum created by the clinician's nonscoping hand. At this point, it is important that the clinician's gaze be fixed on the computer screen rather than in the patient's oral cavity, as the visual feedback on the screen will aid the clinician in maneuvering the scope and achieving a proper placement. The scope should be advanced until the clinician sees initial landmarks such as the base of the tongue, the pyriform sinus, and the arytenoid cartilages on the screen. The landmarks generally become visible when the scope tip reaches the region where the hard and soft palates unite.

Scope Maneuvering

Once in position, the scope will need to be maneuvered *slightly* during the exam to ensure optimal viewing of the vocal folds. The examiner should be aware that a very small movement of the hand creates a larger movement at the tip of the scope. Once again, the clinician will find it helpful to use the nonscoping hand as a fulcrum. This allows the clinician to make subtle changes in the scope's position without losing his or her basic position and without bothering the patient. Finally, it is important that the scope be kept in the middle of the oral cavity, away from the tongue, palate, and teeth. Placing the scope too near the tongue and palate can trigger a gag reflex in some patients, and allowing the metal shaft to touch the teeth can be quite bothersome to others (**Fig. 12.3**).

When at all possible, achieve all necessary views on the first attempt at scoping, as repeated episodes of placing and removing the scope often increase patient anxiety and make the patient more aversive to the scope. Consequently, subsequent views may not be as optimal as early views. Verbally encouraging the patient during the exam and allowing moments of quiet breathing can often extend the exam and eliminate the need for repeated scopings.

The Voice Sample

Once the scope has been optimally positioned, the patient should be asked to perform a series of vocal tasks. Though the sequence may vary across clinicians, it is important that the chosen protocol allow visualization of the laryngeal structures in a variety of postures (eg, abducted, adducted) and appreciation of the vocal folds during an array of vibratory modes (eg, modal, falsetto). The following sequence is helpful in achieving a comprehensive assessment of laryngeal function during the rigid exam*:

- Modal pitch at comfortable loudness, loud, and soft
- High pitch at comfortable loudness, loud, and soft
- Low pitch at comfortable loudness, loud, and soft
- Glide upward
- Glide downward
- Production of /hi-hi-hi/ and /i-i-i/ for laryngeal diadochokinesis
- Forceful inhalation/exhalation
- Panning of the laryngeal region during quiet breathing

While working through the above protocol will give the clinician a comprehensive understanding of the patient's vocal physiology, the formal assessment of vibratory parameters (eg, amplitude, mucosal wave) should be made from samples obtained at a modal pitch and comfortable loudness. Once the protocol has been completed, the scope can be reinserted a second time for modal pitch examination to confirm the results of the previous sample.

Finally, it is important to note that some patients use a disengaged manner of voicing during the procedure, failing to contract the thyroarytenoid muscle and producing a breathy, weak tone. If this occurs, it is important to remind the patient to "engage" the voice or to encourage a louder production, modeling the proper tone for the patient as needed.

◆ Overcoming Problems

The above discussion has presented the ideal protocol for the patient who is typically cooperative, anatomically normal, and can tolerate

*The flexible scope permits observation during a wider range of voicing tasks (eg, connected speech, singing). However, this list of basic tasks should still be documented during flexible examinations to allow a comprehensive understanding of laryngeal function.

the procedure well. However, not all patients fit the mold for the typical evaluation technique and protocol. Age, cognition, anatomy, and physical restrictions may all play a role in the successful examination. Below are some thoughts on each of these areas.

Age and Cognition

There are very few individuals who cannot be successfully examined through stroboscopy using a rigid scope. However, as individuals approach the extremes of age, both the very young and some in the elderly population, the challenge may become greater. A good approach with young children is to take the time to desensitize them to both the instruments and the technique prior to the actual exam. To accomplish this, the clinician should first talk about why the doctor and their parents want them to have the exam. The clinician may then discuss the voice and the fact that it comes from the throat. The child is told that a special television camera can be used to look in the mouth and see how the vocal folds are vibrating. The clinician may then hold the child's hand over his or her own larynx and let the child feel the vibrations—repeating the same procedure with the child feeling his or her own vibrations. The clinician may then show the child the scope, explaining that it will go in the mouth to look at the vocal cords while they make sound. Additionally, the clinician might turn on the light source and permit the child to watch the monitor to see how the camera can visualize his or her fingers, hair, and so forth. During this time, the child will become familiar with the noise and the light that accompany the strobe exam. Next, using a gauze pad and a tongue blade, the clinician may hold the child's tongue and place the tongue blade in the mouth while they say "eeee." Almost all children have had a tongue blade in the mouth with the only new sensation being that of having the tongue held and saying the sound. Having taken the time to desensitize the child to these new experiences, the examiner has a greater chance of successfully completing the stroboscopic examination.

Even after this slow seduction, clinicians often have only a single opportunity to complete the exam with a young child. Consequently, clinicians should make sure their technique is solid and that they move deliberately. Clinicians should continue the exam even if the child begins to protest and cry. Some of the best views of the vocal folds might be gained when the child takes a deep breath to cry. Many children have been spared a direct laryngoscopy because of the view obtained of the vocal folds during a less than adequate stroboscopic examination. Chronological age is not the issue with children but rather maturity and cooperation. Experienced clinicians can attest to the fact that they have examined some 4-year-old children with complete exam protocols while not being able to get near some 10-year-old children. A final suggestion is to try to accomplish the examination without the parent in the room. Children often put up a much braver front without their parents to console them.

Most elderly individuals do not present unusual challenges to completing a successful examination. One issue to consider is what to do with dentures. Dentures that fit well and that stay firmly in place when the mouth is opened widely may remain in the mouth during the exam. Loose-fitting dentures must be removed for fear of becoming dislodged and interfering with the examination.

Individuals who are cognitively impaired at any age should be examined with a caregiver in the room. These authors would advise that clinicians speak directly to the person being examined, giving all of the typical information/protocol but with the understanding that the information is being shared with the caregiver as well. At times, the caregiver can be a great help in comforting the patient and actually assisting the clinician during the examination by controlling interfering head and hand movement.

Anatomic Challenges

Some individuals present anatomic challenges to completing the successful stroboscopic examination. These individuals may include those with a short thick neck, individuals with reduced oral opening or a short frenulum, and those with an omega-shaped epiglottis. These individuals often require that the examiner

deviate from the normal exam protocol. For example, the individual with the short neck may best be viewed by tilting the head back instead of forward. The examiner should not hesitate to position the head and neck of this individual multiple ways in an attempt to view the folds. Finally, for patients in whom the mouth opening is restricted (eg, temporomandibular joint syndrome, scleroderma), it can be helpful to use a 90-degree scope that does not require the upward angle of the 70-degree scope. Otherwise, visualization with a rigid scope may not be possible.

Considering the discussion of tongue issues earlier in this chapter, the reader is aware of how careful the examiner should be with the tongue. Some individuals have a short frenulum making holding the tongue nearly impossible in the normal manner. When this is the case, clinicians may try asking the patient to hold his or her own tongue with the gauze. The patient is not likely to cause himself or herself discomfort. If the patient is not successful in doing this, the examiner may place his or her fingers behind the lower front teeth with the gauze on top of the tongue and with the thumb placed below the jaw. With this technique, the examiner is controlling the tongue and lower jaw.

Finally, the omega-shaped epiglottis is a unique challenge. When present, the examiner must carefully place the 70-degree scope as closely to the tip of the epiglottis as possible and peer between the lateral edges of the epiglottis into the interior of the larynx. At times, this placement requires firm pressure to be applied to the base of the tongue with the middle of the scope as a means of mechanically moving the epiglottis forward. This is a challenge even for the experienced examiner.

Physical Challenges

Some individuals are referred for stroboscopic evaluations who present the examiner with physical challenges. Perhaps the easiest with which to deal is the patient confined to a wheelchair. If at all possible, safely transfer this patient to the examination chair and proceed as normal. When transfer is not possible, position the wheelchair in an adequate position to conduct the examination while sitting on a stool; this may require that you move the examination chair from the room. In the authors' experience, a patient that was brought into the facility by ambulance for the examination. He was confined to a supine position on a gurney and could not be transferred to any other position. The stroboscopic examination was conducted with the examiner standing on a chair positioned above the patient with the scope pointing toward the ground. Thus, with flexibility and ingenuity, even the most challenging physical restrictions can be overcome and successful examinations completed.

◆ Conclusion

The serious voice care team of the 21st century relies upon high-quality laryngeal visualization for the diagnosis and management of voice concerns. When performed properly, laryngeal videostroboscopy can offer a wealth of information to team members. For physicians, the procedure may offer vital diagnostic information and additional guidance for managing the condition. For speech-language pathologists, stroboscopy may offer insight into the patient's manner of voice production and subsequently guide the clinician in goal setting, treatment planning, and the monitoring of progress. The successful stroboscopic exam begins well before the patient is seated in the exam chair and encompasses much more than the physical management of a scope. The clinician who is attentive to detail at all phases of the exam process—from scheduling to examination—will reap optimal benefits of his or her study.

Reference

1. American Speech-Language-Hearing Association. Training guidelines for laryngeal videoendoscopy/ stroboscopy. 1998. Available at: http://www.asha.org/ docs/html/GL1998-00064.html

13

Interpreting the Videostroboscopic Examination

Nicolas E. Maragos

Videostroboscopy is a distinctive tool used in the study of vocal dysfunction and laryngeal disorders. Refinements of equipment over the past two-plus decades has made the examination of the larynx easier, better, and more precise than ever before. In spite of these improvements, the diagnosis of many problems is often illusive, primarily because the laryngologic community is still in the process of learning how to interpret the videostroboscopic results, but also at times because the exam itself is deficient in uncovering an underlying problem. This chapter, then, will attempt to give insight to those who may be asked to perform this exam so that at least the evidence of disorder may be captured on electronic media. It is up to the laryngologist and the speech-language pathologist to look closely for the clues hidden in that media to effectively diagnose and eventually treat the patient. Performing a videostroboscopy is usually not a difficult task, but the goal is not just to do the exam but also to make sure the clinician gets all the information he or she requires for good patient care.

◆ General Observations

Before looking specifically at the vocal folds and their function, we can make several general observations while first examining the laryngopharynx. These observations should be noted in a separate area of the videostroboscopy report so they may be easily identified. General observations include mucosal coloration and swelling, presence or absence of chronic infection (whitish mucus and debris) of the laryngopharynx, pooling of secretions in the piriform sinuses, and silent aspiration (saliva going in and out of the posterior glottis without reflex coughing).

One of the most common causes of dysphonia today is infection of the laryngopharynx with either fungal or bacterial (*Staphylococcus aureus*, mostly methicillin sensitive) organisms. The incidence of chronic throat infections with these organisms has skyrocketed in the past 10 to 15 years primarily because of the changes in treatment of all types of infections with antibiotics that kill normal throat flora in addition to treating the infection. The signs of chronic bacterial or fungal infection that should be noted during the general observations of the larynx include a more generalized erythema/edema affecting the larynx as a whole (false cords, epiglottis, aryepiglottic folds) as well as the hypopharynx (posterior pharyngeal wall, piriform sinuses). Erythema and/or edema of the posterior larynx (arytenoid and interarytenoid mucosa) are more likely to be secondary to acid reflux from the stomach up into the larynx (laryngopharyngeal reflux). This should be differentiated from the generalized signs of infection and noted as such in the report.

Pooling of secretions in the piriform sinuses may signify difficulty swallowing from any cause and can involve structures extending from the oral musculature to the esophagogastric junction. Documenting this in the videostroboscopy report should be followed by a suggestion that a referral for a swallow evaluation be made. Finally, silent aspiration is the end stage of severe laryngopharyngeal dysfunction. It usually includes both anatomic and neurologic deficits of the laryngopharynx that result in great impairment of swallowing.

◆ Visualizing the Larynx

We know intuitively that everyone's voice is a little bit different. How then is it possible to examine the human larynx and know what we need to see? The best approach to accomplish this is to go back to the basics of voice production, for therein lie the clues necessary to understand what we need to see. Consideration of the patient's chief complaint, listening to the voice before doing any physical examination, and understanding how voice is produced are paramount to understanding how to examine a voice-disordered larynx. Even so, it must be kept in mind that the pre-examination information is not always specific. Some vocal symptoms may be classified as general, because that symptom can result from a variety of underlying problems. For example, a softer-than-normal voice may be generated by a whole host of underlying pathology including generalized systemic weakness, diaphragmatic paralysis, chronic obstructive pulmonary disease, subglottic or tracheal stenosis, vocal fold paralysis, arytenoid subluxation, and so forth. Vocal softness, then, is not very helpful in pointing the clinician in the direction of where to look for possible laryngeal problems, and the exam must evaluate for a broad range of possible problems. On the other hand, a "graty" sound to the voice is almost always indicative of a problem at the arytenoids cartilages. So in this case, we have real clues that indicate where we need to look for trouble. With experience, the voice clinician understands the implications of the pre-examination information and

uses it effectively to guide the examination itself.

Instrumentation

Instrumentation used in videostroboscopy includes a telescopic device (rigid or flexible), a light source, a camera, a microphone, a strobe unit linked to the microphone's audio signal, and a video unit typically linked to a computer for digital or analog capture. Finally, the information recorded during video and audio capture needs to be saved in a format and in such a way that it is categorized and easily retrievable. Before digital capture was readily available, the recorded material was usually saved in either VHS or Hi-8 format. With digital recordings, this information is now saved on either DVD media or hard drives.

Laryngologists today use either a rigid telescope (70 or 90 degree) or a flexible endoscope connected to the videostrobe system. Rigid endoscopy remains the gold standard for clear and precise video capture and is usually well tolerated with or without local anesthesia to the pharynx. With the recent advent of distal chip flexible scopes (the camera resides at the far end of the scope), endoscopic examination is available with less distortion of the laryngopharynx from pulling forward on the tongue. In addition, we can now visualize laryngeal function more fully and naturally (see later), putting the larynx through its paces while capturing a very good picture of this organ. Some clarity is sacrificed, but the functional information gained is better overall.

The Vocal Folds

As a review, voice is produced when the lining tissue of the anterior vocal folds, the mucosa, is put into oscillation and changes a steady stream of air into a rhythmically interrupted air stream.[1] We may separate the vocal folds into their two distinct but interactive parts: the anterior vocal fold (membranous soft tissue) and the posterior vocal fold (arytenoid cartilage). The arytenoids are connected to their respective vocal fold ligaments and thyroarytenoid muscles at their vocal processes and along their anterior faces. For all intents and purposes, the medial arytenoid mucosa does not vibrate enough to contribute to the voice under normal conditions but it may in some dysphonias. Please refer to Chapters 2 and 3 for a more detailed discussion of laryngeal anatomy, histology, and physiology.

Anterior Membranous Vocal Folds

The anterior vocal folds include the vocal ligaments, the medial and lateral thyroarytenoid muscles, the overlying vocal fold mucosa, and the connective tissue holding everything together. Dysphonia occurs most often when the vocal fold mucosal waves are disturbed. Thus, observation of the mucosal waves with videostroboscopy is a must. Mucosal waves are described as being present or absent and as having amplitude and speed. In addition, the mucosal waves of one vocal fold must be compared with and described in relation to their counterpart waves on the opposite vocal fold. These latter observations are most important as normal sound production depends upon mucosal waveforms that are nearly identical from side to side. The best voices are generated when mucosal waves are equal, symmetric, and in phase bilaterally.

Videostroboscopy should be aimed, in part, at obtaining enough visual information to describe the mucosal waves completely. This includes:

- A clear picture of both vocal folds at rest and during phonation.
- Release of enough supraglottic tension to see the vocal folds as completely as possible.
- Observation of the mucosal waves bilaterally with phonation. This requires good tracking of the vocal sound by the stroboscopic machine.

Once the video and audio signals are captured, they can be stored within the computer or, more commonly, on removable storage data (DVD, large-capacity hard drive). The most common commercially available hardware and software include ways to store and recover data rather easily and quickly.

After the pictures are captured, saved, and stored, they should be replayed in both normal-speed and slow-speed modes to further examine what is happening during phonation.

With this review, we want to look for and comment on:

- Specific areas where the mucosal waves may be absent on one or both vocal folds.
- The relative sizes of the mucosal waves on each side (normal, too large, or too small).
- Whether the mucosal waves are starting and traveling at the same time or whether one side is going "early" and the opposite side lags behind. This is described as either symmetric (normal and equal) or asymmetric (different and unequal).
- An estimate of the percentage of phonatory time spent with symmetric/asymmetric mucosal waves.

Information gathered about the specifics of the mucosal waves will aid the laryngologist in the search for causes of the patient's dysphonia. For more information on the specifics of each vibratory parameter, please see subsequent chapters.

Posterior Cartilaginous Vocal Folds

Even though the anterior vocal folds are the area of sound generation, dysphonia may also be caused by posterior vocal fold abnormalities. Close observation of the positions, movements, and interactions between the arytenoid cartilages are also an important part of a videostroboscopic exam. Once we begin to closely pay attention to the posterior larynx and the movements of the arytenoids, we will uncover a whole host of things that could be causing phonatory problems and that were never thought of before.

Arytenoid Position

The normal position of the arytenoid cartilages is sitting upright on the posterior cricoid rim. When viewing during videostroboscopy, we see the arytenoids from above. Thus under the mucosa at the posterior end of each aryepiglottic fold lies the superior process of the arytenoid. The medial face of the arytenoid should be fully observable, and the posterior and medial extent of each arytenoid with the smaller corniculate cartilage attached directly to the superior arytenoid may be seen. The

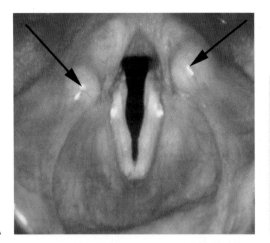

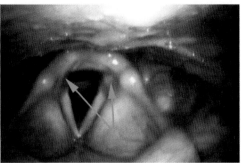

A

B

Fig. 13.1 (A) Normal larynx. The *arrows* indicate cuneiform cartilages in the aryepiglottic folds. Folds are in a partially adducted position. Both vocal folds are seen in their entirety. The medial surfaces of the arytenoids are slightly visible, which is normal. The posterior arytenoids (and corniculates) are equal bilaterally and not excessive. Superior processes are equal (left partially covered by cuneiform).

Cuneiforms: right slightly anterior to left. Aryepiglottic folds and false cords are equal. The epiglottis is deformed. **(B)** Normal larynx. The *arrows* demonstrate how the medial surfaces of the arytenoid cartilages are easily visible. Folds are abducted, and the entire length of both membranous vocal folds is visible.

right and left cuneiform cartilages are frequently mistaken for the superior apex of the arytenoid. The cuneiforms look somewhat like a flattened sphere residing at the posterior end of the aryepiglottic fold, and aside from being a "curiosity" in humans, they do add some weight to those folds (**Fig. 13.1A**).

The "position" of the arytenoids is actually described in relation to the normal (upright) position of the cartilage in the cricoarytenoid joint. At rest, we should be able to see the medial surface of the arytenoids easily, and in addition we should see the entire membranous vocal fold as well (**Fig. 13.1B**). Deviations from this relationship occur when the arytenoid is tilted in any direction away from its normal vertical location. The position may be described as being normal, too effaced (falling laterally and posteriorly), or too far medial and anterior (covering a portion of the vocal fold).

Arytenoid Movement

Examination of the posterior larynx continues with the gross movements of the arytenoid cartilages. These movements may be described individually for their speed (brisk/fast, sluggish/slow), regularity (smooth, hesitant), and excursion (full, limited in either adduction or abduction). These descriptions give us clues to underlying problems but also make us think constantly about what is happening in the posterior larynx. In the past, the posterior larynx and the movement of the arytenoid cartilages have been an area much overlooked because we did not have the videostrobe in most of our offices, but those times are past.

After examining the individual arytenoid movements, we should then compare one side with the other just as we did with the anterior vocal folds and the mucosal waves. In this regard, we should ask the following questions and describe our results in the overall report:

1. Did the arytenoid movements begin at the same time? Stepping through the stroboscopy frame by frame allows us to make this determination.
2. Is there underrotation or overrotation of one arytenoid cartilage during phonation?
3. Do the vocal folds "line up" at the vocal processes of the arytenoids or is there a vertical height difference between the vocal folds?

Differences in movement onset from side to side and rotational deviations of an arytenoid usually signify synkinetic reinnervation after nerve injury. Disparity in the vertical height of the vocal folds with phonation is sometimes difficult to see in a two-dimensional video. However, it is very important to look for this because an uneven closure of the glottis will cause a voice that sounds worse than it appears during laryngeal visualization from above.

◆ Observing Voice Production

There is something special about good vocal production. The voice is an intimate part of an individual's personality, the way one interacts with others, and a beacon of an individual's health. It is no wonder then that the perception of a voice being "abnormal" raises immediate questions in the listener. As we have outlined earlier, there are specific irregularities of both the anterior and posterior vocal folds that may generate a dysphonic voice and be observed directly. There are also, however, aspects of voice production that are directly responsible for dysphonia that could go unnoticed if we are not thinking of them all the time. It is sometimes helpful to the physician ordering the video to mention these possibilities, not in a long and exhaustive list but as something one has observed during the testing.

The final observations needed from a videostroboscopic examination are those telling us how the vocal folds are working together to produce a sound. For this we need to put the vocal mechanism through its paces with more than just a sustained "a" or "i" sound. Several specific vocal tasks have been found useful, helping to uncover and observe laryngeal function during voicing. With time and practice, we may find equally good or better methods of "stretching the limits" of the voice to uncover somewhat hidden vocal deficiencies, but for now we mention those that have been helpful to date.

Glissando

Voicing from low pitch to high pitch approximates the patient's vocal range. More importantly, however, observation of the vocal fold stretching during this exercise may uncover a unilateral or bilateral superior laryngeal nerve weakness. Mild weaknesses are not easily identified, so performing this task on every patient gives us a sense of what is normal and what is not. Close observation of shifting or twisting of the larynx (posterior glottis deviation in relation to the horizontal plane of the epiglottis) is still easier to detect than a difference in vocal fold stretching, but if both are present, then the diagnosis may be made (**Fig. 13.2**).

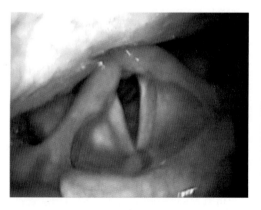
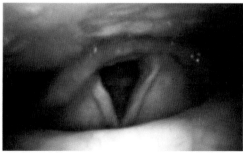

A

B

Fig. 13.2 (A) Left superior laryngeal nerve weakness. Notice the asymmetry of tension between the right and left vocal folds. **(B)** Left superior laryngeal nerve weakness. Note the shift of posterior glottis to the left. The left vocal fold is thinner than the right.

Humming

Producing a humming sound with lips closed usually releases a lot of tension during vocal output. This allows better visualization of the vocal folds with less supraglottic closure from the false cords. In addition, the patient will generally hum in a lower tone, making it easier to see the mucosal waves and any variability from one side to the other. This task is not possible to perform, however, with a rigid endoscope through the mouth but is something that can be done when stroboscopy is being performed with a flexible scope through the nasal cavity.

Voicing at Different Pitches

As just mentioned, the mucosal waves are most easily seen at lower pitches where the amplitude of vibration is greater. At higher pitches, however, we may uncover more disparity between the vocal folds and their mucosal waves. The vocal folds are elongated, thinner, and farther apart during phonation. We may then make observations between the vocal fold mechanism at high pitch when compared with that of low pitch.

Intermittent Voicing

When the voice is produced with short bursts in quick succession, we can see the interactions of the arytenoid cartilages upon each other and how easily the arytenoids move over the cricoarytenoid joints. We can also observe whether or not the internal laryngeal muscles relax quickly or whether there is a delayed relaxation phase. If we suspect or see some delayed relaxation, then we should try at that time to corroborate that finding with possible delayed relaxation of the entire larynx after swallowing. Normal laryngeal movement with swallowing includes a quick upward movement of the larynx of at least 2 to 3 cm followed by a quick relaxation back to baseline. If relaxation is delayed greater than 1 second, then that should be noted in the report. Delayed relaxation is usually caused by neurologic disease, so a consultation with a neurologist should be suggested to the ordering physician in the report if that has not already been done.

◆ Comments

Up to this point, we have discussed extensively what needs to be included in a videostroboscopy report to the laryngologist. Because it is not the purview of this chapter to completely explain what the laryngologist will do with this material, one may wonder why all these details were believed to be important at all! Therefore, a short example is given to demonstrate how the information gathered during videostroboscopy is vital to good patient care. This detailed examination may be used not only for uncovering the cause of a vocal problem but also for planning the medical and surgical care necessary for its improvement. We will illustrate this process with a very common problem seen in laryngology, dysphonia secondary to unilateral vocal fold immobility.

Unilateral Vocal Fold Immobility

When a patient presents with immobility of one vocal fold, the physician immediately thinks of a list of possible causes for this abnormality. Problems leading to vocal fold immobility generally include dysfunction of the laryngeal muscle(s), the arytenoid cartilage, or the cricoarytenoid joint. Thus the list includes, but is not limited to, vocal fold paralysis, arytenoid cartilage subluxation (arytenoid cartilage in its joint but out of place), and cricoarytenoid joint arthrodesis (fixation). Videostroboscopy can give us valuable clues in differentiating between these conditions. For instance, an immobile vocal fold with noticeable movement of the muscles attached to the lateral arytenoid (muscular process) may signal an arytenoid subluxation (the arytenoid cartilage being displaced anteromedially or posterolaterally) or a cricoarytenoid joint or joint capsule fixation (trauma, arthritis, fixation after paralysis) (**Fig. 13.3**).

On the other hand, no noticeable internal laryngeal muscle movement usually signifies a real vocal fold paralysis, and then it becomes important to identify the resulting deficits after muscle atrophy, synkinetic reinnervation, and patient compensations are complete. These factors will determine what kind of

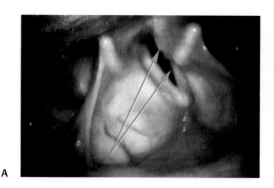

A

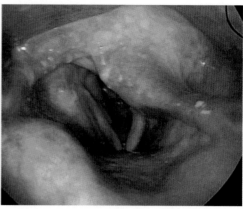

B

Fig. 13.3 **(A)** Left arytenoid subluxation anteriorly. The *arrows* point out that the medial surface of the left arytenoid cartilage cannot be seen and that the full length of the left vocal fold cannot be visualized. **(B)** Another case of arytenoid subluxation. The left arytenoid is falling forward. Again, the medial surface of the left arytenoid cartilage cannot be seen, and the posterior part of the left vocal fold is obscured by the left arytenoid cartilage. Over 50% of the left vocal fold is obscured by the upper arytenoid. The upper rim of the left posterior cricoid is visible. Of note, the patient has fungal laryngopharyngitis.

surgery is needed for the best laryngeal rehabilitation. In this regard, we are interested in essentially three observations: any opening at the anterior glottis, any opening at the posterior glottis, and any pooling of secretions (mucus) in the piriform sinuses. An open anterior glottis alone may be treated with either injectable materials into the vocal fold or an anterior vocal fold medialization procedure (eg, type I thyroplasty). If the posterior glottis is open during phonation, however, the voice will be very breathy (phonation with one breath lasts for about four syllables), and the patient will have intermittent penetration/aspiration with swallowing (choking, coughing). These symptoms stem from posterior laryngeal incompetence, and closing the anterior glottis alone will not completely rehabilitate the voice and will do nothing to improve swallowing. Something will most likely need to be done to the posterior larynx (arytenoid) to obtain the best surgical outcome, and the operations that best handle posterior glottic deficiencies are the arytenoid adduction procedure (rotating, sliding, and stabilizing the arytenoid cartilage at the midline) or the adduction arytenopexy (a suture fixation of the arytenoid cartilage at the midline). These arytenoid procedures are almost uniformly done in combination with an anterior vocal fold medialization because if the posterior glottis is open, then the anterior glottis will

also be open, and past experience and studies have shown that a "direct" approach to both the posterior and the anterior vocal folds gives the highest patient satisfaction.[2]

Lastly, the presence of pooled secretions (saliva, mucus) in the piriform sinus signals real problems with swallowing. Vagal nerve involvement may be just the recurrent laryngeal nerve, resulting in nonrelaxation of the cricopharyngeus muscle (upper esophageal sphincter) or possibly a combination of the recurrent laryngeal nerve plus the pharyngeal branches of the vagus. Whatever the case, a cricopharyngeal myotomy may be added to a combination arytenoid adduction and type I thyroplasty for attempted complete rehabilitation of the patient presenting with a very breathy or aphonic voice and dysphagia. Thus by paying attention to the details seen on clinical examination of the voice and larynx, we now have a more complete picture of why the voice is dysphonic and how we can proceed to help our patient regain more normal laryngeal function.

◆ Conclusion

Our ability to visualize laryngeal anatomy and physiology to a fine degree has opened up our diagnostic capabilities with disease and dysfunction in this area. Knowledge of what is valuable and important for the laryngologist's diagnostic workup and what is necessary to capture on a detailed videostroboscopic examination is vital in the overall care of the patient. In the final analysis, a well-done videostroboscopic exam will hasten the time to correct diagnosis, allow for a more thorough laryngeal evaluation, and help uncover the root cause of the dysphonia.

References

1. Hirano M. Phonosurgery: Basic and Clinical Investigations. Nara, Japan: Otologia (Fukuoka); 1975:239–298
2. Slavit DH, Maragos NE. Arytenoid adduction and type I thyroplasty in the treatment of aphonia. J Voice 1994;8:84–91

14

Normal Glottic Configuration

Edie R. Hapner

Glottal configuration and *glottal closure* are terms often used interchangeably in the literature to describe the spatial characteristics of the vocal folds during phonation when viewed stroboscopically. *Glottal configuration* is defined as the shape of the glottal aperture during phonation. In describing glottal configuration, one is actually referring to the shape of the glottis. Whereas the term *glottis* is frequently used when referring to the vocal folds, the true definition of the term *glottis* is the space between the vocal folds (**Fig. 14.1**).

Glottal closure refers to the extent of vocal fold closure during the closed phase of phonation. Glottal closure is generally described as complete, incomplete, or inconsistent. The duration of glottal closure, relative to the rest of a single vibratory cycle, normally changes with the mode of vibration. Hirano described three typical vocal fold vibratory modes: falsetto, modal, and fry.[1] In falsetto, there is incomplete glottal closure of the vocal folds throughout the cycle (**Video Clip 4**). During modal phonation, the vocal folds close completely during the closed phase of the vibratory cycle (**Video Clip 1**). In vocal fry, there is an extended duration of vocal fold closure relative to the rest of the vibratory cycle. The duration of vocal fold opening divided by the duration of the entire glottal cycle is called the open quotient and describes the percentage of time during a single vibratory cycle that the folds are in the open phase. (One minus the open quotient = the percentage of time during a single vibratory cycle that the folds are in the closed phase.) Vocal folds that never completely close, such as during falsetto, have an open quotient of 1. Modal phonation has an open quotient of 0.5. Glottal fry has an open quotient trending toward 0.[2]

Stroboscopic evaluation of the vocal folds is a frequently used method to assess glottal configuration and closure during phonation. While stroboscopy is the most clinically friendly, cost-effective method of viewing glottal configuration and closure during phonation, several factors must be taken into consideration during the examination. Gender and age have an impact on glottal configuration during phonation.

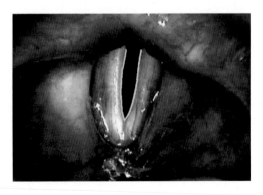

Fig. 14.1 The glottis.

Changes in pitch, loudness, vocal register, phonemic variations, and prosodic emphasis also have an effect on glottal configuration. Technical issues associated with the stroboscopic examination can further play a role in determining glottal configuration and glottal closure.

This chapter will describe (1) normal glottal configuration and the research to date on normal variations in glottal configuration, (2) methods to measure glottal configuration, (3) phonatory behaviors that influence the examination, and (4) technical pitfalls during stroboscopy that can affect an accurate assessment of glottal configuration.

◆ Normal Glottal Configuration

Casper et al. wrote the following:

> We sometimes think about the normal larynx as if that idealized state of perfection actually exists

although we know that the term "normal" does not describe a single condition with set boundaries. Indeed given the opportunity to create the perfectly normal larynx, we probably could not agree on the elements of its design.[3]

It is generally assumed that normal glottal configuration is marked by complete glottal closure during the closed phase of phonation.[4] However, in studies of "normal" larynges, the pivotal finding of most is the variety of glottal configurations identified.[5–8] Casper et al. caution that in the absence of vocal fold pathologies, the difference between a normal larynx and one that is thought to be the cause of a voice disorder is indeed difficult to assess with use of stroboscopy alone.[3]

There is a need for a standardized nomenclature to describe glottal configuration. **Figure 14.2** demonstrates several glottal configurations often referred to in the literature. It is important to recognize that the assessment of glottal configuration remains perceptual

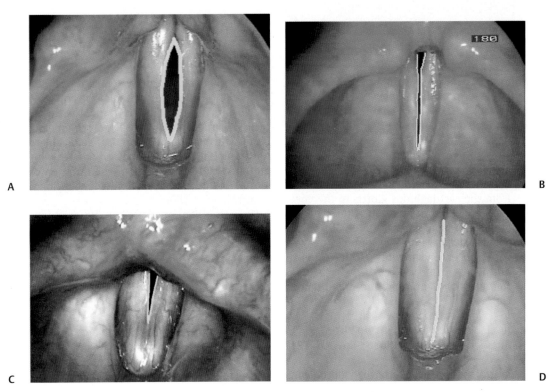

A · B · C · D

Fig. 14.2 Common glottal configurations: spindle **(A)**, incomplete **(B)**, posterior glottal chink **(C)**, complete **(D)**, (Continued on page 130)

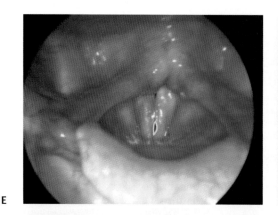

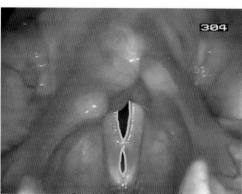

E

F

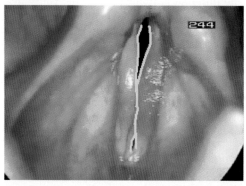

G

Fig. 14.2 (*Continued*) anterior glottal gap **(E)**, hourglass **(F)**, irregular **(G)**.

at best and, as such, is subject to interrater differences and confusion, due to the use of multiple terms and multiple descriptive rating systems. The seven most common glottal configurations plus complete glottal closure are listed here:

- *Complete closure* (**Video Clip 1**)
- *Posterior glottal chink* (triangular opening from the cartilaginous glottis to the vocal processes that may extend anteriorly into the membranous glottis) (**Video Clip 15**)
- *Spindle shape* (anterior commissure and vocal process closure only) (**Video Clips 16 and 17**)
- *Hourglass configuration* (mid-membranous closure only) (**Video Clip 18**)
- *Irregular closure* (**Video Clip 19**)
- *Incomplete closure* (**Video Clip 20**)
- *Anterior glottal chink* (**Video Clips 3 and 21**)

Several authors have described glottal configurations seen during stroboscopy, though there is no consensus on nomenclature to describe the glottis, and no universally accepted glottal configuration scale exists to date.[9–12] Hirano proposed a rating system that included a description of glottal configuration and glottal closure.[1] He recommended that the examiner determine if the glottis is ever completely closed during phonation and, if so, evaluate how long it is closed. His descriptive scale for glottal closure is a rating of the duration of glottal closure as follows: a, very long; b, long; c, fairly long; d, short; or e, very short.

He also recommended that the examiner draw the shape of the glottis during maximum closure.

Bless et al. used seven line drawings of glottal configuration during phonation to develop a clinical evaluation tool to be used to rate the stroboscopic studies.[10] The drawings represented frequently encountered glottal configurations and included complete closure; posterior glottal chink; anterior chink; spindle shape; incomplete closure; hourglass closure; and irregular closure patterns. Gelfer and Bultemeyer attempted to test the reliability of this system but included a measure of degree of glottal closure that was

III Videostroboscopy

130

based on a three-point rating scale with 1 indicating complete closure and 3 indicating that the vocal folds never closed. They found that intrarater reliability was experience-dependent and perhaps related to the examiner's visual-spatial skills. Their study also attempted to provide data on vocal fold vibratory patterns in normal adult females. Notably, they found that glottal configuration and glottal closure demonstrated the most intersubject variability of the stroboscopic parameters tested.[6]

Another system used in the literature to rate glottal configuration and glottal closure is found in studies by Södersten and Lindestad and Södersten et al. using a rating scale for judging vocal fold closure during phonation with line drawings of glottal configuration and scalar points for degree of closing. The six-point scale is as follows:

1. Complete closure the full length of the vocal folds.
2. Incomplete closure of the cartilaginous portion of the folds.
3. Triangular incomplete closure extending into the membranous fold past the vocal processes.

4. Triangular incomplete closure extending to include the posterior third of the vocal folds.
5. Incomplete closure of the posterior two thirds of the vocal folds.
6. Incomplete closure the full length of the folds.

There are an additional four descriptions including spindle-shaped closure with closure only at the vocal processes, spindle-shaped closure of the posterior third of the vocal folds with closure at the vocal process, spindle-shaped closure at the anterior third of the vocal folds, and spindle-shaped closure of the anterior third and the posterior third of the vocal folds with mid-membranous closure present.[7,12,13]

It is important when describing glottal configuration that the assessment of the shape of the glottis is made during the closed phase of the cycle. Glottal configuration changes as the phase of the glottal cycle changes.[9] **Figure 14.3** demonstrates the changes in glottal configuration and closure as the vocal folds move through the phases of modal phonation.

In the American Speech-Language-Hearing Association (ASHA) consensus document

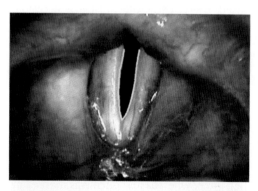

A

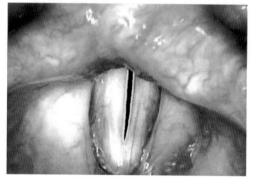

B

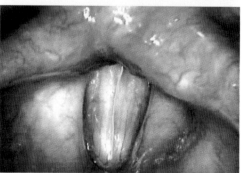

C

Fig. 14.3 Glottal configuration during glottal cycle in modal phonation: open phase (**A**), closing phase (**B**), closed phase (**C**).

"Knowledge and Skills for Speech Language Pathologists with Respect to Vocal Tract Visualization and Imaging," the working group suggested vocal fold closure during stroboscopy be rated as complete (open quotient normal, open quotient increased, open quotient decreased) or incomplete (posterior glottal gap, anterior glottal gap, elliptical, hourglass slit, or incomplete).[14]

A method to quantitatively measure glottal configuration was described by Secarz et al.[15] Frames from the stroboscopic examination that represent the most open glottal width and those representing the most closed glottal width are first identified. A reference mark is made somewhere near the middle of the glottis, and measurements in pixels are made between the reference mark and the glottal edge. Woo used a method of drawing the glottal edge and measuring the glottal area.[16] A similar procedure using a laser beam to identify a reference point on the vocal folds to assist with standardizing scope distance from the vocal folds and then using a method to measure glottal width was described by Patel (R. Patel, personal communication, 2008).

◆ Demographic Factors That Affect Glottal Configuration

Gender

Multiple studies in the late 1980s and early 1990s examined the gender differences in glottal configuration during stroboscopy. There was a consensus that there is a difference in the incidence of various glottal configurations between the genders.[5,6,12,17] Men demonstrate complete glottal closure more often than women. Women demonstrate a greater incidence of posterior glottal chink, whereas, if present in men, the chink tends to be located toward the mid-membranous or anterior portions of the vocal folds.

Age

Age has an impact on glottal configuration. Biever and Bless found a high incidence of glottal gap in elderly women aged 60 to 77 years, and Linville found a high incidence of glottal gap in elderly women aged 72 to 87 years in a second study.[5,18] The shape of the gap varied from a posterior glottal gap to a mid-membranous gap to an anterior glottal gap. In both studies, young women in their twenties were also found to have a higher incidence of posterior glottal gap. Most studies agree that normal age-related changes to the vocal folds are marked by atrophy and a resulting mid-membranous glottal gap. Varying degrees of spindle-shaped gaps are generally described in the aging larynx with a bowed appearance to the vocal folds themselves.

◆ Psychoacoustic Effects on Glottal Configuration

Pitch, mode of phonation, loudness, and register will impact glottal configuration. One must consider muscle activation used to produce differences in phonation. Bonilha and Deliyski noted that glottal width irregularities should be expected when examining the vocal folds in any mode other than modal/habitual phonation even in normal, nondysphonic speakers.[2] As an example, when the pitch is raised, the cricothyroid muscle is activated and pulls the thyroid and cricoid cartilage together thus lengthening and tensing the vocal folds. Clinicians generally believe that the result of this cricothyroid muscle activity is to prevent complete adduction during phonation thereby producing a complete mid-line glottal gap during phonation. However, Gelfer and Butlemeyer found glottal configuration was idiosyncratic within subjects at different pitches. They noted complete, incomplete, hourglass, and spindle configuration at high pitch, whereas low pitch was marked by complete, incomplete, and posterior glottal gap configurations.[6]

Loud phonation is produced by increasing subglottal pressure and glottal closure. It should not be a surprise that glottal closure is increased and glottal configuration tends toward more closed as loudness increases in normal speakers.

Register of phonation, or vibratory mode, has been found to impact glottal closure but not glottal shape.[4] This phenomenon has been studied in modal and falsetto phonation.

Though it is generally accepted that glottal closure is complete in modal register, incomplete in falsetto register, and extended in vocal fry, glottal configuration during both falsetto and modal varies between speakers.[4] Once again, glottal configuration appears to be idiosyncratic.

Technical Considerations in the Measurement of Glottal Configuration

The technology of videostroboscopy limits the assessment of degree of glottal closure. Hapner and Johns write that stroboscopy provides only a two-dimensional view of the vocal folds viewed from above, the bird's-eye view.[19] This limits the ability to perceive three-dimensional contours of normal and pathologic tissue.

The type of scope used in laryngeal videostroboscopy can influence glottal configuration.[20] Södersten and Lindestad found that use of a rigid laryngoscope increased the detection of incomplete glottal closure over what was found when using flexible laryngoscopy.[12] This study and other studies used a 90-degree rigid laryngoscope, whereas other studies have used a 70-degree rigid laryngoscope.[17] Different oral, laryngeal, and upper chest postures are used when examining with a 70-degree versus a 90-degree rigid laryngoscope, and the effects on glottal configuration have yet to be established. Therefore, care must be used when applying the results of the studies to clinical practice unless using the same method of examination.

Videostroboscopy has been found to be useful in determining the outcome of medical, surgical, or therapeutic intervention to correct glottic defects. Serial examinations are used to establish outcomes. The problem is that technical issues associated with stroboscopy make it difficult to compare accurately one examination with a repeat examination. Hibi et al.[21] and Peppard and Bless[11] proposed a method to increase the reliability of serial examinations by drawing on transparencies overlaid on the video monitor while the monitor displays a chosen image of the vocal folds and using the drawing in a follow-up examination for positioning of the folds on the monitor during the examination.

Conclusion

Though videostroboscopy remains the most useful clinical tool to examine glottal configuration and glottal closure, care must be taken to avoid common technical pitfalls that impact the results of the examination. Bonilha and Deliyski warn that the extent of irregularity considered to be within normal limits should be determined for each evaluation tool used to assess glottal configuration as it may differ between evaluation tools.[2] It is also important to be cognizant of the age and gender of the patient; the pitch, loudness, register, and mode of phonation during the examination; to establish a protocol of phonatory tasks to allow for better reliability in serial examination; and to understand the limitations of the stroboscopic examination.

Finally, Elias et al. studied stroboscopic variability in normal healthy singers.[22] What was particularly interesting is that they found that 58% of the singers had abnormal videostroboscopy examinations, yet none of the singers reported any problems with vocal performance. In the discussion, the authors note that it is imperative for the examiner to remember that normal can occur in the presence of abnormal findings and that care should be taken before implying causality.

No definitive database of normal, nondysphonic vocal fold behavior has been developed, and most of the research into glottal configuration is at a minimum 10 years old. It behooves the examiner to be educated on normal variability in glottal configuration and glottal closure to prevent overdiagnosing abnormal behavior and referring for intervention.

References

1. Hirano M. Clinical Examination of Voice. New York, NY: Springer-Verlag; 1981
2. Bonilha HS, Deliyski DD. Period and glottal width irregularities in vocally normal speakers. J Voice 2008;22:699–708
3. Casper JK, Brewer DW, Colton RH. Variations in normal human laryngeal anatomy and physiology as viewed fiberscopically. J Voice 1987;1:180–185
4. Murry T, Xu JJ, Woodson GE. Glottal configuration associated with fundamental frequency and vocal register. J Voice 1998;12:44–49
5. Biever D, Bless DM. Vibratory characteristics of the vocal folds in young adult and geriatric women. J Voice 1989;3:120–131

6. Gelfer M, Bultemeyer D. Evaluation of vocal fold vibratory patterns in normal voices. J Voice 1990;4:335–345

7. Södersten M, Hertegård S, Hammarberg B. Glottal closure, transglottal airflow, and voice quality in healthy middle-aged women. J Voice 1995; 9: 182–197

8. Kendall KA. High-speed laryngeal imaging compared with videostroboscopy in healthy subjects. Arch Otolaryngol Head Neck Surg 2009;135:274–281

9. Karnell M. Synchronized videostroboscopy and electroglottography. J Voice 1989;3:68–75

10. Bless DM, Hirano M, Feder RJ. Videostroboscopic evaluation of the larynx. Ear Nose Throat J 1987;66:289–296

11. Peppard RC, Bless DM. A method for improving measurement reliability in laryngeal videostroboscopy. J Voice 1990;4:280–285

12. Södersten M, Lindestad PA. Glottal closure and perceived breathiness during phonation in normally speaking subjects. J Speech Hear Res 1990;33:601–611

13. Södersten M, Lindestad PA. A comparison of vocal fold closure in rigid telescopic and flexible fiberoptic laryngostroboscopy. Acta Otolaryngol 1992;112:144–150

14. American Speech-Language-Hearing Association. Knowledge and skills for speech language pathologists with respect to vocal tract visualization and imaging. ASHA Suppl 2004;24:184–192

15. Secarz JA, Berke GS, Arnstein DA, Gerratt B, Navidad M. A new technique for quantitative measures of laryngeal videostroboscopic images. Acta Otolaryngol 1991;117:871–875

16. Woo P. Quantification of videostrobolaryngoscopic findings: measurements of the normal glottal cycle. Laryngoscope 1996;106(3 Pt 2, Suppl 79)1–27

17. Sulter AM, Schutte HK, Miller DG. Standardized laryngeal videostroboscopic rating: differences between untrained and trained male and female subjects, and effects of varying sound intensity, fundamental frequency, and age. J Voice 1996;10:175–189

18. Linville SE. Glottal gap configuration in two age groups of women. J Voice 1992;35:1209–1215

19. Hapner ER, Johns MM. Recognizing and understanding the limitations of laryngeal videostroboscopy. Perspect Voice 2007;17:3–7

20. Pemberton C, Russell A, Priestley J, Havas T, Hooper J, Clark P. Characteristics of normal larynges under flexible fiberscopic and stroboscopic examination: an Australian perspective. J Voice 1993;7:382–389

21. Hibi S, Bless DM, Hirano M. Distortions of videostroboscopy images. J Voice 1988;2:168–175

22. Elias ME, Sataloff RT, Rosen DC, Heuer RJ, Spiegel JR. Normal strobovideolaryngoscopy: variability in healthy singers. J Voice 1997;11:104–107

15

Normal Vocal Fold Symmetry and Phase Characteristics

Donna S. Lundy and Mario A. Landera

Vocal characteristics and qualities are determined by fine-tuning the vocal fold vibratory patterns during phonation. Since Rethi's first reported recognition of the mucosal wave in 1897 and through use of high-speed photography of the vibratory cycle, interest in studying the details of vocal fold oscillation has increased.[1] A variety of vocal fold vibratory parameters have come to the forefront for study, including symmetry and phase.

At the onset of normal vocal fold vibration, the vocal folds are adducted. Evidence from stroboscopic imaging indicates that they begin their displacement away from the midline in unison, achieve their maximum point of displacement at the same time (and to the same extent), and arrive back at the midline at the same time. This mirror-like symmetry pertains not only to vibration in the horizontal plane but also to vibration in the vertical plane. When the vocal folds are closing, contact is made, first, between the lower margins of the folds and then extending to the superior margins. During opening, the same pattern occurs; that is, separation between the folds begins along their lower margins and continues vertically to their superior margins (**Video Clip 3**). The separation, or *opening*, and approximation, or *closing*, components of a vibratory cycle of the vocal folds are described as *phases*, and the

symmetry of fold behavior across these phases is referred to as *phase symmetry*.[2–4]

The portion of a vibratory cycle in which the folds are open (which includes opening and closing) is referred to as the *open* phase of vibration, and the portion when the folds are approximated is defined as the *closed* phase of vibration. At comfortable pitch and loudness (or modal voice), the open and closed phases are approximately equal in duration (see Chapter 10, **Fig. 10.3A**). The actual extent of displacement and the time spent in displacement and return to midline may vary according to several factors. For example, the amount of time the vocal folds are open, opening, closing, and closed in each cycle is related, in part, to the regulation of airflow through the glottis. The extent of displacement is influenced by other factors, including vocal intensity (**Video Clip 6**).[5,6] These differences notwithstanding, the "mirroring" of the two vocal folds in amplitude and timing has generally been considered characteristic of normal vibration and normal voice.[2–4] Similarly, significant deviations from such symmetry have been associated with abnormal vibration and voice.[2]

Most authors rate symmetry dichotomously as either present or absent; symmetric versus asymmetric. Colton and colleagues describe a more detailed rating system including normal versus open phase predominates sometimes or always; or normal versus closed phase predominates sometimes or always.[7] The significance of phase determination is that greater glottal efficiency with improved flow conversion is seen when the cycle is in-phase.[6]

◆ Clinical Relevance

Symmetric movements of the vocal folds are an indication that the mechanical properties of the tissues are equivalent, just as asymmetric vibration implies possible lack of equivalence with the position, shape, mass, elasticity, and/or viscoelastic properties of the vocal folds. For example, in vibratory cycles that are out-of-phase, the vocal folds may not oppose at the same time, allowing for increased air loss and the potential perception of breathiness (**Video Clips 22 and 23**).

◆ Methods of Evaluation

The evaluation of finer vocal fold vibratory qualities like symmetry and phase is not possible when viewing the vocal folds with a constant light source. Stroboscopy uses high-speed flashes of light that are synchronized on sequential parts of the vibratory cycle and allow for an illusion of motion and the ability to appreciate whether the cycle is symmetric and/or in-phase. Careful review of the virtual slow-motion recordings made during stroboscopy allows the clinician to evaluate the extent and timing of movement of the right and left vocal folds relative to each other (**Video Clip 7**). Vocal folds that begin to open simultaneously, that move laterally at the same speed and to the same extent, then begin to close at the same time, move to the midline at the same speed, and then come together simultaneously, through several cycles of vibration, are considered to be vibrating symmetrically (**Fig. 15.1; Video Clips 1, 3, 5, 6, 15, and 21**).

Dejonckere and colleagues studied the reliability of experienced clinicians in rating a variety of vibratory parameters, including symmetry.[8] Low reliability in rating symmetry was found when seven experienced laryngologists and/or phoniatricians rated 30 stroboscopic images. Thus, whereas symmetry is an important factor of vocal fold vibration, the reliability of assessing it, at least via stroboscopy, is not completely clear.

To determine the phase characteristics of vibration using stroboscopy, the "montage"

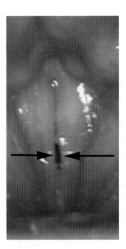 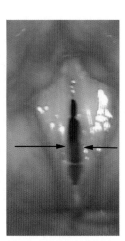 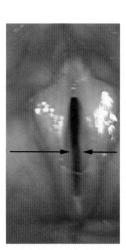 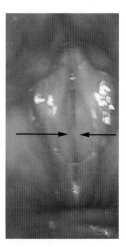

A,B

C,D

Fig. 15.1 **(A)** Symmetric vocal fold vibration begins as the vocal folds begin to open at the same time and at the same speed. **(B)** Symmetric vocal fold vibration requires that both vocal folds reach maximal opening at the same time and that they both open to the same extent. **(C)** Both vocal folds begin to close at the same time and at the same speed. **(D)** The vocal folds reach the midline simultaneously and close together.

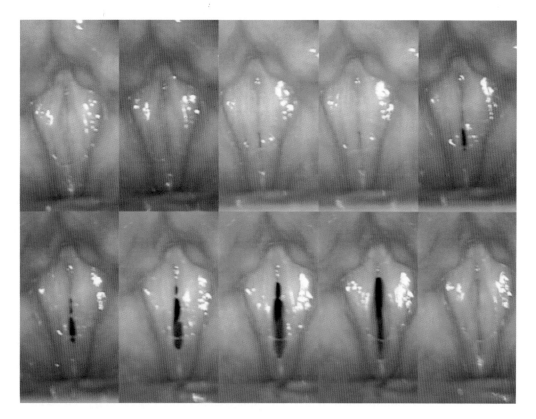

Fig. 15.2 Example of a montage with 50% open phase.

function is often used. This feature allows the clinician to choose a representative sample of vibration from the study. The software then places 10 images from that point in the study, representing one cycle of vibration, on the screen simultaneously. The number of images with the vocal folds open during the cycle can be counted and compared with the number of images with the vocal folds closed during the cycle. Normal open phase during phonation at a comfortable pitch and loudness is 50% (**Fig. 15.2**).

◆ Variations in Healthy Individuals

As vocal fold vibration is dependent not only on the myoelastic properties of the vocal fold epithelium and lamina propria but also on control of the laryngeal intrinsic musculature and on coordinated pulmonary support, it is

not unexpected that some variations would exist in otherwise asymptomatic individuals. Doellinger and colleagues assessed the effect of vocal load on symmetry of vibration in a normal subject via phonovibrogram and found asymmetric, left versus right, movement at the end of the day, indicating that "fatigue" in otherwise healthy individuals may result in "abnormal" symmetry.[9] Likewise, Shaw and Deliyski assessed 52 healthy subjects via stroboscopy, high-speed videoendoscopy, and kymography. They found asymmetry of vocal fold vibration during modal and pressed phonation leading them to question the clinical utility of this vibratory parameter.[10] In another study of normal subjects, Elias and colleagues evaluated 65 asymptomatic, classically trained singing students. They found that four of the students had prominent asymmetry of horizontal or lateromedial vocal fold excursion despite a lack of symptoms. The authors concluded that some degree of variability in vibratory symmetry did not appear to have a significant impact on the subjects' perceptions of their voice, possibly owing to technical training.[11] Kendall studied 50 healthy volunteers and found periods of asymmetric vibration in 26%.[12]

The effect of pitch on symmetry has also been evaluated (**Video Clip 5**). Haben and associates studied videostroboscopic images in 57 normal subjects (30 females and 27 males) and found 33% of subjects exhibited lateral phase asymmetry in their upper registers with 10.5% demonstrating asymmetry in both chest and upper registers.[3] However, Fong assessed symmetry at different pitch levels (modal, vocal fry, falsetto) (**Video Clip 4**) in 15 normal subjects with high-speed videography and found no significant difference in the incidence of asymmetry based on pitch.[13] In addition, Jiang and colleagues studied the effect of physiologic alterations on pitch and symmetry. They studied vocal fold vibration from an infraglottic view and found that thyroarytenoid muscle contraction resulted in larger amplitudes of vibration with a concurrent decrease of the vibratory frequency and increased vibratory asymmetry. In contrast, increased airflow through the glottis resulted in smaller amplitudes of vibration and minimized vibratory asymmetry while increasing vibratory frequency. Vocal fold lengthening was also shown to decrease vibration amplitude with a resultant increase in vibratory frequency and decreased asymmetry.[5] This conflicting evidence, even in normal subjects, underscores the importance of accurate interpretation of asymmetry associated with pitch or frequency in dysphonic patients. In short, some asymmetry may be "normal," and asymmetry may not always explain an individual patient's dysphonia.

Pontes and colleagues evaluated the effect of age on phase symmetry.[14] They reviewed 50 laryngeal imaging studies from young (20 to 45 years) individuals and compared them with 50 imaging studies performed in older (65 to 85 years) individuals. The results of the study revealed abnormal vibratory patterns predominately in the older group. Specifically, phase and amplitude asymmetry was seen more frequently in the older group despite a lack of vocal complaints among subjects. Biever and Bless also looked at the effect of aging on vibratory patterns. They evaluated 40 asymptomatic females, 20 young versus

20 old, and found that older women demonstrated 15% asymmetry versus no asymmetry in the younger group.[15]

Woo studied 65 normal subjects with simultaneous stroboscopy and EGG at different pitch and loudness levels (**Video Clips 5 and 6**).[6] When vocal intensity or loudness was increased, males in the study demonstrated a slight increase in the amount of asymmetric vibration for all pitch levels. Males also demonstrated a longer closed phase for all pitch levels when compared with the females in the study. Both groups had an increase in the closed phase as vocal intensity increased. In general, Woo concluded that the open phase of the cycle tends to vary with variations in the frequency of phonation, while the closing phase of the cycle changes with variation in the intensity of phonation.

The importance of hydration for vocal health is emphasized throughout the voice literature with varying amounts being recommended. However, the impact of hydration on vibratory symmetry and phase closure has not been established. Fujita and colleagues looked at the effects of hydration on vibration via videokymography and found that individuals that were better hydrated demonstrated an increase in the closed phase of the cycle.[16]

Thus, the presence of asymmetric vibration and phase closure changes is not always the cause of vocal symptoms and needs to be considered carefully. The impact of vocal pitch and loudness on vibratory symmetry is unclear. The impact of vocal pitch and loudness on phase is well established.

◆ Conclusion

The intricate vibratory patterns of the vocal folds are subject to many different influences. Contractions of the intrinsic laryngeal musculature interact with steady airflow from the pulmonary system, with support from the abdominal musculature, to create vibration. As described by Woo, "good vocal function requires symmetric vibration with the vocal folds on the same vertical level, good phase symmetry, and the ability to open and close rapidly to modulate airflow."[6] In general, vocal folds vibrate in a mirror image of each other in terms of symmetry and phase properties.

Asymmetric, out-of-phase vibration is more frequently seen in pathologic states, in particular, where there is a differential in the mass or tone between the two vocal folds, as seen with lesions and unilateral vocal fold paralysis or with neurologic voice disorders such as spasmodic dysphonia. On the other hand, the evaluation of specific vibratory factors like symmetry and phase in patients with voice symptoms must consider the variations observed in healthy individuals prior to deciding that any one abnormality seen on examination is the cause of specific voice complaints. Some variations in normal individuals are found with changes in register, vocal intensity, fatigue, and advancing age. Thus, abnormalities observed in symmetry and phase on laryngeal examination need to be considered with the rest of the physical findings, acoustic measures, and the patient's symptoms to determine whether this finding alone is indicative of underlying pathology.

References

1. Rethi L. Experimentelle Untersuchungen uber den Stimmbander bei der falsettstimme. Wein Klin Rundschau 1897;11:88
2. Bless DM, Hirano M, Feder RJ. Videostroboscopic evaluation of the larynx. Ear Nose Throat J 1987;66:289–296
3. Haben CM, Kost K, Papagiannis G. Lateral phase mucosal wave asymmetries in the clinical voice laboratory. J Voice 2003;17:3–11
4. Thompson DM, Maragos NE, Edwards BW. The study of vocal fold vibratory patterns in patients with unilateral vocal fold paralysis before and after type I thyroplasty with or without arytenoid adduction. Laryngoscope 1995;105(5 Pt 1):481–486
5. Jiang JJ, Yumoto E, Lin SJ, Kadota Y, Kurokawa H, Hanson DG. Quantitative measurement of mucosal wave by high-speed photography in excised larynges. Ann Otol Rhinol Laryngol 1998;107:98–103
6. Woo P. Quantification of videostrobolaryngoscopic findings: measurements of the normal glottal cycle. Laryngoscope 1996;106(3 Pt 2, Suppl 79)1–27
7. Colton RH, Woo P, Brewer DW, Griffin B, Casper J. Stroboscopic signs associated with benign lesions of the vocal folds. J Voice 1995;9:312–325
8. Dejonckere PH, Crevier L, Elbaz E, et al. Quantitative rating of video-laryngostroboscopy: a reliability study. Rev Laryngol Otol Rhinol (Bord) 1998;119:259–260
9. Doellinger M, Lohscheller J, McWhorter A, Kunduk M. Variability of normal vocal fold dynamics for different vocal loading in one healthy subject investigated by phonovibrograms. J Voice 2009;23:175–181
10. Shaw HS, Deliyski DD. Mucosal wave: a normophonic study across visualization techniques. J Voice 2008;22:23–33
11. Elias ME, Sataloff RT, Rosen DC, Heuer RJ, Spiegel JR. Normal strobovideolaryngoscopy: variability in healthy singers. J Voice 1997;11:104–107
12. Kendall KA. High-speed laryngeal imaging compared with videostroboscopy in healthy subjects. Arch Otolaryngol Head Neck Surg 2009;135:274–281
13. Fong R. High Speed Laryngoscopic Study of Vocal Fold Vibratory Patterns in Normal and Dysphonic Subjects [unpublished dissertation]. Hong Kong: University of Hong Kong; 1995
14. Pontes P, Yamasaki R, Behlau M. Morphological and functional aspects of the senile larynx. Folia Phoniatr Logop 2006;58:151–158
15. Biever DM, Bless DM. Vibratory characteristics of the vocal folds in young adult and geriatric women. J Voice 1989;3:120–131
16. Fujita R, Ferreira AE, Sarkovas C. Videokymography assessment of vocal fold vibration before and after hydration. Rev Bras Otorrinolaringol 2004;70:742–746

16

Normal Vocal Fold Vibratory Amplitude and Mucosal Wave

Heather Shaw Bonilha

◆ Amplitude of Vibration

Amplitude of vibration can be defined as the extent of lateral movement of each vocal fold during phonation. It is judged as the displacement of the medial edge of the vocal fold from its position at the closed phase of the vibratory cycle to its position at the maximal open point of the cycle. Amplitude of vibration is judged separately for the right and left vocal folds.

The term *glottal width* has been used to describe a phenomenon with characteristics that overlap those of amplitude of vibration. Glottal width, however, does not look at the right and left vocal folds individually. It is defined as the size of the largest opening between the vocal folds during the vibratory cycle and depends on the extent of lateral movement of *both* vocal folds.

In perfect vocal fold vibration, glottal width and amplitude of vibration should provide the same information. In that scenario, the glottal width should be twice the vocal fold amplitude of one vocal fold because the amplitude of vibration for each vocal fold is equal. However, if the vocal folds are not moving symmetrically (at the same time), these two parameters may be different. For example, if the right vocal fold reaches the maximal open point prior to the left vocal fold, yet both vocal folds move the same distance, the glottal width would be smaller than normal whereas the amplitude of vibration for each vocal fold would still be normal. In a clinical situation, amplitude of vibration combined with an assessment of vibratory symmetry is better at defining the extent of vocal fold excursion than either measurement alone, because it takes into account the difference in both timing and extent of movement between the two vocal folds. For many research experiments, the specifics of the extent of movement of the right versus the left vocal fold are not of interest, and the pertinent information is the glottal area available for outward flowing air. However, because the amplitude of vibration is more commonly used in a clinical setting and is related to vocal quality, we will confine our discussion to amplitude of vibration.

The amplitude of vibration depends on the pliability of the vocal fold tissues, the subglottal pressure, and the force of medial compression. These factors can either increase or decrease the amplitude of vibration. Increased tissue pliability increases the amplitude of vibration because pliable tissues are more easily displaced by the force of the outflowing air. Tissue that is less pliable requires stronger airflow to move it the same distance that more pliable tissue moves with a weaker airflow. In situations of stable tissue pliability, increased subglottal pressure results in larger amplitudes of vibration, whereas decreased subglottal pressure results in smaller amplitudes of vibration. Increased subglottal pressure can occur in two ways: (1) by increasing the volume of air exhaled and (2) by increasing the medial compression of the vocal folds. Medial compression of the vocal folds occurs secondary to increased laryngeal muscular contraction. During normal phonation, there is a relationship between subglottal pressure and medial compression. Increased medial compression results in an increased resistance to airflow through the glottis and requires that increased subglottal pressure be generated to overcome that resistance, thus initiating and maintaining vocal fold vibration. To produce a typical amplitude of vibration, the medial compression and subglottal pressure need to be carefully balanced. Increasing medial compression, without a substantial increase in breath support, generally produces smaller amplitudes of vibration. In addition to the physiology of producing a habitual voice, other typical voice changes such as a pitch increase or decrease or a change in loudness also are linked to changes in the amplitude of vibration (**Video Clips 5 and 6**).

High-pitched phonation is associated with smaller amplitudes of vibration, and conversely, low-pitched phonation is associated with larger amplitudes of vibration (**Video Clip 5**). Clinicians should expect smaller amplitudes of vibration in high-pitched phonation as a result of a decrease in the availability of pliable tissue. This phenomenon is mediated by the stretching action of the cricothyroid muscle on the vocal folds. The cricothyroid muscle pulls the vocal folds anteriorly and medially, making them taut, and, as this happens, the tension on the vocal fold tissues increases and lateral movement is impeded. In lower-pitched phonation, the thyroarytenoid muscle relaxes and decreases the tautness and tension on the vocal fold tissues. This allows the vocal fold tissues to easily move laterally in the outflowing air and results in amplitudes of vibration that are larger than those seen with habitual pitch and loudness.

This principle holds true for vocally normal speakers voluntarily increasing or decreasing the pitch of their phonation and should not be applied to persons with voice disorders that cause high- or low-pitched phonation. One can expect this relationship between pitch and amplitude of vibration to be altered with certain types of vocal fold pathology. A key example of the difference can be found in persons who have a low-pitched voice due to vocal fold edema. These individuals may demonstrate a smaller than normal amplitude of vibration, rather than the larger amplitude expected with low pitch, because there is expansion of the tissues with fluid. The fluid under the vocal fold mucosa makes it taught and thus prevents the mucosa from "blowing in the wind" of the exhalation.

The relationship between amplitude of vibration and loudness is not as clear as that of amplitude of vibration and pitch. Loud phonation is mediated by high subglottal pressure (**Video Clip 6**). As discussed above, there are two ways to increase subglottal pressure. These two ways have different effects on the amplitude of vibration. If one phonates loudly by increasing the volume of expired air, as we hope one would, then the amplitude of vibration increases relative to the increase in loudness of the individual's speech. However, if phonation is made louder by increasing medial compression of the vocal folds rather than by increasing expiratory volume, then the amplitude of vibration is restricted by the muscular contraction. Clinicians need to evaluate the method of increasing loudness in their patients prior to judging the normalcy of the change in the amplitude of vibration with changes in loudness. If it is difficult to determine the role of medial compression on the amplitude of phonation after eliciting a natural loud phonation, further instructions regarding the production of loud phonation can be given to the patient. Most patients can easily be instructed to take a larger than normal breath prior to a loud phonation, which should result in an appropriate sample of phonation upon which to judge increased amplitude.

Luckily, softer phonation is less complicated with regard to the amplitude of vibration. Softer phonation is associated with smaller amplitudes of vibration due to the smaller force of the exhaled air on the vocal fold tissues. One should remember that this discussion regarding amplitude of vibration holds true for vocally normal speakers voluntarily increasing or decreasing the volume of their phonation and cannot be applied to persons with voice disorders that cause loud or soft phonation. An example of the difference between vocally normal speakers and those with a voice disorder can be found in persons who have a soft voice due to vocal fold atrophy (**Video Clips 16 and 17**). These persons may have larger than normal amplitude of vibration as there is less tension on the vocal fold tissue to impede the mucosa from moving laterally by the force of the exhaled air (**Video Clip 24**). It is important to remember that what causes a loud or soft voice in persons without voice disorders may be very different than what causes it in persons with voice disorders.

Amplitude of vibration is judged during stroboscopy of phonation at a normal pitch and loudness. Amplitude of vibration should also be judged during high- and low-pitched phonation and during loud and soft phonation to ensure that the changes in amplitude, which we may expect from our knowledge of physiology, do occur. Given that amplitude of vibration is judged at the relatively short open phase of the vibratory cycle, we need stroboscopy, kymography, or high-speed videoendoscopy to be able to see this feature of vocal fold vibration.

Typical amplitude of vibration has been defined for stroboscopy by Bless et al. as one third the width of the visible portion of the vocal folds.[1] In the clinic, a five-point scale of severely decreased, decreased, typical, increased, and severely increased is commonly used (**Fig. 16.1**). Quantitative measures of vibration amplitude are available when using high-speed videoendoscopy and the resulting kymography. Because of the restrictions of stroboscopy, measurements of vibratory features using stroboscopy are not accurate or reliable.

◆ Mucosal Wave

The mucosal wave is the wave-like movement of the vocal fold cover (epithelium and superficial layer of the lamina propria) during vibration. An exact, agreed upon definition of

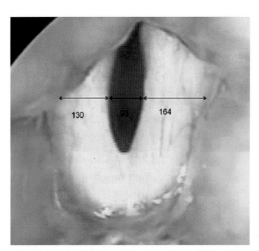

Glottal width (130) / Total width of vocal folds (296) = 0.31

A

Habitual

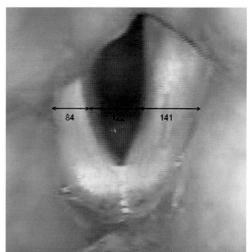

Glottal width (83) / Total width of vocal folds (308) = 0.54

Pressed

B

Fig. 16.1 (A) Amplitude of vibration measured from stroboscopic recordings of habitual pitch and loudness. Measures represent the number of pixels. The glottic opening is approximately one third of the total width of the superior surface of the vocal folds.

(B) Amplitude of vibration measured from stroboscopic recordings of pressed phonation. During pressed phonation, the amplitude of vibration is approximately one half of the total width of the superior surface of the vocal folds.

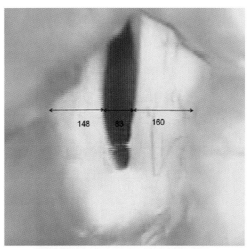

Glottal width (83) / Total width of vocal folds (308) = 0.27

Glottal width (119) / Total width of vocal folds (296) = 0.40

C

High

Low

D

Fig. 16.1 (*Continued*) **(C)** Amplitude of vibration measured from stroboscopic recordings of high-pitch phonation. As the vocal folds are stretched and vibrate at a higher frequency, the amplitude of vibration decreases and is approximately one quarter of the total width of the superior surface of the vocal folds. **(D)** Amplitude of vibration measured from stroboscopic recordings of low-pitch phonation. At lower frequency of vibration, the amplitude of vibration is relatively larger, approximately 40% of the total width of the superior surface of the vocal folds.

mucosal wave is difficult to find, as there seems to be some disagreement among experts in the field. That being said, the mucosal wave is generally agreed to encompass the differential between the lower and upper margins of the vocal folds as can be seen during the closing phase of vibration. There is disagreement about whether the movement of the mucosa on the superficial aspect of the vocal fold during the closed phase of vibration should be included in the term *mucosal wave*, although many clinicians do include an evaluation of this movement in their assessment of the mucosal wave. Furthermore, there is an upward swelling or vertical motion of the mucosa prior to the opening phase that some have included in their definition of mucosal wave (**Fig. 16.2**; **Video Clip 7**).

The pliability of the vocal fold mucosa has been considered one of the most important endoscopic indicators of vocal fold health and is directly reflected by the characteristics of the mucosal wave. Furthermore, the mucosal wave depends on the ability of the superficial vocal fold tissues to vibrate independently

from the deeper structures and requires that the relationship of the vocal fold histologic layers be in balance. (See Chapter 3 for a more in-depth discussion of vocal fold histology.) The mucosal wave is therefore not just an indicator of the health of the superficial tissue. It also provides information regarding the underlying layers of the lamina propria and the thyroarytenoid muscle.

The mucosal wave can be impacted by not only the vocal fold anatomy but also by changes in the loudness and pitch of phonation. High-pitched phonation is associated with a smaller mucosal wave, and conversely, low-pitched phonation is associated with a larger mucosal wave. Clinicians should expect the mucosal wave to decrease when gliding from habitual to high-pitched phonation (**Video Clip 5**). This occurs with lengthening of the vocal folds due to contraction of the cricothyroid muscle. The superficial vocal fold tissues are placed on stretch at higher frequencies of vibration leading to a decrease in the amount of available movable tissue. The cricothyroid muscle acts like a person pulling

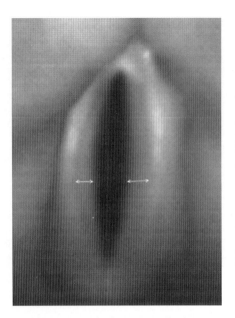

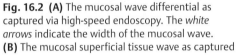

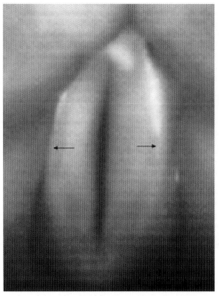

A B

Fig. 16.2 (A) The mucosal wave differential as captured via high-speed endoscopy. The *white arrows* indicate the width of the mucosal wave. **(B)** The mucosal superficial tissue wave as captured via high-speed endoscopy. The *black arrows* indicate the position of the wave as it travels over the superficial surface of the vocal fold.

on two ends of a rubber band: as the rubber band stretches, the rubber gets thinner. The reduction in mass of the vibratory portion of the vocal folds, which causes them to vibrate faster, also reduces the tissue available for production of the mucosal wave. The opposite is true for lower-pitch phonation. When a person purposefully phonates in a lower pitch, he or she relaxes the thyroarytenoid muscles and allows for an increase in pliable mucosa that can "blow in the wind" of exhalation.

One thing to remember is that the above discussion regarding mucosal wave holds true for vocally normal speakers voluntarily increasing or decreasing the pitch of their phonation and should not be applied to persons with voice disorders that cause high- or low-pitched phonation. The same example used to illustrate this point for the amplitude of vibration can be applied to illustrate this point for mucosal wave. Persons who have a low-pitched voice due to vocal fold edema may have smaller than normal mucosal waves because there is fluid in the lamina propria tenting the mucosa of the vocal fold and preventing the mucosa from "blowing in the wind" of the exhalation. It is important to remember that what causes a high- or low-pitched voice in persons without voice disorders may be very different than what causes a low-pitched voice in persons with a voice disorder.

Louder phonation is associated with a larger mucosal wave, and conversely, softer phonation is associated with a smaller mucosal wave (**Video Clip 6**). Clinicians should expect an increased mucosal wave with louder phonation as a result of the build-up of greater subglottal pressure. The larger subglottal pressure is required to initiate and sustain vocal fold vibration in the presence of increased medial compression of the vocal folds mediated by the lateral cricoarytenoid, thyroarytenoid, and the interarytenoid muscles. Softer phonation is associated with less medial compression and less subglottal pressure. Thus, softer phonation does not have the physical properties that would create a larger mucosal wave.

Mucosal wave is judged with stroboscopy during phonation with a normal pitch and loudness. Mucosal wave should also be judged during high- and low-pitched phonation and during loud and soft phonation to ensure that the changes in mucosal wave, which we may expect from our knowledge of physiology, do occur. Given that the mucosal wave is generally defined as the differential between the lower and upper margins of the vocal folds, as can be seen during the closing phase of vibration, we need stroboscopy, kymography, or high-speed videoendoscopy to be able to see the mucosal wave.

A typical mucosal wave has been defined for stroboscopy by Bless et al. as a differential that is as wide as one-half of one of the vocal folds.[1] In the clinic, a five-point scale of severely decreased, decreased, typical, increased, and severely increased is commonly used. There are some clinics and researchers that use a six-point scale of 0 = typical mucosal wave to 5 = absent mucosal wave. Given the valuable information available from larger than typical mucosal waves, there may be a benefit to evaluating mucosal wave as being typical, larger than normal, or smaller than normal. Currently, there are no clinically viable quantitative measures of mucosal wave.

◆ Conclusion

Amplitude of vibration and mucosal wave tend to vary in a similar pattern as they are mediated by similar factors such as medial compression, subglottal air pressure, and tissue pliability. During an endoscopic examination, it is helpful to make sure that there is a rationale for similarities and differences in

how the amplitude of vibration and mucosal wave are varying. Because amplitude of vibration and mucosal wave can vary with pitch and loudness, it is quite important to ensure that the phonation being evaluated under endoscopy is of habitual pitch and loudness. One particular consideration is the tendency for some persons to increase pitch and loudness when phonating with a rigid endoscope in their oral cavity. Additional samples of purposefully produced high- and low-pitched phonation and loud and soft phonation are helpful in evaluating and understanding the phenomena associated with amplitude of vibration and mucosal wave.

Reference

1. Bless DM, Hirano M, Feder RJ. Videostroboscopic evaluation of the larynx. Ear Nose Throat J 1987;66: 289–296

Additional Suggested Reading

Hirano M, Bless DM. Videostroboscopic Examination of the Larynx. San Diego, CA: Singular; 1993

Poburka BJ. A new stroboscopy rating form. J Voice 1999;13:403–413

Shaw H, Deliyski D. Comparison of glottal configuration and glottal width recorded with stroboscopy and high-speed videoendoscopy in normophonic speakers. Presented at: 36th Symposium of The Voice Foundation: Care of the Professional Voice; June 2007; Philadelphia, PA

Shaw HS, Deliyski DD. Mucosal wave: a normophonic study across visualization techniques. J Voice 2008; 22:23–33

IV

Vibratory Abnormalities

17

Persistent Glottic Opening

Glendon M. Gardner

Glottic closure is the ability of the vocal folds to make contact along their medial edges. Videostroboscopy provides an effective tool for measurement of closure. In general, during the closed phase of the glottic cycle, the vocal folds should make complete contact along their length. In females, there is often a small gap posteriorly, which is considered normal (**Fig. 17.1**).

With normal closure and normally vibrating vocal folds, air is released through the glottis in discrete puffs. This periodic pulsatile airflow is the glottic sound source.[1,2] Incomplete vocal fold closure during voicing allows for

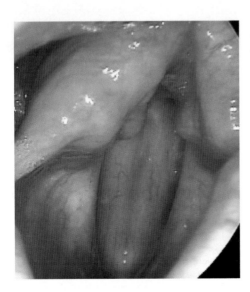
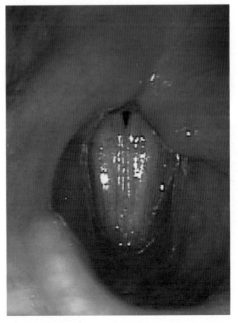

A
B

Fig. 17.1 **(A)** Normal complete glottic closure in a male. **(B)** Small normal posterior gap in a female.

leakage of air through the glottis in an uncontrolled manner. Often this escaping air creates noise that is perceived by the listener as breathiness or a hiss. Due to air escape, less air is available for voice production, which may cause the voice to be weaker than normal. Thus, in cases of glottic inefficiency, more air is required to create the same amount of sound. Also, more effort is usually employed by the speaker in an attempt to squeeze the vocal folds together and achieve complete closure. These last two factors may lead to vocal fatigue, a very common complaint in patients who suffer from incomplete glottic closure.

In the normal larynx, the vocal folds are straight, taut, and fully mobile. These characteristics allow the vocal folds to come together fully during phonation. Pathology that interferes with any of these characteristics can affect the closure, including abnormalities of the vocal fold margin (medial tissues available for vibration) and abnormalities of the laryngeal musculature (medial compressive forces). In some cases of unilateral pathology, compensation by one vocal fold for abnormalities of the other can yield normal closure.

The role of videostroboscopy in the assessment of closure cannot be overestimated. For years we had judged closure with the naked eye, viewing vocal folds vibrating over 100 cycles per second. At that speed, the edges of the vocal folds appear fuzzy and blurred to the eye, and whereas we can know if the vocal processes (where vibration does not occur) are in contact, we cannot know whether the membranous folds are truly making contact (**Fig. 17.2**). With stroboscopy, the apparent motion of the vocal folds is slowed down, and the rate of vibratory motion and the amount of time the vocal folds are in contact can be

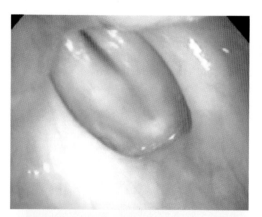

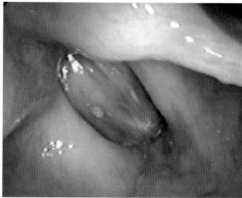

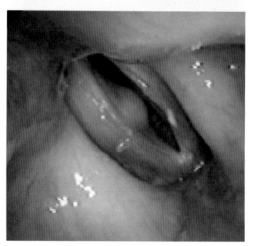

Fig. 17.2 **(A)** Right vocal fold cyst viewed with halogen light and without stroboscopy during phonation. Although we would expect closure to be incomplete, the image does not clearly demonstrate the status of the closure. **(B)** Right vocal fold cyst viewed with xenon light and with stroboscopy. Closure is noted to be complete during the closed phase of vibration. **(C)** Right vocal fold cyst viewed with stroboscopy. The cyst itself is much better defined during the open phase of vibration.

A

B

C

assessed. The technique of laryngeal stroboscopy is covered elsewhere in this book. Be aware that the pitch at which the subject is phonating can affect glottic closure. Remember to test patients at different pitches.

The various configurations of a glottal gap (in incomplete closure) have been described by Bless et al.[3] Note that some authors have described the pattern of closure rather than the shape of the gap, which may reverse the meaning of the descriptors.[4] In this chapter, the descriptor relates to the shape or location of the gap rather than which part of the vocal folds are in contact.

Closure can be affected by three basic problems:

1. An inability to bring the musculomembranous vocal folds together at any site along their length because of a mobility problem or bowing of one or both vocal folds (**Fig. 17.3**; **Video Clips 16, 17, 24, and 25**).

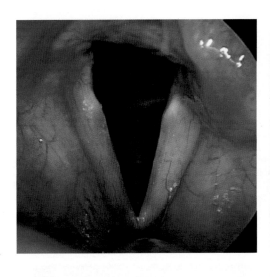

A

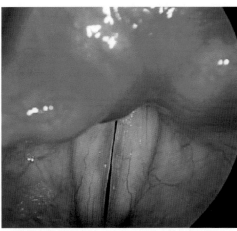

B

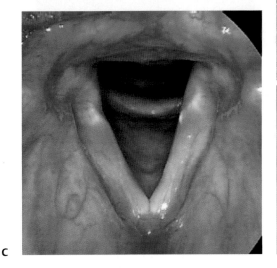

C

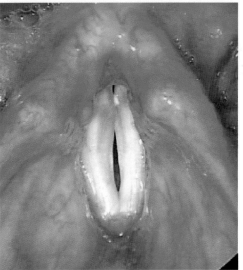

D

Fig. 17.3 **(A)** Left vocal fold paralysis. View of larynx with vocal folds abducted. **(B)** Left vocal fold paralysis with vocal folds adducted. Closure is incomplete along the entire length of the vocal fold, although the posterior glottis is difficult to see during phonation. **(C)** Bilateral vocal fold bowing viewed with vocal folds abducted. **(D)** Bilateral vocal fold bowing viewed with vocal folds adducted. Note that the vocal processes make contact, but the musculomembranous vocal folds cannot.

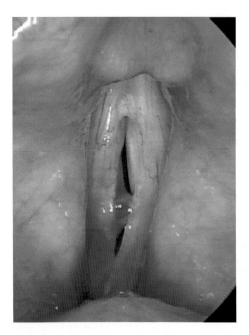

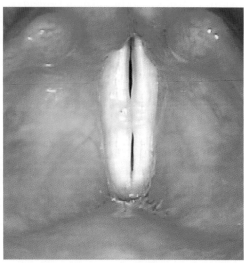

A

B

Fig. 17.4 (A) Right vocal fold polyp prevents complete closure. The glottic gap is shaped as half an hourglass.
(B) Vocal fold nodules cause incomplete closure in an hourglass configuration.

2. One or more mass lesions that make premature contact and prevent the remainder of the musculomembranous folds from making contact (**Fig. 17.4**; **Video Clips 18, 19, and 26**).

3. A defect in one or both vocal folds. The vocal folds make complete contact except at the site of the defect(s) (**Fig. 17.5**).

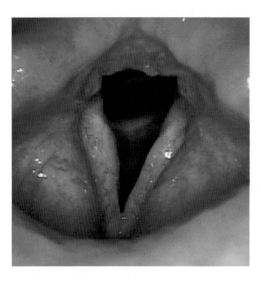

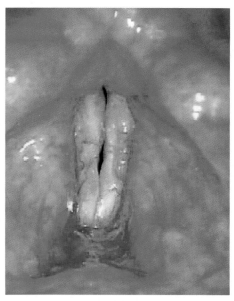

A

B

Fig. 17.5 (A) Scarred vocal folds during abduction.
(B) Scarred vocal folds during adduction with defect causing incomplete closure at site of defect. Edema of

remainder of vocal folds contributes to inability to close at defect site.

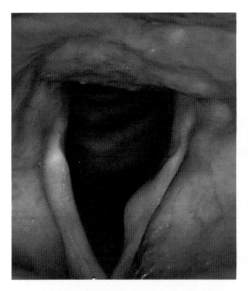

A

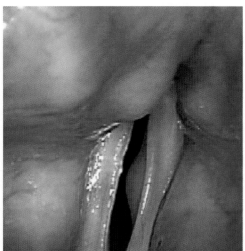

B

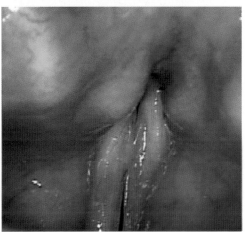

C

Fig. 17.6 (A) Left vocal fold cyst and bilateral vocal fold bowing viewed with vocal folds in abduction. **(B)** Left vocal fold cyst and bilateral vocal fold bowing viewed with vocal folds in adduction during the open phase of vibration. **(C)** Left vocal fold cyst and bilateral vocal fold bowing viewed with vocal folds in adduction during the closed phase of vibration. Closure is incomplete because of the bowing, not the cyst. Removal of the cyst would not improve closure.

The information obtained with videostroboscopy helps us determine which type of lesion is present and which procedure or treatment is necessary to improve closure. With mass lesions, excision of the lesion will usually lead to improved closure. However, stroboscopy will sometimes reveal that closure would be incomplete even in the absence of the lesion (**Fig. 17.6**). In these cases, a significant improvement in voice may not result from excision, and the patient can be counseled accordingly, or the lesion may be left alone.

◆ Mobility Problems

Vocal Fold Paralysis

Vocal fold immobility is due to either paralysis of the musculature that moves the vocal fold or fixation of the cricoarytenoid joint. An immobile vocal fold may rest in the midline or in a paramedian or even lateral position. If the vocal fold is not in the midline, incomplete closure is likely to result (**Fig. 17.3A, B**). In the case of a paralyzed vocal fold, as opposed to a fixed cricoarytenoid joint, the muscle is often

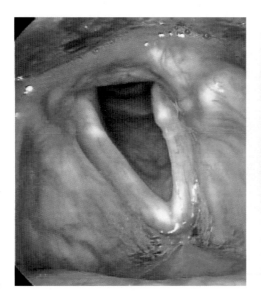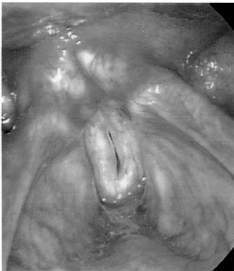

A

B

Fig. 17.7 **(A)** Left vocal fold paralysis viewed with vocal folds in abduction. **(B)** Left vocal fold paralysis with flaccidity seen with vocal folds in adduction.

flaccid and the vocal fold is bowed (**Fig. 17.7**). The bowed configuration of the paralyzed vocal fold further contributes to the open glottic configuration (**Video Clip 27**).

In some cases of unilateral vocal fold immobility, the mobile contralateral vocal fold may be able to cross the midline to make contact with the immobile vocal fold and achieve complete closure. (However, the open phase may still predominate during the vibratory cycle in modal phonation [**Video Clip 28**]. In that case, the patient may complain of a soft, breathy voice, despite complete closure.) Similarly, complete closure may occur in cases of vocal fold paralysis where a certain degree of reinnervation has occurred. Unfortunately, this does not always result in a mobile vocal fold, as synkinesis often results. This means that both abductor and adductor muscles contract at the same time so that the vocal fold remains immobile but has tone. The synkinetic vocal fold is an immobile, straight vocal fold that may rest in the midline, making it easy for the mobile vocal fold to make full contact and achieving complete closure.

When vocal fold closure is incomplete due to vocal fold paralysis, there is usually a gap from the anterior commissure to the vocal process of the arytenoid cartilage or even to

the posterior aspect of the glottis (**Fig. 17.8**). With an isolated recurrent laryngeal nerve lesion (superior laryngeal nerve and cricothyroid muscle functioning), a subject may be able to attain better closure at high pitch when the cricothyroid muscle is active. Hence, some patients with a paralyzed vocal fold will speak at an unusually high pitch to compensate for the weak voice at normal pitch (**Video Clip 25**).

The effect on the mucosal wave of an immobile vocal fold depends on the glottal gap. If closure is normal and there is good vocal fold tone, the mucosal wave may be normal, and vibration may be symmetric with the normal fold. With a large gap, there may be no observable wave or the voice may be so aperiodic that stroboscopy is unable to reliably demonstrate the wave (**Video Clips 29 and 30**). With a small gap, the wave of the immobile fold is likely to lag behind that of the normal fold (**Video Clip 28**).[5]

In cases of immobility, the initial workup is aimed at determining the cause of the mobility problem. A computed tomography (CT) scan from the skull base to below the arch of the aorta will detect most neoplasms involving the vagus or recurrent laryngeal nerves. Laryngeal electromyography (EMG) with testing of the

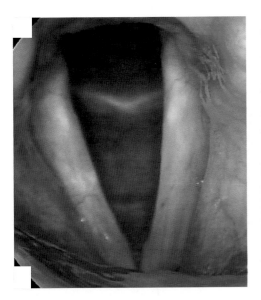 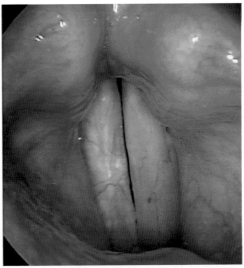

A   B

Fig. 17.8 **(A)** Right vocal fold paralysis seen with vocal folds abducted. **(B)** Right vocal fold paralysis with straight vocal fold and better closure on adduction.

intrinsic laryngeal muscles (usually thyroarytenoid and cricothyroid muscles) can help locate the site of the lesion (recurrent laryngeal and/or superior laryngeal nerve or vagus nerve) and may provide information regarding the prognosis for recovery. If the EMG is normal, then the vocal fold is mechanically fixed. This can be confirmed with direct microlaryngoscopy and palpation of the arytenoid cartilage.[6–8] Careful examination of the subglottis is critical to ruling out causes of fixation, such as the rare chondroid tumor of the cricoid cartilage (which would also been seen on the CT scan done earlier).

There are also many other, less common neurologic disorders that will result in impaired vocal motion and glottic closure. These must be considered when the etiology is not due to some other obvious cause.[9]

If accommodation does not occur and the vocal fold does not recover normal motion, closure will remain incomplete, and the voice will remain abnormal. There are surgical options to improve the voice. Closure can be improved by bulking up the immobile vocal fold with injection laryngoplasty, medialization of the vocal fold with framework surgery, with or without arytenoid adduction or arytenoidopexy, or reinnervation of the paralyzed vocal fold (**Fig. 17.9**). Restoration of normal closure may yield normal vibration and mucosal wave propagation in the paralyzed vocal fold despite lack of reinnervation (**Video Clip 31**).[10,11]

Vocal Fold Bowing and Vocal Fold Paresis

As we age, muscles and ligaments may become less taut. In the vocal fold, this results in bowing. The vocal folds are still mobile but cannot come completely together. Because there is no paralysis, the arytenoid cartilages are still fully mobile, and the vocal processes will make contact but the musculomembranous folds do not, resulting in a lentiform-shaped persistent glottic opening (**Fig. 17.3C, D; Video Clips 16, 17, and 24**). Atrophy of the vocalis muscle as a result of a paresis will also result in lack of bulk and bowing of the vocal fold and incomplete closure. With the vocal fold mobile, the workup is usually not as aggressive, as a neoplastic etiology is less likely. EMG can confirm a paresis. Voice therapy may result in improved closure and voice. As with the immobile vocal fold, surgery can be done to improve closure in cases of bowing or paresis. With a bowed but otherwise mobile vocal fold, the musculomembranous vocal fold should be medialized, but movement of the

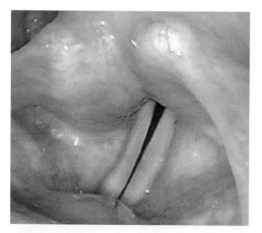

A

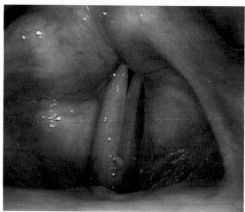

B

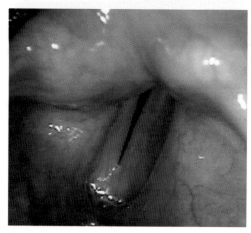

C

Fig. 17.9 **(A)** Closure prior to medialization of paralyzed left vocal fold. **(B)** Closure after medialization of paralyzed left vocal fold. **(C)** A mucosal wave can be seen on the paralyzed left vocal fold after medialization.

arytenoid should not be impaired. The size of the glottic gap can be documented with videostroboscopy, and this information can be used to judge the amount of medialization necessary.

◆ Mass Lesions That Prevent Closure

Most benign vocal fold masses occur on the musculomembranous vocal folds. With phonation, these masses often make initial contact and prevent the remainder of the vocal folds from making contact, preventing complete closure. The location, size, shape, and consistency of the various lesions will determine how closure is affected.

Nodules, cysts, pseudocysts, and polyps are all masses that may develop on the musculomembranous vocal folds. They are sometimes difficult to differentiate.[12,13] Classic vocal fold nodules are symmetric masses in the midportion of the musculomembranous vocal folds, and their premature contact results in a glottic opening in the shape of an hourglass (**Fig. 17.4B**; **Video Clip 18**). Often, other benign lesions such as cysts and pseudocysts will be associated with a contralateral reactive nodule that may be close to the same size as the original lesion. Again, an hourglass-shaped glottic opening will result (**Fig. 17.10**). If there is only a unilateral lesion, such as a polyp or cyst, glottic closure will be shaped as half an hourglass (**Fig. 17.4A**; **Video Clip 26**). Higher pitch will stretch the vocal folds and accentuate the effect of a lesion of the vocal fold. At lower pitch, a lesion may not even be visible and closure may be normal, whereas at high pitch the lesion becomes apparent and

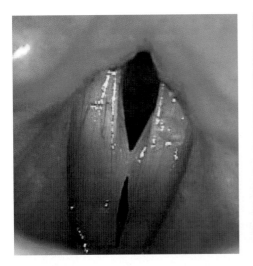

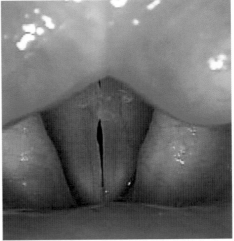

A   B

Fig. 17.10 (A) Left vocal fold polyp or pseudocyst and reactive swelling of the right vocal fold. Vocal fold tissue makes early contact at this site prior to reaching maximal closure. **(B)** Left vocal fold polyp or pseudocyst and reactive swelling of the right vocal fold. Closure is incomplete during the closed phase of vibration in an hourglass configuration.

closure is incomplete. This point stresses the importance of testing all patients along their full dynamic range.

Granulomas are benign inflammatory masses that almost always occur on the vocal process of the arytenoid cartilage. When they are small, they do not affect closure at all, and the contralateral vocal process fits into a notch in the granuloma (**Fig. 17.11**). Even large granulomas often do not affect closure (**Fig. 17.12**).

◆ Defects in the Vocal Fold

A fortunately less common cause of incomplete closure is a defect of the musculomembranous vocal fold. This is usually a result of surgical excision of a mass from the vocal fold. Videostroboscopy demonstrates the exact configuration of closure and the location of the defect (**Fig. 17.5**). It also shows whether

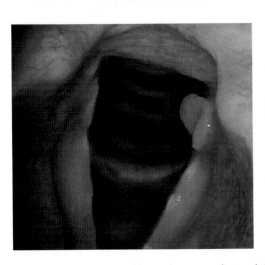

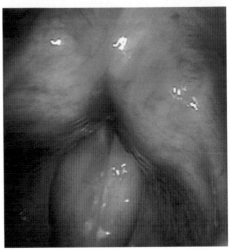

A   B

Fig. 17.11 (A) Left vocal fold granuloma seen during abduction of vocal folds. **(B)** During adduction, left vocal fold granuloma does not affect closure.

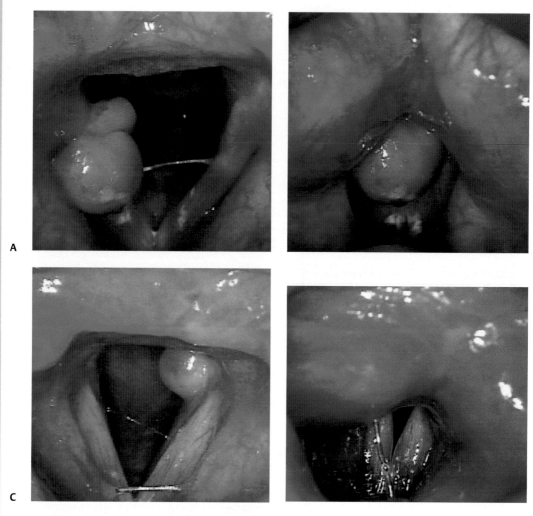

Fig. 17.12 **(A)** Large, right-sided granuloma seen with vocal folds abducted. **(B)** The same large, right-sided granuloma does not affect closure, which is complete. **(C)** Large, left-sided granuloma in another patient seen during vocal fold abduction. **(D)** The left-sided granuloma in this patient seems to prevent closure posteriorly.

the tissue at the site of the defect vibrates normally or not. This is very important, as surgery to improve closure at the defect may not achieve a normal voice if the tissue was not vibrating properly preoperatively. Surgical procedures, such as fat graft implantation into the defect, have been designed both to improve closure and hopefully restore vibration to the vocal fold edge. If the tissue at the site of the defect vibrates normally (mucosal wave is present) and closure is incomplete, surgery should be focused on improving closure without disrupting the architecture of the edge of

the vocal fold, which might yield a nonvibrating segment.

Sulcus Vocalis

Sulcus vocalis is a condition in which there is a longitudinal scar on the medial edge of the vocal fold with adherence of the mucosa to the underlying vocal ligament (**Fig. 17.13**).[14] This is thought to be due to chronic voice abuse/overuse or perhaps to the rupture of an intracordal cyst. These patients present with rough, breathy

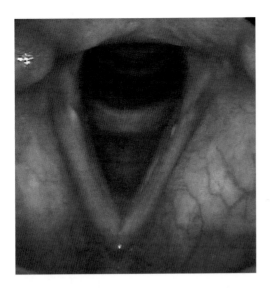
A

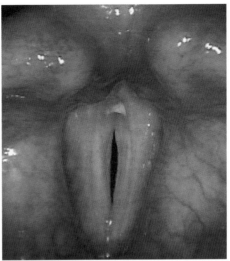
B

Fig. 17.13 (A) Bilateral sulcus vocalis and vocal fold bowing seen with the vocal folds abducted. **(B)** Bilateral sulcus vocalis and vocal fold bowing with incomplete closure during adduction.

voices and voice fatigue. The initial impression on physical examination is that the vocal folds are bowed, and closure is usually incomplete. Videostroboscopy reveals a groove on the medial edge of the vocal fold that is usually not detected without stroboscopy. Also, the mucosal wave is absent. The surgical approach to these patients is somewhat controversial.

Improving closure with framework surgery or injection is often the first step. A stronger voice with less fatigue usually results, but it is still not a normal voice (**Fig. 17.14**). Addressing the sulcus itself is, in this author's opinion, a technically much more challenging procedure than improving closure and carries higher risk.

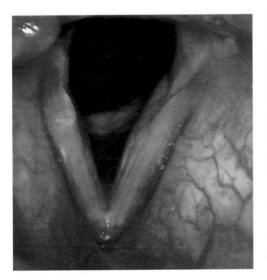
A

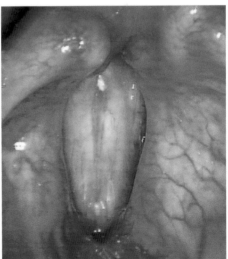
B

Fig. 17.14 (A) Bilateral sulcus vocalis and vocal fold bowing seen with the vocal folds abducted after bilateral medialization. **(B)** Bilateral sulcus vocalis and vocal fold bowing. There is improved closure and voice after medialization of both vocal folds.

◆ Conclusion

The differential diagnosis of a persistent glottic gap during phonation includes lesions that affect the medial tissues of the vocal fold margin and lesions that affect the compressive abilities of the vocal folds. Lesions of the medial tissues of the vocal fold include benign vocal fold lesions due to trauma and scarring of the vocal folds from any cause. These lesions prevent complete closure of the glottis during voicing by the change they impart to the shape of the vocal fold margin. Lesions that affect the compressive abilities of the vocal folds include vocal fold paralysis and paresis and prevent closure by their effect on the position of the vocal fold during phonation.

References

1. Hirano M. Clinical Examination of the Voice. New York, NY: Springer-Verlag; 1981
2. Colton RH. Physiology of phonation. In: Benninger MS, Jacobson B, Johnson A, eds. Vocal Arts Medicine: The Care and Prevention of Professional Voice Disorders. New York, NY: Thieme Medical Publishers; 1993:30–60
3. Bless DM, Hirano M, Feder RJ. Videostroboscopic evaluation of the larynx. Ear Nose Throat J 1987;66:289–296
4. Gelfer MP, Bultemeyer DK. Evaluation of vocal fold vibratory patterns in normal voices. J Voice 1990;4:335–345
5. Sercarz JA, Berke GS, Ming Y, Gerratt BR, Natividad M. Videostroboscopy of human vocal fold paralysis. Ann Otol Rhinol Laryngol 1992;101:567–577
6. Altman JS, Benninger MS. The evaluation of unilateral vocal fold immobility: is chest X-ray enough? J Voice 1997;11:364–367
7. Benninger MS, Crumley RL, Ford CN, et al. Evaluation and treatment of the unilateral paralyzed vocal fold. Otolaryngol Head Neck Surg 1994;111:497–508
8. Terris DJ, Arnstein DP, Nguyen HH. Contemporary evaluation of unilateral vocal cord paralysis. Otolaryngol Head Neck Surg 1992;107:84–90
9. Benninger MS, Gardner GM, Schwimmer C. Laryngeal neurophysiology. In: Rubin J, Sataloff R, Korovin G, eds. Diagnosis and Treatment of Voice Disorders, 2nd edition. Clifton Park, NY: Thomson Delmar Learning; 2003:107–113
10. Gardner GM, Parnes S. Status of the mucosal wave post Teflon vocal cord injection vs. thyroplasty. J Voice 1991;5:64–73
11. Kokesh J, Flint PW, Robinson LR, Cummings CW. Correlation between stroboscopy and electromyography in laryngeal paralysis. Ann Otol Rhinol Laryngol 1993;102:852–857
12. Woo P, Colton R, Casper J, Brewer D. Diagnostic value of stroboscopic examination in hoarse patients. J Voice 1991;5:231–238
13. Sataloff RT, Spiegel JR, Hawkshaw MJ. Strobovideolaryngoscopy: results and clinical value. Ann Otol Rhinol Laryngol 1991;100(9 Pt 1):725–727
14. Ford CN, Inagi K, Khidr A, Bless DM, Gilchrist KW. Sulcus vocalis: a rational analytical approach to diagnosis and management. Ann Otol Rhinol Laryngol 1996;105:189–200

18

Decreased Vibratory Amplitude

C. Blake Simpson

The amplitude of vocal fold vibration is defined as the degree of horizontal displacement of the vocal folds during vibratory activity as viewed on videostroboscopy. During normal phonation, the vocal folds remain closed, while subglottal pressure builds with continued exhalation, until subglottal pressure increases enough to blow them apart. As air flows through the glottis, medial to lateral excursion of the vocal folds occurs. The amplitude of vibration is generally measured as the degree of displacement from the midline to the maximum lateral point of excursion in the vibratory cycle. Although there is no "normal" value for amplitude, it is generally accepted that an excursion of roughly one third of the width of the vocal fold should occur in normal subjects at a habitual pitch and loudness (**Video Clip 3**). The amplitude of vibration can vary due to physiologic factors (pitch, intensity) and pathologic factors (vocal fold lesions/stiffness, paresis, and vocal fold tension) (**Video Clips 5 and 6**). Both of these factors will be addressed in this section (see also Chapter 16).

Decreased vibratory amplitude is one of the most common findings associated with vocal fold pathology. When the amplitude of vocal fold vibration is asymmetric (specifically, a reduction in amplitude on one vocal fold compared with that of the "normal" side), this is almost always associated with vocal fold pathology. Certain general factors, however, have an influence on vibratory amplitude of the vocal folds, and they can be broken down into physiologic and pathologic factors (**Table 18.1**).

◆ Physiologic Factors Associated with Reduced Vibratory Amplitude

Normal Reductions in Vibratory Amplitude

When assessing vibratory amplitude, it is helpful to first observe for symmetry. Symmetrically reduced vibratory amplitude can, and often is, due to normal variations in pitch and intensity of phonation. For example, when a singer is demonstrating his or her full vocal range during a typical videostroboscopic exam, one should expect the amplitude of vibration to decrease an equal amount in both vocal folds as the patient sings progressively higher notes on the scale (**Video Clips 4 and 5**). This is due to a tightening or stiffening of the vocal fold as pitch is increased, resulting in reduced excursion of the vocal fold from the midline during phonation. One must always be cognizant of the pitch of the patient's voice when assessing amplitude of vibration and take this into account.

Table 18.1 Physiologic and Pathologic Factors That Result in Reduced Vibratory Amplitude

Physiologic factors that result in reduced vibratory amplitude:

◆ Decreased subglottal pressure (usually due to reduced intensity/volume of vocalization)

◆ Increased fundamental frequency/pitch

Pathologic factors that result in reduced vibratory amplitude:

◆ Shortening of the vibratory portion of the membranous vocal fold

◆ Stiffness of the vocal folds

◆ Increased mass of the vocal folds

◆ Increased tension of the vocal folds

◆ Incomplete vocal fold closure

In the same way, as the patient phonates in a softer voice (lower intensity), the amplitude should be reduced in a symmetric fashion. Reduced volume/intensity is associated with a reduction in the subglottal pressure generated during phonation. As subglottal pressure decreases, the amplitude of vibration is reduced. In essence, the reduction in airflow causes a decrease in the displacement of the vocal folds in a medial to lateral direction (**Video Clip 6**).

If one takes into account both of the two factors discussed above (intensity and fundamental frequency), then one should expect that the maximum amplitude of vibration would be expected to occur with loud, low-pitched phonation (low fundamental frequency at a high intensity). This is an excellent method to observe the maximum pliability of the vocal folds. Conversely, a patient using a soft, high-pitched voice (low intensity at a high frequency) is going to demonstrate a maximum reduction in vibratory amplitude. This is especially true if there is incomplete closure as well—as seen in falsetto voice (**Video Clip 4**).

The wide variation in vibratory amplitude observed in the *same patient* over the full spectrum of his or her phonatory range and intensity sometimes makes absolute determinations of "normal" vibratory amplitude problematic. As stated before, if there appears to be no pathology of the vocal folds present and the amplitude "reduction" appears symmetric, it is probably just due to increased pitch and/or reduced intensity of the patient's phonation. The exceptions to this rule are the disorders of muscle tension, such as adductor spasmodic dysphonia and muscle tension dysphonia (discussed later).

◆ Pathologic Factors That Result in Reduced Vibratory Amplitude

Shortening of the Vibratory Portion of the Membranous Vocal Folds

This is not commonly seen clinically and is usually related to a congenital or traumatic anterior glottic web. The formation of an anterior web between the vocal folds creates a nonvibratory segment, as vocal fold approximation cannot occur in this region. This results in a shortened segment of the remaining membranous vocal fold. This shortened segment is incapable of achieving the extent of excursion during vibration that a longer, normal vocal fold can achieve. As a result of this, the amplitude of vibration is dampened.

Stiffness of the Vocal Folds

This condition is one of the most common reasons for a reduction in vibratory amplitude. The stiffness can be due to several pathologic factors including scarring, infiltration by carcinoma, and submucosal benign lesions that are tightly bound to the epithelium and/or vocal ligament such as cysts or fibrous bands. It is generally easy to differentiate between these different entities (**Video Clips 32 to 35**).

One of the most concerning findings on a videostroboscopy examination is a vocal fold with an epithelial lesion (leukoplakia/erythroplakia/papillomatous changes) that demonstrates severely reduced or absent amplitude/mucosal wave. The surface changes of the epithelium are generally obvious on routine laryngoscopy. In these cases, the findings on videostroboscopy are potentially important clinically. The reduction in amplitude is suggestive of carcinomatous infiltration into the lamina propria, which creates a stiff, nonvibratory vocal fold. Another possible reason for the reduction of amplitude in these cases involves the increase in mass due to the epithelial lesion (see later), therefore both potential factors should be kept in mind when examining these patients (**Video Clip 35**).

A scarred vocal fold can frequently appear "normal" on routine laryngoscopy because of the lack of epithelial changes. A scarred vocal fold results in stiffness because of deposition of fibrous tissue in the superficial lamina propria. The elimination of this potential space and the resulting loss of pliability leads to a reduction or loss of vibratory amplitude on stroboscopy. Loss of vibratory activity in the context of a suggestive history (laryngeal biopsy, aggressive resection of a benign lesion, external beam radiation) is critical in making the clinical diagnosis of scar (**Video Clips 32 and 33**).

Certain submucosal lesions (cyst and fibrous band) can be subtle on routine laryngoscopy, in contrast with more common and obvious benign vocal fold pathology (polyps, nodules). With vocal fold cysts, the lesion is either on the infraglottic (mucous retention) or superior surface (epidermal inclusion) of the vocal fold, and its outline may be indistinct. Vocal fold cysts are located in the superficial lamina propria and are frequently adherent to the epithelium and/or vocal ligament, resulting in stiffness and a substantial reduction in vibratory amplitude and mucosal wave (**Video Clips 26 and 34**). Fibrous bands are another form of vocal fold pathology, and these lesions represent an accumulation of fibrous tissue within the superficial lamina propria. This material is typically amorphous in nature and often has thin extensions anteriorly and posteriorly within the vocal fold giving it a fusiform shape. The deposition of fibrous tissue is similar to scar formation, but the tissue is organized into a lesion that is discrete from the surrounding tissue. Because this tissue behaves much like scar in terms of vibratory activity, there is a reduction or (more typically) a complete absence of vibratory amplitude.

Increased Mass of the Vocal Folds

Increased mass of the vocal folds is typically related to more extensive vocal fold pathology of either the epithelium or of the superficial lamina propria. Typical examples are large mass lesions such as papilloma, large hyperkeratotic plaques, and polyps. The lesion acts as a resistive force in the displacement of the vocal folds, and this effect is magnified when the lesion also causes incomplete closure of the vocal folds (which is quite common) as is discussed later. Another example of a lesion that may lead to reduced or absent vibratory amplitude is Reinke's edema (also referred to as polypoid corditis). Interestingly, the mucosal wave in these lesions is often increased because of the increased pliability of the polypoid/myxoid component of the superficial lamina propria. When the polypoid degeneration results in significant increase in mass, this may reduce the amplitude of vibration (**Video Clip 36**). In a similar fashion, acute edema of the vocal folds due to infection or inflammation will lead to a reduction of vibratory amplitude (**Video Clip 37**).

Increased Tension of the Vocal Folds

Unlike all of the previously mentioned causes of reduced vibratory amplitude, the category of increased vocal fold tension consists principally of muscle tension disorders and not an actual pathophysiologic derangement of the vocal fold itself. Examples include adductor spasmodic dysphonia and muscle tension dysphonia. Adductor spasmodic dysphonia (adductor SD) is a neurologic disorder (dystonia) that results in excessive and forceful closure of the vocal folds during most phonatory tasks. The effect is most marked on words beginning with vowels and nasal consonants. Muscle tension dysphonia (MTD) is a functional disorder that presents with a consistently strained voice across phonatory tasks (**Video Clip 20**). With videostroboscopic studies, the amplitude of vibration with adductor SD and MTD is markedly diminished or completely absent. It is often difficult to assess vibratory parameters in many of these cases due to the lack of vocal fold visualization during phonation secondary to supraglottic compression. The excessive lateral compressive forces prevent displacement of the vocal fold and thus dampen or completely extinguish vibratory amplitude. During singing, patients with adductor SD may have normal vibratory amplitude, as the spasmodic activity can be absent during activities outside of the realm of connected speech. In addition, patients with MTD may have a normalization of vibratory amplitude if the muscle tension patterns are eliminated using voice therapy techniques that "unload" the abnormal muscular compressive forces. (See Chapter 25 for a full discussion of these conditions.)

Incomplete Vocal Fold Closure

Incomplete vocal fold closure can be caused by vocal fold paralysis and paresis. In severe cases, there may be a large (3 mm or more) glottal gap during phonation, and this may prevent any vibration whatsoever. In less severe cases, incomplete vocal contact results in diminished subglottal pressure buildup, so that the displacement force of the vocal folds during phonation is decreased. The reduction in displacement of the vocal folds during phonation results in diminished amplitude of vibration in the vocal fold (**Video Clips 25, 27, and 28**).

◆ Conclusion

The amplitude of vocal fold vibration depends on the interaction between the superficial tissues at the margin of the vocal fold (superficial lamina propria), the mass of the vocal fold, the length of the vocal fold, the subglottic pressure, and the medial compressive forces generated by muscular contraction. The differential diagnosis of a decrease in vibratory amplitude includes pathology that impacts any of these factors.

Suggested Reading

Hirano M, Bless DM. Videostroboscopic Examination of the Larynx. San Diego, CA: Singular Publishing Group; 1993

19

Vibratory Asymmetry

Adam D. Rubin and Cristina Jackson-Menaldi

The evaluation of a patient with hoarseness begins with the clinician listening to the patient's voice. As soon as the patient vocalizes, the clinician begins to gather clues about the source of the pathology. A raspy or rough voice suggests irregular or aperiodic vibration of the vocal folds. Even small changes in vocal fold vibration can result in large changes in vocal quality.[1–5] To determine if vibratory abnormalities are the source of vocal changes, an evaluation of vocal fold vibration with videostroboscopy is required.

Symmetry of vocal fold vibration is defined as the degree to which the vocal folds are mirror images of one another during vibration. Asymmetry of vibration can occur due to asymmetry in the timing (phase) or amplitude of the mucosal wave (**Fig. 19.1**).[6] Although asymmetry, particularly phase asymmetry, is not specific and does not always signify pathology, asymmetry of vocal fold vibration usually suggests a difference in the viscoelastic or mechanical properties of the vocal folds. This includes differences in mass, shape, position, tension, and elasticity.[6–8] Often more than one property is affected. Very commonly, asymmetry of vibration is the result of a decrease in the amplitude of vibration of one of the vocal folds relative to the other due to unilateral vocal fold pathology (**Video Clips 32 to 34**).

Sometimes the reason for vibratory asymmetry is obvious, such as a large mass on one vocal fold, or it may be subtle, as in the case of unilateral submucosal fibrosis. If one vocal fold vibrates normally and the other one does not, asymmetry should be easy to identify. When pathology involves both vocal folds, asymmetry may be more difficult to recognize, but doing so will help the clinician to make appropriate treatment decisions. For example, a patient with unilateral Reinke's polyposis and a poorly vibrating contralateral vocal fold should be treated more conservatively than a patient with a normal contralateral vocal fold. Overaggressive resection of the polyp or poor healing at the site of resection could result in scar, which, along with an abnormal contralateral vocal fold, would require high phonation pressures to vocalize and result in a very rough, strained voice. It might be more prudent to avoid surgery in such cases or perform a very conservative excision. In addition, asymmetry of vibration in patients with bilateral Reinke's polyposis may suggest unilateral sulcus or scar that should also lead to caution on the part of the surgeon (**Fig. 19.2**).

◆ Coupling

Vocal folds with different viscoelastic properties can still appear to vibrate synchronously through a process called *coupling*. Because of

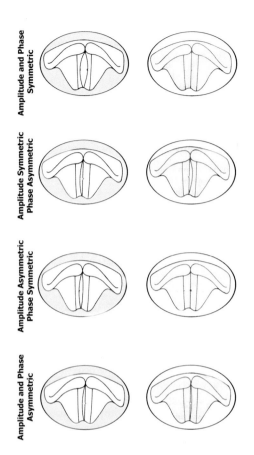

Fig. 19.1 Phase and amplitude asymmetry.

the coupling effect, subtle asymmetry may not be detected either in vocal quality or on videostroboscopic examination. More severe viscoelastic asymmetry and asymmetry in vocal fold position can compromise coupling and yield only partial synchronization of vibration resulting in bifurcations or modulations (**Video Clip 23**). Clinically, this may manifest as diplophonia or the perception of two or more simultaneous pitches in the patient's voice. Diplophonia occurs through quasi-periodic variations in vocal fold vibration. The acoustic structure of diplophonia can be appreciated with narrow-band spectrography. Spectrography demonstrates subharmonics and perturbation within vibratory cycles (**Fig. 19.3**). Subglottic pressure and airflow contribute to the efficiency of coupling and can mask vocal fold asymmetry.[7,9–11] It is important, therefore, to have the patient phonate at different volumes and pitches during the videostroboscopic examination to illicit subtle asymmetry in vibration (**Video Clips 38 and 39**).

◆ Interpretation of Vibratory Asymmetry

When asymmetric vibration is observed during videostroboscopy, the examiner needs to consider the differences in the mechanical

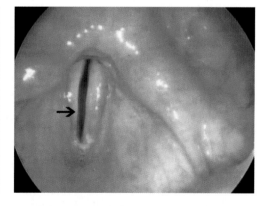

Fig. 19.2 (A) Bilateral Reinke's polyposis in a patient who presented 15 years after having a unilateral polypectomy. The right vocal fold has a sulcus superior to the remaining Reinke's polyposis. The mucosal wave was impaired on the right. Extra care must be taken to avoid sulcus on the contralateral side or the patient might be left with a worse voice.

In fact, the surgeon may operate on only the right vocal fold polyp and wait to decide if contralateral surgery is necessary after allowing the patient to heal. Double arrows point to a sulcus superior to the remaining Reinke's polyposis on the right vocal fold. **(B)** Scarring of the right vocal fold is more apparent during phonation.

IV Vibratory Abnormalities

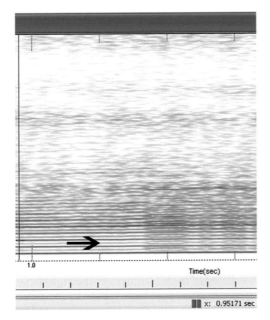

Fig. 19.3 Spectrogram: Narrow-band sustained vowel /a/ with subharmonics. The *arrow* points to subharmonics.

properties of each vocal fold that are likely contributing to the asymmetry. A unilateral decrease in vibratory amplitude will result in asymmetric vocal fold vibration. As a result, when considering the differential diagnosis of asymmetric vocal fold vibration, there is significant overlap with the differential diagnosis of decreased vibratory amplitude.

Vocal Fold Masses

Although, in general, an increase in the mass of the vocal fold will result in a reduction of the vocal fold vibration amplitude (and, in cases of a unilateral change in mass, result in vibration asymmetry), distinct vocal fold masses affect vibration differently. Zhang and Jiang developed a unilateral vocal fold polyp model and demonstrated that the larger the polyp, the larger the degree of vocal fold vibration asymmetry. In addition, the larger the polyp, the greater its nonlinear effect on vocal fold vibration and the more likely it is for chaotic vibration to occur.[4,12] Although it seems logical that the size of a vocal fold mass will contribute to the degree of asymmetry,

other properties of the mass, such as firmness, shape, and depth, will also have ramifications on vocal fold vibration. It is difficult to define the effects of a mass on vocal fold vibration based on its etiology and nomenclature alone.

Small unilateral superficial lesions such as vocal fold polyps, papilloma, and noninvasive leukoplakia may not have a dramatic affect on the amplitude of horizontal vocal fold excursion. It is the localized effect of the lesion on the stiffness of the vocal fold cover that determines the impact of the lesion on vibration at that location. This will depend on how firm or fibrotic the lesion is or if there is surrounding submucosal fibrosis or invasion. A long-standing vocal fold polyp may become firm and fibrotic or develop significant fibrosis at the base, which will result in a localized hypodynamic segment (**Video Clip 19**). This is important to note, to appropriately counsel patients and temper expectations, if surgical intervention is necessary. Leukoplakia and papilloma tend to increase the stiffness of the cover and result in decreased vibration. However, significantly reduced vibration in the presence of leukoplakia must raise suspicion for an invasive process, such as carcinoma (**Video Clip 35**). Of course, the degree of invasion can be assessed at the time of surgery with palpation and hydrodissection, but preoperative recognition is important for patient counseling and preparation. The surgeon can prepare the patient for the possible necessity of a wider excision than might be required for dysplasia or hyperkeratosis, involving more than only the superficial epithelium.

If superficial bilateral masses exist, asymmetry of vibration will be determined by the different morphologic characteristics of the masses and how the masses interact. For example, true vocal fold nodules are symmetric and will likely affect the vibratory characteristics of each respective vocal fold to the same degree, so that vibration will remain symmetric (**Video Clips 18 and 40**). A soft, small hemorrhagic polyp and a firm fibrotic contact mass, however, will likely result in asymmetric vibration. If the lesions interfere with each other, vibration will be chaotic bilaterally.[6]

Lesions that extend deeper into the vocal fold tend to affect vibration more significantly then superficial lesions. Reinke's polyposis involves the entire superficial layer of the lamina propria, increasing the mass of the vocal fold and resulting in reduced vibratory amplitude. The consistency of the Reinke's stroma will determine how vibration is affected. If the stroma is more fluid, vibration amplitude may not be compromised and may even appear to be increased. If the stroma is more dense and fibrotic, the amplitude of vibration will be reduced or chaotic. As mentioned, a sulcus within Reinke's polyposis will also affect vibration (**Fig. 19.2**). Submucosal cysts usually result in a more dramatic effect on vibration than do superficial lesions. Amplitude and mucosal wave are decreased and vibration is impaired at the site of the cyst (**Video Clips 26 and 34**). In general, deeper cysts, particularly if they abut the vocal ligament, will severely impair vibration (**Fig. 19.4**). Invasive malignancies will reduce vibration, increasing mass and stiffness of the vocal fold. As they invade the

vocal ligament and vocalis muscle, vibration becomes severely compromised, and vibratory asymmetry becomes more pronounced (**Video Clip 35**).

As any asymmetry in the mass of the vocal folds results in vibratory asymmetry, a unilateral decrease in mass (as opposed to an increase in mass as a result of vocal fold pathology) may also present with vibratory asymmetry. This situation might occur after recovery from vocal fold paralysis or persistent paresis (**Video Clips 41 and 42**).

Vocal Fold Stiffness

Scar and Sulcus Vocalis

A difference in the stiffness of the superficial tissues of one vocal fold relative to the other will result in vibratory asymmetry. Stiffer

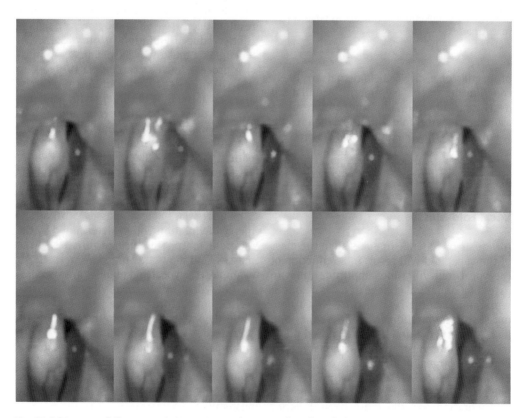

Fig. 19.4 Montage of vibratory cycle in a patient with a large right submucosal cyst and a soft, left hemorrhagic polyp. The amplitude of vibration is more compromised on the side with the cyst as it involves the deeper layers of the vocal fold.

tissues are not displaced as much as normal tissues during vibration. A unilateral or localized reduction in vibratory amplitude and mucosal wave, in the absence of a discreet mass, is often a result of increased tissue stiffness due to scar or a sulcus vocalis lesion. The injury may be localized, such as in the site of a previous surgical excision, or involve the entire length of the vocal fold. In general, location and depth of the lesion will determine its effect on vibration and voice. Deep scars and scars involving the mid-membranous portion of the vocal fold will be more symptomatic than superficial scarring or scars in the posterior third of the vocal fold (**Video Clips 32, 33, and 43**). Furthermore, voice manifestations will be less severe in the setting of unilateral stiffness involving the entire vocal fold. If the contralateral vocal fold is pliable and glottic closure is good, voice is usually not as severely affected as it would be in the case of bilateral vocal fold scar.

The terms *scar* and *sulcus* are often used interchangeably. Both contribute to irregular or decreased vibration secondary to a loss of pliability and bulk of the vocal fold cover. In general, *sulcus* refers to a groove within the medial edge of the vocal fold. The etiology is unknown, but there appears to be migration of epithelium into the lamina propria. *Scar* results from replacement of normal superficial lamina propria with disorganized collagen fibers. The voice impact of both entities results from irregularity in vibration and glottic insufficiency.[13-16]

Ford et al. described three types of sulcus. Type I, or "physiologic sulcus," is a depression along the entire length of the vocal fold, resulting from migration of the epithelium into the superficial lamina propria, but not all the way to the vocal ligament. Type II also involves the entire length of the vocal fold, but the epithelium migrates to the vocal ligament or deeper. Type III is a localized deep "pit."[4] It may easily be missed on videostroboscopy.[15,16]

On videostroboscopic evaluation, scar or sulcus may result in decreased or aperiodic vocal fold vibration, a concavity or groove along the medial edge, "spindle-shaped" glottis, a whitish-hue to the vocal fold, and a thickened appearance to the cover of the vocal fold. Again, findings will depend on the severity and size of the lesion. A small sulcus or scar will result in a localized hypodynamic segment, and more diffuse scarring will result in a generalized reduction in the mucosal wave (**Fig. 19.5**). Asymmetry may become more apparent at different pitches. Localized hypodynamic segments often present more clearly at higher pitches when the vocal fold is stretched, resulting in a stiffer cover.

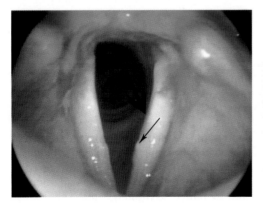

A

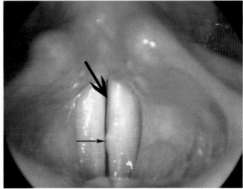

B

Fig. 19.5 (A) A 40-year-old woman who presented 5 months after having a left Reinke's polyp removed by another surgeon. She was still dysphonic. The surgeon told her she had a recurrent mass on her left vocal fold that needed excision (*thin arrow*). She presented for a second opinion. Videostroboscopy showed asymmetric vibration with a severely reduced amplitude of vibration of the left vocal fold. The vocal fold was severely hypodynamic along the entire medial edge due to scarring along the entire length of the vocal fold (*thick arrow*). The patient was advised in our clinic that the scarring was the main reason for her dysphonia. **(B)** Patient during vocal fold adduction.

Acute Phonotrauma

Vocal fold tears and vocal fold hemorrhages result from acute phonotrauma. Vocal fold tears are subtle mucosal disruptions, typically at the mid-membranous portion of the vocal fold. On videostroboscopy, they are often unilateral and present as a hypodynamic segment. A linear disruption in the mucosa can often be visualized when the videostroboscopy recording is played back frame by frame. At other times, a focal area of inflammation around the tear is appreciated.[17,18]

Vocal fold hemorrhages occur because of a ruptured blood vessel. When superficial, they may have little-to-no effect on vocal fold vibration. However, deeper hemorrhages increase both the mass and stiffness of the vocal fold resulting in decreased amplitude of vibration and mucosal wave (**Video Clip 44**). Identifying and treating hemorrhages and tears appropriately is important to avoid long-term vocal fold scarring and mass formation.[17,18]

Vocal Fold Tension

Superior Laryngeal Nerve Paralysis

Asymmetry in the tension of each vocal fold often manifests as asymmetry in both the phase and amplitude of vibration during phonation.[8] Vocal fold tension is primarily the result of contraction of the vocalis muscle and the viscoelastic properties of the vocal ligament. It contributes to medial compressive forces needed to create resistance to air flow through the glottis.[19]

Secondarily, an increase in vocal fold tension occurs as a result of cricothyroid muscle contraction. Contraction of the cricothyroid muscle alters the angle between the thyroid and cricoid cartilages, increasing the distance between the vocal processes of the arytenoid cartilages and the anterior commissure of the thyroid cartilage. This process elongates the vocal fold, thus increasing vocal fold tension, vibratory frequency, and vocal pitch. The cricothyroid muscle is innervated by the external branch of the superior laryngeal nerve. If this nerve is injured, the vocal fold of the affected side will be lax at higher pitches relative to the unaffected side (**Fig. 19.6**). Increased vocal fold

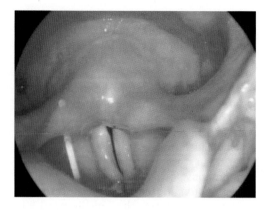

Fig. 19.6 Rigid videostroboscopy of a patient with right superior laryngeal nerve paresis. Right vocal fold is flaccid with increased vibration amplitude. The posterior larynx tilts to the right.

laxity results in an increased vibratory amplitude and more chaotic vibration during phonation. The lax vocal fold is more sensitive to changes in subglottic pressure and airflow, which increases voice perturbation.[1,7–9,20,21]

Superior laryngeal nerve paresis or paralysis can be difficult to diagnose by videostroboscopic examination. Phase and amplitude asymmetry, though they may be the only findings in superior laryngeal nerve palsy, are not specific to the diagnosis. Other findings that may occur, and therefore help to confirm the diagnosis, include vocal fold lag, posterior glottic tilt, and vocal fold height discrepancy.[7,20,21]

Recurrent Laryngeal Nerve Injury

Injury to the recurrent laryngeal nerve will result in denervation of the thyroarytenoid muscle. A flaccid paralysis results and the vocal fold appears bowed. However, spontaneous reinnervation is common after recurrent laryngeal nerve injury. Because of synkinesis, vocal fold movement may not be restored in cases of reinnervation, but tone will improve, and vibratory asymmetry may not be as prominent. If vocal fold paresis or paralysis occurs because of an upper motor neuron injury, vocal fold tone may be paradoxically increased or "spastic." Increased tone results in a decreased amplitude of vibration, whereas decreased tone results in an increased amplitude of vibration (**Fig. 19.7**).[20,21]

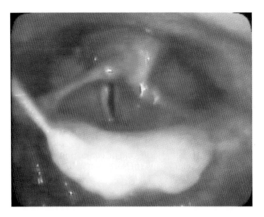 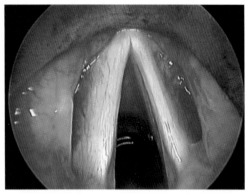

A   B

Fig. 19.7 (A) Flexible (distal chip) videostroboscopy demonstrating flaccid right vocal fold in a patient with a RLN paralysis. **(B)** Operative view prior to injection laryngoplasty. Note the severe atrophy of the right vocal fold.

The vibratory effect from a unilateral vocal fold paralysis is largely determined by the degree of glottic insufficiency, in other words, the size of the glottic gap. Vocal fold coupling is less efficient with a large glottic gap, resulting in more chaotic vibration. Increased airflow can compensate for glottic insufficiency, but this too becomes less effective as the gap widens (**Video Clips 25, 27, and 28**). Additionally, asymmetry in vocal fold height (another feature that may be seen with unilateral vocal fold paralysis or paresis) can result in more chaotic vibration.[1,8,11] Vocal fold height is best evaluated using a 70-degree rigid telescope during videostroboscopy.[20,21] Recognizing height discrepancy is important, as it may need to be addressed in addition to improving glottic closure during laryngeal framework surgery.

◆ Conclusion

Evaluation of vibratory symmetry is an important aspect of a videostroboscopic examination. Asymmetric vibration may be the result of differences in the amplitude of horizontal vocal fold excursion or the timing of vocal fold excursion. Although not always pathologic, asymmetry suggests a difference in the mass, tension, or viscoelastic properties between the two vocal folds. When there is not an obvious mass, asymmetry in vocal fold vibration may be the only visible clue to the etiology of the voice problem. It may be suggestive of a submucosal process such as scar or muscle weakness.

References

1. Plant RL. Aerodynamics of the human larynx during vocal fold vibration. Laryngoscope 2005;115:2087–2100
2. Herzel H. Possible mechanisms of vocal instabilities. In: Davis P, Fletcher N, eds. Vocal Fold Physiology: Voice Quality Control Controlling Complexity and Chaos. San Diego, CA: Singular Publishing Group; 1996:63–75
3. Titze IR, Baken RJ, Herzrl H. Evidence of chaos in vocal fold vibration. In: Titze IR, ed. Vocal Fold Physiology: Frontiers in Basic Science. San Diego, CA: Singular Publishing Group; 1993:143–182
4. Jiang JJ, Zhang Y, McGilligan C. Chaos in voice, from modeling to measurement. J Voice 2006;20:2–17
5. Berry DA, Herzel H, Titze IR, Krischer K. Interpretation of biomechanical simulations of normal and chaotic vocal fold oscillations with empirical eigenfunctions. J Acoust Soc Am 1994;95:3595–3604
6. Hirano M, Bless DM. Videostroboscopic Examination of the Larynx. San Diego, CA: Singular Publishing Group; 1993
7. Maunsell R, Ouaknine M, Giovanni A, Crespo A. Vibratory pattern of vocal folds under tension asymmetry. Otolaryngol Head Neck Surg 2006;135:438–444
8. Isshiki N, Tanabe M, Ishizaka K, Broad D. Clinical significance of asymmetrical vocal cord tension. Ann Otol Rhinol Laryngol 1977;86(1 Pt 1):58–66
9. Giovanni A, Ouaknine M, Guelfucci R, Yu T, Zanaret M, Triglia JM. Nonlinear behavior of vocal fold vibration: the role of coupling between the vocal folds. J Voice 1999;13:465–476
10. Berry DA, Herzel H, Titze IR, Story BH. Bifurcations in excised larynx experiments. J Voice 1996;10:129–138
11. Hong KH, Kim HK. Diplophonia in unilateral vocal fold paralysis and intracordal cyst. Otolaryngol Head Neck Surg 1999;121:815–819

12. Zhang Y, Jiang JJ. Chaotic vibrations of a vocal fold model with a unilateral polyp. J Acoust Soc Am 2004;115:1266–1269

13. Pontes P, Behlau M. Treatment of sulcus vocalis: auditory perceptual and acoustical analysis of the slicing mucosa surgical technique. J Voice 1993;7:365–376

14. Bouchayer M, Cornut G, Witzig E, Loire R, Roch JB, Bastian RW. Epidermoid cysts, sulci, and mucosal bridges of the true vocal cord: a report of 157 cases. Laryngoscope 1985;95(9 Pt 1):1087–1094

15. Dailey SH, Ford CN. Surgical management of sulcus vocalis and vocal fold scarring. Otolaryngol Clin North Am 2006;39:23–42

16. Ford CN, Inagi K, Khidr A, Bless DM, Gilchrist KW. Sulcus vocalis: a rational analytical approach to diagnosis and management. Ann Otol Rhinol Laryngol 1996; 105:189–200

17. Klein AM, Johns MM III. Vocal emergencies. Otolaryngol Clin North Am 2007;40:1063–1080, vii

18. Sataloff RT, Spiegel JR, Hawkshaw M. Acute mucosal tear and vocal fold hemorrhage. Ear Nose Throat J 1994;73:633

19. Titze IR. Control of fundamental frequency. In: Titze IR, ed. Principles of Voice Production. Englewood Cliffs, NJ: Prentice-Hall; 1994

20. Rubin AD, Sataloff RT. Vocal fold paresis and paralysis. In: Sataloff RT, ed. Professional Voice: The Science and Art of Clinical Care, 3rd ed. San Diego, CA: Plural Publishing; 2005

21. Rubin AD. Neurolaryngologic evaluation of the performer. Otolaryngol Clin North Am 2007;40:971–989

20

Abnormalities of the Mucosal Wave

Mona M. Abaza

No characteristic of laryngeal imaging is more dependent on the unique capacity of videostroboscopy than the mucosal wave evaluation. Still images, or even recorded normal light fiberoptic examinations, cannot provide the data necessary to evaluate the mucosal wave. The use of stroboscopic light or high-speed image capture (such as high-speed video or videokymography) is needed to evaluate this parameter.

One important limitation of videostroboscopic examinations should be mentioned here. Because videostroboscopy requires a periodic voice to trigger a stroboscopic light source, videostroboscopy is not always capable of recording the mucosal wave information in all patients. Furthermore, severely dysphonic voices, significant pitch breaks, glottal insufficiencies, and large mass effects can make visualization of a mucosal wave with videostroboscopy difficult or even impossible.

High-speed imaging systems eliminate the need for a periodic voice by capturing real-time images but come with their own constraints (**Fig. 20.1**).[1] The high cost of videostroboscopic systems often limits their availability, but the even higher cost of high-speed imaging systems makes their availability more rare. In addition, the large quantity of data that high-speed systems record, for which discrete clinical protocols do not exist, makes the routine use of these imaging systems uncommon.

Videokymography is another alternative for imaging vocal fold vibration in patients with nonperiodic voicing. Widely viewed as a more economical way to achieve real-time images, it can record, in real time, a single selected line across the vocal folds, providing an opportunity to look at the mucosal wave form produced at that point of the vocal fold margin (**Fig. 20.2**). Looking at several points on the vocal fold edge

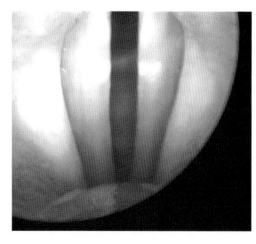

Fig. 20.1 A high-speed video image.

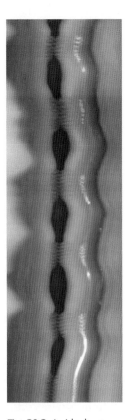

Fig. 20.2 A videokymography image.

or at the site of a lesion requires several evaluation passes. Videokymography is considered to be more capable of identifying subtle differences in the mucosal waveform from side to side, and its use should be considered in complicated diagnostic situations.[2]

It is important to remember that the image of a mucosal wave on the screen is a two-dimensional representation of the three-dimensional movement of the vocal fold mucosa and the superficial lamina propria over the deeper vocal fold structures. As such, the mucosal wave is the best vocal fold vibratory parameter for providing information about the state of the histologic layers of the vocal fold and the disorders affecting them. It can be impacted, however, by other components of the vibratory system, in addition to the state of the superficial vocal fold tissue. The degree of tension present in the entire laryngeal system affects the mucosal wave, with increasing tension often, but not always, decreasing vibration. In addition, because vocal fold vibration and

mucosal wave are the result of pulmonary pressure and airflow rates, abnormalities in these parameters can affect the wave as well. The overall glottal configuration also plays a role in the vibratory pattern. We will discuss each of these components individually.

◆ Respiratory Effects on Mucosal Wave

The inability to generate adequate respiratory support, intentionally or unintentionally, causes the vibratory component of vocal fold movement during phonation to decrease and results in a decrease of the mucosal wave. For example, in a patient with a tracheotomy and no vented airflow to the larynx, no vocalization is present due to lack of a power source, so no mucosal wave is present. Pathologic etiologies such as asthma, emphysema, and other pulmonary disorders that decrease glottal airflow can decrease the mucosal wave by the same mechanism.

Neurologic disorders affecting respiratory strength, such as post-polio syndrome and other central neurologic pathologies, can also decrease pulmonary function and subsequent vibration. Furthermore, abnormalities of glottal function linked to abnormal "respiratory" patterns can cause decreases in the mucosal wave, such as paradoxical vocal fold motion, spasmodic dysphonia, and other dystonias or neurologic disorders. In addition, hypofunctional and aphonic vocalization created by poor functional respiratory effort will produce a lack of airflow and, therefore, cause a decrease or absence of the mucosal wave.

◆ Glottal Configuration Effects on Mucosal Waves

Glottal configuration patterns also play a role in mucosal wave development. Hypofunctional or hyperfunctional patterns of closure will affect the vibratory edge and can be shown to change the mucosal wave. In situations where a lack of contact between the vocal folds takes place, such as presbyphonia (**Fig. 20.3**; **Video Clips 16, 17, and 24**), vocal fold paralysis (**Fig. 20.4**; **Video Clips 25, 27,**

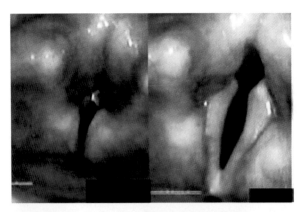

A

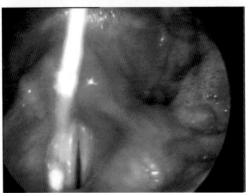

B

Fig. 20.3 **(A)** Presbyphonia. On the left, supraglottic tension obscures view of the vocal folds. On the right, the concave contour of the folds is better appreciated.
(B) Presbyphonia with the vocal folds at maximum adduction. Note the persistent glottic opening.

and 28), and hypofunctional muscle tension dysphonia (**Fig. 20.5**; **Video Clip 20**), the mucosal wave can be decreased or absent. In these situations, inadequate forces opposing the vocal folds alter the vibratory pattern by decreasing the build-up of subglottal pressure.

◆ Medial Compressive Forces

Decreases in the mucosal wave can be seen in situations of hyperfunction when the muscular tension on the vibratory edges of the vocal folds becomes too great for the subglottal air pressure to overcome. This phenomenon is most typically seen in hyperfunctional muscle tension dysphonia (**Fig. 20.6**) but is also seen in disorders such as spasmodic dysphonia (**Fig. 20.7**) and central neurologic disorders. It is important to remember that normal vibratory structures likely exist in these patients and that it is the forces at the glottal level that limit airflow and vibratory function. Additionally, extreme hyperfunction can prevent the visualization of the vocal folds,

making evaluation of vocal fold vibration impossible (**Fig. 20.8**).

Studies have shown that specific muscle activation and firing patterns alter the vocal fold vibratory pattern and that certain sequences increase the stresses on the vibratory margin.[3] However, quantifying or distinguishing the forces causing the decrease of the mucosal wave in various muscular patterns seen clinically is not currently readily achievable. As most models now being used to quantitatively describe the impact of changes in the various components of the laryngeal vibratory system are theoretical models, their use in the clinical setting is problematic.

◆ Superficial Lamina Propria and Mucosal Effects on Mucosal Wave

The limitation of many theories about vocal fold injury and healing is the fact that they are based on studies using animal and in vitro

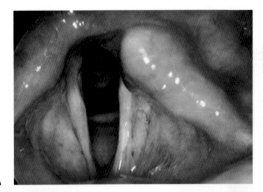

A

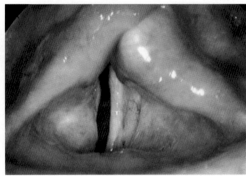

B

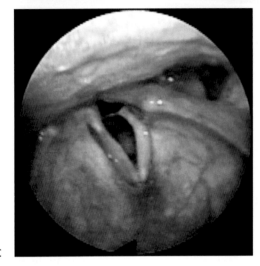

C

Fig. 20.4 **(A)** Left vocal fold paralysis with the vocal folds in an abducted position. **(B)** Left vocal fold paralysis with the vocal folds adducted. A persistent glottic opening is apparent even at maximal adduction. **(C)** Vocal fold paralysis and contralateral hemorrhage. The lateralized position of the left vocal fold prevents closure despite medial movement of the right vocal fold.

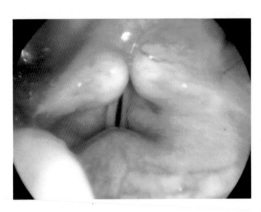

Fig. 20.5 Hypofunctional dysphonia with a persistent glottic opening.

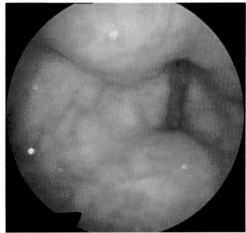

Fig. 20.6 Hyperfunctional dysphonia. Notice medialization of ventricular folds secondary to squeezing.

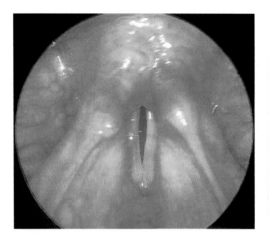

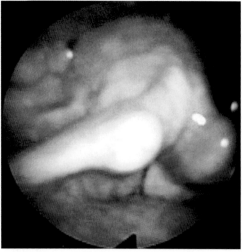

Fig. 20.7 Adductor spasmodic dysphonia. The vocal folds appear normal but the mucosal wave is less than one half of the width of the vocal fold. The short green line depicts the width of the right mucosal wave, and the longer green line depicts the width of the right vocal fold. Normally, the short green line should be about half the length of the long green line.

Fig. 20.8 Severe hyperfunctional dysphonia. The ventricular folds obscure the true vocal folds, preventing evaluation of their vibratory characteristics.

models, so direct data on human disease processes is not available. What we do know is that the role of the superficial lamina propria in the development and resolution of glottal edema is likely related to its role in the development of vocal fold fibrosis, both in short-term and long-term outcomes. Increased intravascular pressure at the vocal fold edge has been shown to affect vocal vibration and is theorized to be a component of the response to injury of vocal folds.[4] In addition, the vibration of vocal fold fibroblasts increases the production of matrix proteins in the lamina propria, such as fibronectin and collagen type 1.[5] Changes in collagen types and quantity are an important factor in scarring in any tissue and are critical at the vocal fold vibratory margin. This type of alteration of the balance of the lamina propria components can result in changes to mucosal wave patterns. One of the more important inferences that can be made from the evaluation of the mucosal wave during a diagnostic videostroboscopy concerns the health of the superficial lamina propria and overlying mucosa.

It is important to remember that the progression of a patient along the spectrum of edema, stiffness, and frank scarring is not absolute or irreversible. The acute mass effects caused by fluid or blood due to edema and hemorrhage can cause a decease in the mucosal wave patterns by themselves (**Fig. 20.9**). Following the mucosal wave recovery through repeated videostroboscopic examinations can be an effective way to monitor the recovery of the vocal fold in these processes. Persistent decrease of a mucosal wave can indicate a fibrotic reaction and cause concern about potential scarring (**Fig. 20.10**).

Scarring and the associated loss of the normal superficial lamina propria structure represents

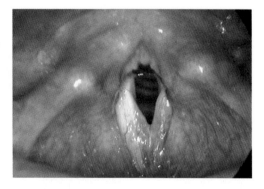

Fig. 20.9 Vocal fold edema. The swelling of the superficial lamina propria secondary to fluid in the interstitial space results in a decreased mucosal wave.

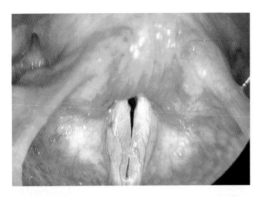

Fig. 20.10 Fibrotic reaction resulting in scarring and a decrease in the mucosal wave.

one of the most common diagnoses indicated by a decreased mucosal wave. The complete absence of a mucosal wave implies that the superficial lamina propria has been completely eradicated (**Video Clips 32 and 33**). The results of vocal fold stripping procedures are an extreme example of this problem (**Fig. 20.11**). Affected patients demonstrate no mucosal wave throughout the vibratory edge, indicating that the superficial lamina propria was likely removed with the surgical procedure and has now been replaced with more fibrotic tissue.

A decreased mucosal wave can also provide information about the state of mass lesions on the vocal fold vibratory edge, such as the degree of associated fibrosis (**Video Clip 40**). Changes in the mucosal wave can indicate the depth of the lesion, as in premalignant lesions, as well as provide information about how amenable a benign lesion is to nonsurgical and surgical intervention. Leukoplakia, a white keratotic patch, is a lesion in which the decrease of mucosal wave can be concerning, as a cancer diagnosis can be more likely when a decreased mucosal wave indicates involvement of the superficial lamina propria (**Fig. 20.12**; **Video Clip 35**). The status of vocal nodules can be aided by the evaluation of the mucosal wave over them. The presence of a continuous, normal mucosal wave over the nodules indicates they are probably not fibrotic and, therefore, more likely to resolve with voice therapy (**Fig. 20.13**; **Video Clip 18**).

◆ Limitations and Concerns about Mucosal Wave Interpretation

There is sometimes difficulty in interpreting the implications of differences in the mucosal wave between the vocal folds. Whereas this type of difference may represent unilateral pathology, such as paralysis or a mass lesion, left-right differences in the mucosal wave are also seen in normal individuals. The relationship of these differences to fatigue and other components are not known.[6] Changes found in a normal population with the more detailed videokymographic techniques indicate that some of these changes may not be clinically significant and may not represent a cause of dysphonia.[7]

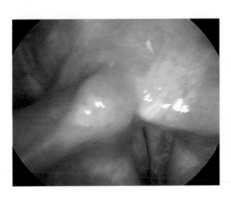
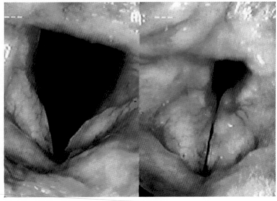

A

B

Fig. 20.11 **(A)** Scarring after vocal fold stripping of the left vocal fold. **(B)** Severe bilateral vocal fold scarring.

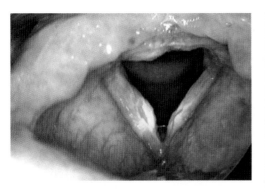

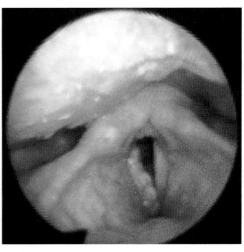

Fig. 20.12 (A) Leukoplakia of both vocal folds that may result in a decrease of the mucosal wave depending on the involvement of the superficial lamina propria. **(B)** Extensive leukoplakia of the right vocal fold with complete loss of the mucosal wave.

A

B

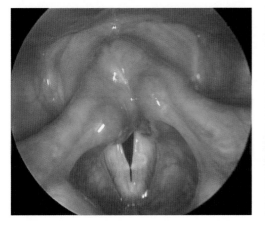

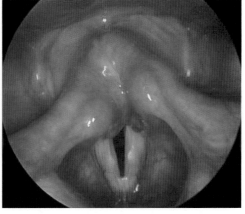

Fig. 20.13 (A) Nodule: View with superior surface of vocal folds approximated before the onset of the mucosal wave. **(B)** Nodule from **A** with mucosal wave flowing over the nodules indicating that they are soft and likely to respond to speech therapy.

A

B

Although the mucosal wave provides significant information about the state of the multilayer vocal fold structure, it is only one element of the overall evaluation of a videostroboscopic examination and must be taken in context of the entire clinical picture. Several different components of the vocal tract can cause the decrease of the mucosal wave, so it is important to look at all components and their role. Disorders affecting the respiratory power source of vibration, glottal configuration changes both organic and functional, and vibratory edge lesions can all play a role in decreasing the vibratory effect.

References

1. Patel R, Dailey S, Bless D. Comparison of high-speed digital imaging with stroboscopy for laryngeal imaging of glottal disorders. Ann Otol Rhinol Laryngol 2008; 117:413–424
2. Svec JG, Sram F, Schutte HK. Videokymography in voice disorders: what to look for? Ann Otol Rhinol Laryngol 2007;116:172–180

3. Lowell SY, Story BH. Simulated effects of cricothyroid and thyroarytenoid muscle activation on adult-male vocal fold vibration. J Acoust Soc Am 2006;120:386–397

4. Czerwonka L, Jiang JJ, Tao C. Vocal nodules and edema may be due to vibration-induced rises in capillary pressure. Laryngoscope 2008;118:748–752

5. Wolchok JC, Brokopp C, Underwood CJ, Tresco PA. The effect of bioreactor induced vibrational stimulation on extracellular matrix production from human derived fibroblasts. Biomaterials 2009;30:327–335

6. Lohscheller J, Eysholdt U, Toy H, Dollinger M. Phonovibrography: mapping high-speed movies of vocal fold vibrations into 2-D diagrams for visualizing and analyzing the underlying laryngeal dynamics. IEEE Trans Med Imaging 2008;27:300–309

7. Shaw HS, Deliyski DD. Mucosal wave: a normophonic study across visualization techniques. J Voice 2008;22:23–33

V

Vocal Fold Pathology and Vibratory Characteristics

21

Vocal Fold Nodules

Glendon M. Gardner

Vocal fold nodules are relatively symmetric areas of mucosal thickening located in the midportion of the musculomembranous vocal fold (**Fig. 21.1**).[1,2] The cause of nodules is thought to be phonotrauma, which consists of excessive or loud voice use, excessively forceful glottic closure, and other inappropriate voicing techniques.[3] Though this seems like a fairly straightforward definition, nodules can be easily confused with other benign swellings that occur in the midportion of the vibrating portion of the vocal fold, including polyps, cysts, pseudocysts, reactive nodules (opposite one of the other benign lesions), and simple edema (**Figs. 21.2 to 21.4**).

Stroboscopy helps us differentiate between these various lesions because different lesions affect vocal fold vibration and mucosal wave propagation in different ways. Mucosal lesions (as opposed to submucosal) may dampen the mucosal wave but usually do not eliminate the wave. Lesions that involve the superficial layer of the lamina propria (submucosal, Reinke's space) may abolish the wave altogether. Scarring, sulcus vocalis, and true cysts are the more common causes of an abolished wave because

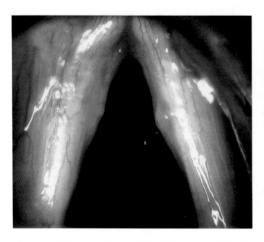
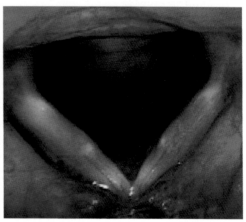

A   B

Fig. 21.1 **(A)** Surgical view of hard fibrotic nodules. **(B)** Softer nodules located at the midportion of the musculomembranous vocal folds.

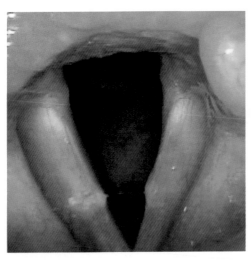

Fig. 21.2 Left vocal fold cyst with reactive swelling of right vocal fold. Mucus is adherent to the right vocal fold swelling.

Fig. 21.3 Left vocal fold polyp or pseudocyst with reactive swelling of right vocal fold.

they effectively connect the mucosa to the underlying ligament (**Fig. 21.5**).

The masses most often confused with classic vocal fold nodules are small cysts and pseudocysts and small polyps.[4] These lesions are covered in other chapters in detail. It should be noted, however, that even laryngologists, much less general otolaryngologists, cannot agree on the definition of these various lesions.[1,5] Pathologists have not helped the situation. They will diagnose most benign vocal fold lesions microscopically as "nodules" even when the surgeon

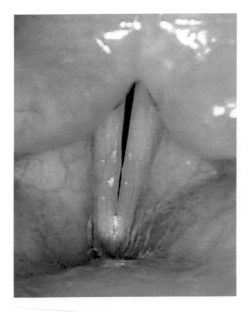

A

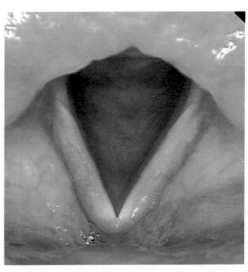

B

Fig. 21.4 **(A)** Mild vocal fold edema at the midportion of the musculomembranous vocal folds. View with vocal folds adducted. **(B)** Mild vocal fold edema at the midportion of the musculomembranous vocal folds. View of patient in **(A)** but with vocal folds abducted.

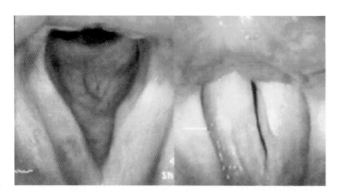

A

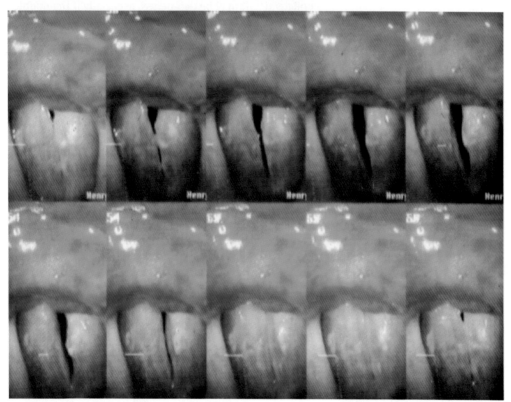

B

Fig. 21.5 **(A)** Left vocal fold cyst. **(B)** In patient from **(A)**, mucosal wave seen on the right, not on the left.

has observed that the lesions are different from each other grossly.[3]

The most basic description of nodules is that they are a thickening of the mucosa in the midportion of the musculomembranous portion of the vocal fold; that is, the vibratory portion. They are, therefore, located halfway between the anterior commissure and the vocal process of the arytenoid cartilage. They are generally very symmetric. Early nodules, or prenodules, may simply be edema of the mucosa, whereas chronic nodules may be fibrotic (**Video Clips 18 and 40**). This is differentiated from a polyp in which the mucosa is generally normal, or thin, and the bulk of the mass is a submucosal gelatinous matrix, although there are many variations of the composition of polyps (**Video Clips 19 and 23**). A true cyst has a well-defined capsule and is either a mucus retention cyst or an epidermoid cyst (**Video Clip 26**). A pseudocyst appears similar to a true cyst, but when dissected out, or examined histologically, there is no true capsule.

Dikkers and Schutte in 1991 suggested the following diagnostic criteria for the most common glottic lesions. This was similar to Kleinsasser's definitions.[6]

◆ *Cyst:* A unilateral lesion with a smooth surface, immobile during phonation, usually on the middle third of the vocal fold and often of a yellowish fluid-like appearance (**Video Clip 26**).

◆ *Reinke's edema:* A condition with a unilateral or bilateral bleach-white swelling of the vocal fold, filled with fluid, is sessile, and very mobile during phonation (**Video Clip 36**).

◆ *Polyp:* A unilateral lesion on the anterior third of the vocal fold, often on the free edge, sessile or pedunculated, and very mobile when pedunculated—a pedunculated polyp on the free edge can sometimes be heard popping through the glottis during the initiation of a phonation (**Video Clips 19, 23, and 46**).

◆ *Nodules:* Small lesions occurring on both sides of the larynx, strictly symmetrical on the border of the anterior and middle third of the vocal folds, and usually immobile during phonation—they can be divided, with the aid of stroboscopy, into the early spindle type (soft) or more chronic, white, cone-like form (hard)[1] (**Video Clips 18 and 40**).

With vocal fold nodules, the superficial layer of the lamina propria and the vocal ligament are normal. The mucosa is free to slide over the underlying vocal ligament, even if the mucosa, itself, is abnormal. Stroboscopy shows the mucosal wave flowing through a nodule (soft early nodule) (**Fig. 21.6**) or the nodule "riding" the wave (harder fibrotic nodules) (**Fig. 21.7**), but the wave is not abolished (**Video Clip 18**). It may be dampened, especially if the nodules are hard and fibrotic or exceptionally large (**Video Clip 40**). A true cyst abolishes the wave at the location of the cyst, although the wave may flow around the cyst (anterior and posterior to the cyst) (**Fig. 21.5**) (**Video Clip 26**). The true cyst, residing in the superficial layer of the lamina propria, is adherent to both the mucosa and the vocal ligament, thereby tethering these two structures and preventing the normal sliding motion of the mucosa over the vocal ligament.[7] Pseudocysts have variable effects on the wave. The mucosal wave flows through a soft polyp, especially the small sessile polyps that appear similar to nodules (**Fig. 21.8**). Harder pedunculated polyps generally interfere so much with closure and vibration that the mucosal wave is difficult to see (**Fig. 21.9**).

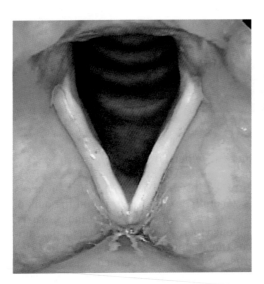 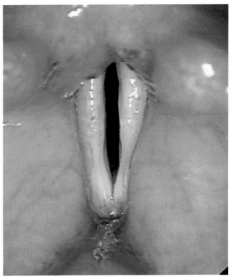

A B

Fig. 21.6 (A) Soft vocal fold nodules during vocal fold abduction. **(B)** Soft vocal fold nodules. Mucosal waves are normal.

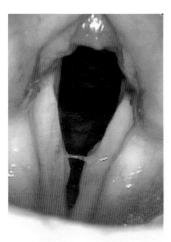
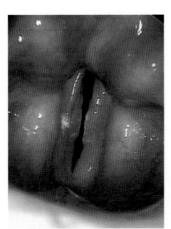
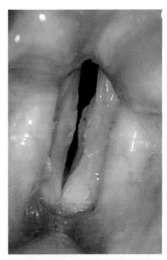

A–C

Fig. 21.7 (A) Large fibrotic nodules with vocal folds abducted. **(B and C)** Large fibrotic nodules "ride" the mucosal waves.

Polypoid vocal folds (Reinke's edema, polypoid degeneration, polypoid corditis), in which the entire vibratory portion of the vocal fold (anterior commissure to the vocal processes) is severely edematous, will have larger than normal mucosal waves, and the appearance is so different from vocal fold nodules that confusion regarding these two entities is rare (**Video Clip 36**). Nodules, however, may be present on the surface of polypoid vocal folds. In this case,

the nodule is seen to ride a very large mucosal wave (**Fig. 21.10**).

Vibration of the vocal folds is also influenced by the mass of the fold and closure. Vocal fold nodules affect both these factors. Vocal fold nodules interfere with closure by making premature contact at the midportion of the folds, resulting in an hourglass configuration. With less than complete closure, air leaks through the open gaps, decreasing the

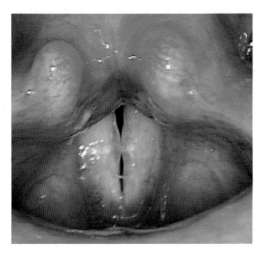
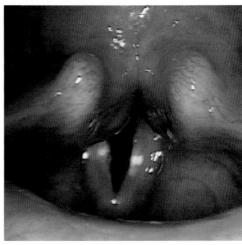

A

B

Fig. 21.8 (A) Right vocal fold pseudocyst or polyp with incomplete closure. **(B)** Right vocal fold pseudocyst or polyp. Mucosal wave is intact.

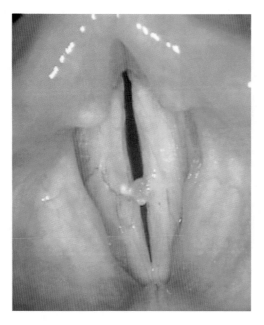

Fig. 21.9 Hard pedunculated left vocal fold polyp.

power transferred to the vocal fold edges and decreasing the amplitude of vibration and the size of the mucosal waves. The increased mass of the vocal fold edge also dampens vibration of the vocal fold. Whereas classic vocal fold nodules are symmetric, slight asymmetries often exist that affect each vocal fold slightly differently. Vibration may become aperiodic or asymmetric if the difference between the sides is significant (**Video Clip 45**). All of the benign lesions of the musculomembranous vocal folds will be more apparent at higher pitch, with the vocal fold stretched out under more tension. It is, therefore, important to view the folds all at aspects of the patient's dynamic range.

The differentiation between vocal fold nodules and similar lesions is not purely academic. Treatment varies for these different lesions. Voice therapy is the primary treatment for vocal fold nodules, whereas surgery is often required for polyps, pseudocysts, and true cysts.[8] Soft vocal fold nodules generally respond better to voice therapy than do the more chronic fibrotic nodules, nevertheless therapy should be tried in all cases of vocal fold nodules. Occasionally, when the diagnosis is not clear, the response to therapy will reveal the nature of the vocal fold abnormalities (**Fig. 21.11**). There are many cases in which the diagnosis of vocal fold nodules was made without stroboscopy, but the patient did not respond to therapy as expected, and the lesions were later found not to be nodules when stroboscopy was used for better evaluation.[4,9] Similarly, a surgeon who thought that he or she was about to remove nodules was instead confronted intraoperatively with a cyst.

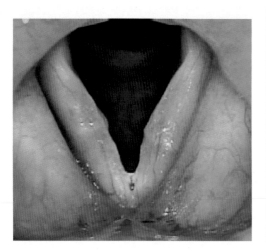

A

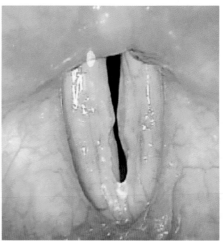

B

Fig. 21.10 (A) Nodules on surface of polypoid vocal folds viewed with vocal folds abducted. **(B)** Nodules on surface of polypoid vocal folds viewed during phonation.

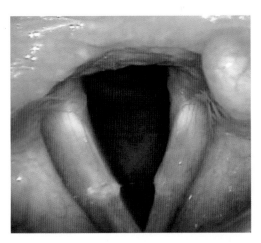

A

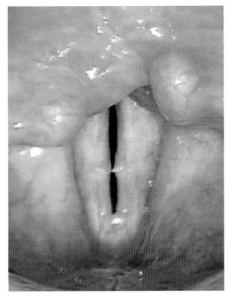

B

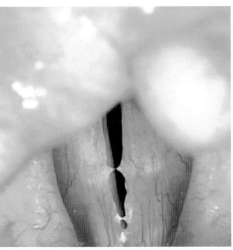

C

Fig. 21.11 (A) The lesions seen in this figure were initially thought to be nodules although mucosal wave was seen on the right only. View with vocal folds abducted. (B) View with vocal folds adducted of bilateral mid-membranous lesions initially thought to be nodules. (C) View during phonation showing mucosal wave on right prior to voice therapy.

In summary, differentiating between classic vocal fold nodules and those other benign vocal fold lesions that have a similar appearance is important for prognosis and treatment decisions and is best done with videostroboscopy. An easy way to remember how to differentiate nodules from cysts is that nodules are located in the midportion of the musculomembranous fold, are bilaterally symmetric, and generally do not affect the mucosal wave, whereas cysts are usually unilateral and abolish the mucosal wave at the site of the cyst. Cysts can be located anywhere on the vocal fold.

◆ Summary: The Effect of Nodules on Vocal Fold Vibratory Characteristics

- Nodules are due to phonotrauma.
- Nodules are bilateral, symmetric, and located in the mid-membranous portion of the vocal fold.
- The mucosal wave is normal with nodules or slightly dampened if the nodules are particularly fibrotic.
- The nodules result in an hourglass glottic configuration.

- The amplitude of vibration will be decreased secondary to the open glottic configuration and the mass of the nodules on the folds.
- If the nodules are symmetric, there is normal symmetric vibration. If the nodules are asymmetric, there may be asymmetry of vibration.

References

1. Dikkers FG, Schutte HK. Benign lesions of the vocal folds: uniformity in assessment of clinical diagnosis. Clin Otolaryngol Allied Sci 1991;16:8–11
2. Rosen CA, Murry T. Nomenclature of voice disorders and vocal pathology. Otolaryngol Clin North Am 2000;33: 1035–1046
3. Rubin JS, Yanagisawa E. Benign vocal fold pathology through the eyes of the laryngologist. In: Rubin JS, Sataloff RT, Korovin GS, eds. Diagnosis and Treatment of Voice Disorders, 2nd ed. Clifton Park, NY: Thomson Delmar Learning; 2003:69–86
4. Woo P, Colton R, Casper J, Brewer D. Diagnostic value of stroboscopic examination in hoarse patients. J Voice 1991;5:231–238
5. Chau HN, Desai K, Georgalas C, Harries M. Variability in nomenclature of benign laryngeal pathology based on video laryngoscopy with and without stroboscopy. Clin Otolaryngol 2005;30:424–427
6. Kleinsasser O. Microlaryngoscopic and histologic appearances of polyps, nodules, cysts, Reinke's edema, and granulomas of the vocal cords. In: Vocal Fold Histopathology, a Symposium. San Diego, CA: College Hill Press; 1986:51–56
7. Alberti PW. The diagnostic role of laryngeal stroboscopy. Otolaryngol Clin North Am 1978;11:347–354
8. Sataloff RT, Hawkshaw MJ. Common medical diagnoses in voice patients: an overview. In: Benninger MS, ed. Benign Disorders of the Voice. Alexandria, VA: American Academy of Otolaryngology—Head and Neck Surgery Foundation, Inc.; 1996:45–71
9. Sataloff RT, Spiegel JR, Hawkshaw MJ. Strobovideolaryngoscopy: results and clinical value. Ann Otol Rhinol Laryngol 1991;100(9 Pt 1):725–727

22

Vocal Fold Polyps and Cysts

Kenneth W. Altman and Melin Tan-Geller

Vocal fold polyps and cysts are considered vocal masses because they add weight and may displace the existing microanatomy. As such, these masses have a direct effect on the vibrating margin, so video or digital stroboscopy is especially helpful in characterizing these lesions. Although the terms *polyp* and *cyst* imply different types of lesions, there is actually a continuum of vocal fold masses with overlap in features between these lesions in some cases.[1] Both types of lesions may be associated with intracordal scarring (within the lamina propria), sulcus deformities (epithelial indentations or defects bridging superficial to the deeper layers of the vocal fold microanatomy), as well as reactive callus or hyperkeratosis on the contralateral vocal fold. In this latter situation, bilateral lesions may initially appear as "nodules" if one were not to have the benefit of stroboscopy. Therefore, an understanding of the pathogenesis of these lesions and an understanding of typical findings on stroboscopy will improve accuracy of diagnosis, surgical planning, and ultimately prognosis to treatment.

◆ Pathogenesis of Polyps and Cysts

Both polyps and cysts are believed to have similar initiating factors involving mucosal injury due to a multiple of factors, although they are believed to have different final steps in their pathogenesis. Vocal overuse and misuse are central to the development of vocal fold masses. This initial trauma is exacerbated by baseline inflammation often caused by laryngopharyngeal reflux. Another source of baseline inflammation may be sinonasal or pulmonary diseases. The resulting mucosal injury leads to increased shearing forces at the midportion of the membranous vocal fold, which is the most common site of vocal fold polyps and cysts.[2] In many cases, the presence of the mass causes impaired glottic closure during phonation resulting in excess air egress, so there is a tendency for the patient to compensate for resulting voice limitations with hyperfunctional voice behavior.[3] This maladaptation further increases shear and prevents the natural healing process.

In the case of *vocal fold polyps*, it is believed that capillary hemorrhage in the superficial lamina propria leads to extravasation of blood, resultant local edema, and ultimate organization with hyalinized stroma.[4] Pathologically, polyps are acellular, with thickened epithelium over superficial lamina propria, and increased vascularity in an abundant delicate fibrin stromal matrix. They have more vasculature and less organized collagen than do nodules, but the distinction may be difficult for the pathologist.[4] Immunohistochemistry studies reveal clustered fibronectin and disruption of laminar pattern suggesting diffuse injury in the region of the polyp.[5]

The resulting mass may be broad-based (sessile) or pedunculated (fusiform) and hemorrhagic versus nonhemorrhagic (**Fig. 22.1**). Hemorrhagic polyps may also have an associated blood vessel or varix. Though the gross appearance may vary, the lesion is generally considered to be an out-pouching of inflamed and organized Reinke's space. Therefore, a superficial nonhemorrhagic, broad-based polyp may be interpreted as a pseudocyst, as a true cyst has an intact epithelial lining.

Vocal fold cysts are subepidermal epithelial-lined sacs located within the lamina propria and may be mucus retention or epidermoid in origin (**Fig. 22.2**). Mucus-retention cysts form when a mucous gland duct becomes obstructed (usually during an upper respiratory infection or with overuse), retaining glandular secretions. Epidermoid cysts develop either from congenital cell rests in the subepithelium (from the 4th and 6th branchial arches) or from healing injured mucosa burying epithelium. A ruptured cyst may result in scarring within the lamina propria or in a sulcus. Varices are also often associated with vocal cysts.

◆ Indications and Usefulness of Stroboscopy

As one may infer from the discussion above, a two-dimensional picture of the vocal folds is not sufficient to characterize features that may be used to distinguish polyps from cysts. Transoral mirror evaluation and traditional indirect laryngoscopy may recognize a vocal fold mass, but the displacement of normal architecture in the vocal fold microanatomy lends itself to characteristic stroboscopic findings in the two lesions.[6] Therefore, in addition to the use of traditional indirect laryngoscopy to visualize the larynx, stroboscopy is uniquely useful and indicated to characterize a lesion and its relationship to the layered microanatomy of the vocal fold and to help determine the etiology of dysphonia in patients when a lesion, or cause, is not apparent.

As these masses have distinct histology, the prognosis is different, and the best treatment is also different. Treatment modalities may include behavioral, medical, surgical, or office-based procedures. For example, a hemorrhagic vocal polyp with associated varix may be amenable to an office-based angiolytic laser treatment, sparing an epithelial dissection and potentially facilitating recovery of the voice.[7] A vocal polyp may be amenable to resolution with strict voice rest and behavior modification in selected individuals.[8] Conversely, a true cyst will not resolve with conservative management.

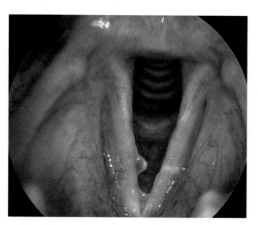

Fig. 22.1 A broad-based sessile polyp with subtle hemorrhagic component on the right vocal fold. Note that signs of posterior inflammation and thick dry mucus from laryngopharyngeal reflux pay tribute to multifactorial contributions to the pathogenesis of the polyp.

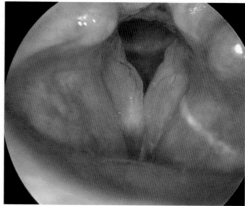

Fig. 22.2 A right vocal fold mucus inclusion cyst. Note that these vocal folds are markedly edematous consistent with polypoid corditis (Reinke's edema), which often occurs as a result of chronic irritation/inflammation.

The phonosurgical approach for cyst removal requires more extensive dissection than does that with a polyp, as the cyst is in the submucosal plane. The cyst may also be associated with intracordal scarring, requiring a more elaborate dissection. Consequently, recovery of the mucosal wave is prolonged and may never return to being completely normal. Furthermore, leaving behind a minute fragment of epithelium in the cyst sac may result in recurrence of the cyst.[9] In a large series of patients, Sataloff et al. recognized the usefulness of videostroboscopy to help distinguish between polyps and cysts and thus improve surgical planning and preoperative patient counseling.[10]

◆ Interpretation: Impact of Polyps and Cysts on Vibratory Parameters

As discussed elsewhere in this text, stroboscopy features may help distinguish polyps from cysts. These features include glottic configuration, amplitude of vibration, mucosal wave phase (closed, open, irregular, hourglass, anterior/posterior chink), mucosal wave symmetry/asymmetry, and periodicity (regular, irregular). Common to both lesions is the impact of the mass on the linearity of the vocal fold, which often results in premature contact at the site of the lesion and subsequently an hourglass or irregular glottic configuration on phonation.

Vocal folds with small *polyps* generally have intact mucosal waves but phase asymmetry due to the impaired phase closure and the mass effect of the polyp (**Video Clips 23 and 46**). Vocal folds with larger polyps may have increased mucosal wave amplitude due to a shearing effect tethering a pedunculated polyp to the normal adjacent mucosa or decreased amplitude due to overwhelming mass effect. As polyps are asymmetric masses of the vocal folds, they are more prone to result in chaotic vibrations and aperiodic mucosal waves.[11] Examples of vocal polyps and their impact on vibratory patterns seen on stroboscopy are shown and discussed in **Figs. 22.3 to 22.6**.

A

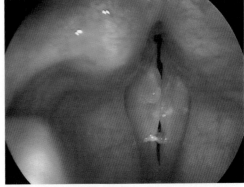

B

C

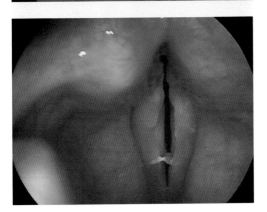

Fig. 22.3 (A) Small pedunculated hemorrhagic polyp involving the medial margin of the left vocal fold, seen on abduction and associated with left sulcus vergeture and tight contact irritation. **(B)** Small pedunculated hemorrhagic polyp involving the medial margin of the left vocal fold seen during phonation showing the mass effect limiting phase closure. **(C)** Small pedunculated hemorrhagic polyp involving the medial margin of the left vocal fold seen during late-phase closure on stroboscopy demonstrating intact left vocal fold mucosal wave. Note the area of contact irritation on the right vocal fold now shows a small area of hyperkeratosis at the inferior margin of the vocal fold striking zone that is apparent only on stroboscopy because the mucosal wave allows visualization of the inferior margin.

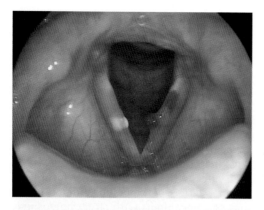

A

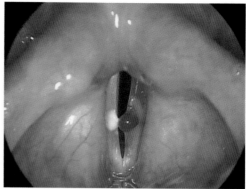

B

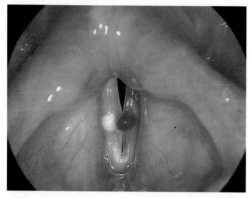

C

Fig. 22.4 (A) Left vocal fold hemorrhagic polyp associated with varices and active vocal fold hemorrhage, seen on abduction. **(B)** Early contact of the polyp with the contralateral vocal fold seen on stroboscopy. **(C)** Late-phase closure of the vocal folds in the case of left vocal fold hemorrhagic polyp. Note that the presence of an intact mucosal wave bilaterally permits the rotation of the polyp superiorly to allow for improved (yet compromised) phase closure on phonation.

The history of a patient with a vocal *cyst* is similar to those of patients with nodules and polyps, but often with less vocal limitation than expected from its size. The voice may sound diplophonic (particularly with epidermoid cysts), where there is great pitch instability and there is splitting of the fundamental frequency overtones.

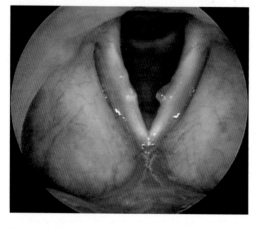

A

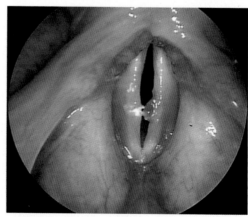

B

Fig. 22.5 (A) Left vocal fold oblong sessile polyp, seen on abduction, with a contralateral (right) reactive callus. **(B)** Early phase closure on phonation demonstrating the typical but irregular hourglass closure in a case of left vocal fold oblong sessile polyp.

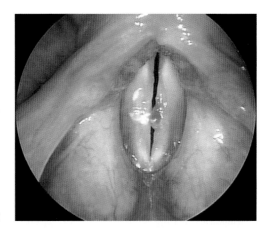

C

Fig. 22.5 (*Continued*) **(C)** Later phase closure seen on stroboscopy with compression of the polyp by the vocal folds. Note that there is poor excursion of the mucosal wave (with decreased amplitude) on both vocal folds associated with chronic inflammation and possible intracordal scarring.

Though it is often possible to distinguish some cysts solely by still-light endoscopy, visualizations of the outline of the cyst, associated capillary patterns, and characteristic changes in the edge or free margin are not always present. On stroboscopy, the vocal folds appear asymmetric with occasional evidence of the subepithelial mass. The free edges of the vocal folds are generally smooth.[12]

Due to displacement of the lamina propria and the fibrosis that frequently occurs around vocal fold cysts, there is a significant

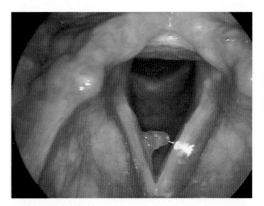

A

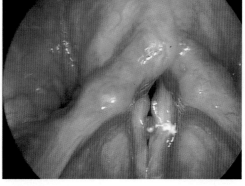

B

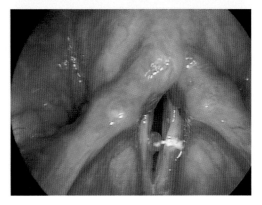

C

Fig. 22.6 (A) Right lobulated polyp with broad-based edema at the vocal fold margin, seen on abduction. **(B)** Initial phase of closure with deformity of the vibratory margin at the site of the lobulated polyp, resulting in the appearance of good phase closure. **(C)** However, the trailing edge of the intact mucosal wave (particularly on the left vocal fold) reveals the impaired closure and reduced right mucosal wave secondary to the mass effect of the polyp.

decreased or absent mucosal wave on the side of the cyst (**Video Clip 26**). Whereas vocal fold polyps have intact mucosal waves in 80% of all cases, Shohet et al. demonstrated the mucosal wave to be diminished or absent in 100% of vocal fold cysts.[13] This can be explained by changes in the elastic coefficient of the lamina propria surrounding the cyst.[14] If light reflection indicates an intact mucosal wave, the vocal fold with a cyst will not reflect light. In contrast with a polyp, a cyst would have a dynamic segment of mucosa adjacent to the cyst, lacking reflected light, with an intact mucosal wave over the contralateral cord-corresponding segment.[13] The amplitude and vibration of the wave are also diminished and absent.[9] Examples of vocal cysts and their impact on vibratory patterns seen on stroboscopy are shown and discussed in **Figs. 22.7 to 22.10**.

◆ Pearls and Pitfalls in the Diagnosis of Polyps and Cysts on Stroboscopy

The general *pearls* that may be assumed from the above discussion follow:

1. Polyps are out-pouchings of Reinke's space, may be pedunculated (fusiform) or broad-based (sessile), and may or may not show signs of hemorrhage.
2. Cysts are epithelial-lined sacs within Reinke's space and may be mucus or epidermoid related.
3. Polyps and cysts result in an hourglass or irregular vocal fold glottic configuration on phonation.
4. The amplitude of the mucosal wave is generally decreased with vocal cysts, whereas

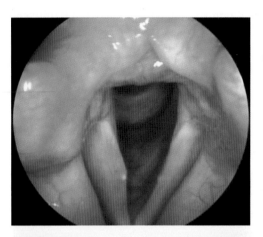

A

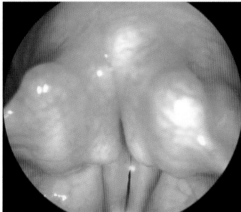

B

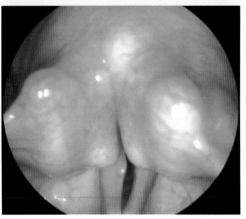

C

Fig. 22.7 **(A)** Right vocal fold cyst, seen on abduction. Although there is not a discrete submucosal mass seen, the appearance of a focal submucosal fullness is a clue to the underlying cyst. **(B)** Initial contact of the vibratory margin on stroboscopy reveals irregular closure and premature contact at the apex of the cyst. **(C)** Later phase closure reveals an intact mucosal wave on the left vocal fold with significantly reduced mucosal wave on the right.

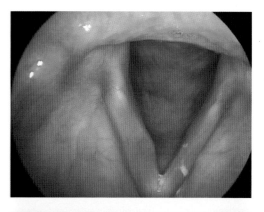

A

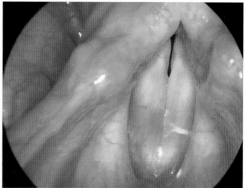

B

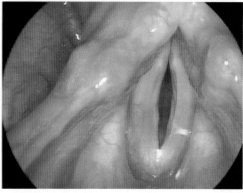

C

Fig. 22.8 **(A)** Subtle right vocal fold cyst, seen on abduction with associated hyperemia. **(B)** There is the initial appearance of linear vocal fold closure with only a minor posterior chink with subtle right vocal fold cyst. **(C)** Later phase vocal fold vibration seen on stroboscopy reveals decreased to absent right mucosal wave, intact left mucosal wave, and more obvious right submucosal contour consistent with the cyst. This is a particularly good example of how a subtle lesion may be missed on still-light two-dimensional endoscopy in the absence of stroboscopy.

it is generally normal or increased with vocal fold polyps.

5. The amplitude of vibration will likely be decreased secondary to the mass of the lesion combined with an incomplete glottic closure.

6. Vocal fold vibration will likely be asymmetric and possibly aperiodic.

Despite these pearls, there are pitfalls in the use of stroboscopy to distinguish vocal fold

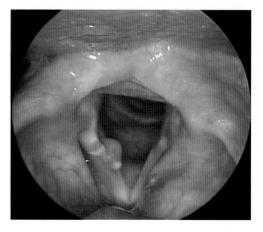

A

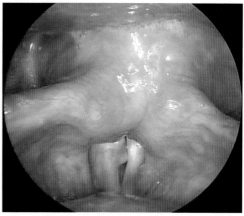

B

Fig. 22.9 **(A)** Large right posterior vocal fold mucus inclusion cyst with hemosiderin deposition superficially (seen as yellow spot) suggestive of prior hemorrhage, seen on abduction. **(B)** Early glottal closure is noted to be poor due to the mass effect of the cysts. (*Continued on page 198*)

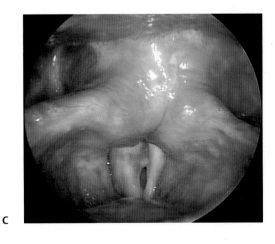

C

Fig. 22.9 (*Continued*) **(C)** Intact left vocal fold mucosal wave with absent mucosal wave on the right, despite the posterior location of the cyst.

polyps from cysts or other lesions. The presence of a polyp or cyst may cause a reactive lesion, or "callus," on the contralateral vocal fold secondary to contact irritation. A unilateral lesion with reactive callus formation may look like bilateral lesions, in other words nodules, which may confound the diagnosis, prognosis, and ultimate management. Also, though the glottic closure of the vocal folds with cysts may often be complete (for example), it depends on the cyst size and whether there is development of the callus on the contralateral vocal fold (**Video Clip 26**).

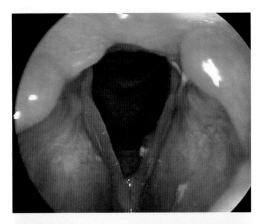

A

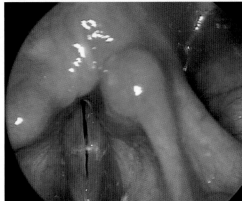

B

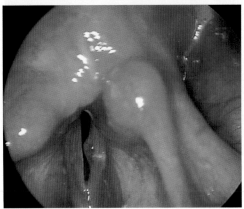

C

Fig. 22.10 (A) Left submucosal cyst with hemorrhage in a patient with severe chronic laryngitis (manifested by edematous and erythematous vocal folds, stagnant secretions, and interarytenoid inflammation), seen on abduction. **(B)** Early phase closure demonstrates only a small margin of the cyst caught tangentially on a vertical plane. **(C)** Intact (but decreased) left mucosal wave reveals eversion of the cyst on late phase closure during phonation, seen on stroboscopy. This example clearly demonstrates that the hemorrhagic component is within the superficial mucosa overlying the cyst and not within the cyst itself.

Rosen et al. evaluated a series of 85 patients with bilateral vocal fold lesions and found 21 to have nodules and 64 to have a unilateral vocal fold lesion with a contralateral reactive lesion (UVFL/RL).[15] When comparing patients with nodules and those with UVFL/RL, they found statistically significant differences in (1) symmetry of vocal fold vibration, (2) amplitude perturbations, (3) estimated subglottic pressure, and (4) voice handicap index, suggesting that these parameters be used as tools to differentiate nodules from UVFL/RL.

Repeated inflammation, vocal trauma, vocal hemorrhage, and the presence of an intracordal cyst predispose to scarring in Reinke's space. Intracordal scarring is often found in association with a cyst, particularly if it is epidermoid in origin and has ruptured. Intracordal scarring is suspected on stroboscopy when there is markedly reduced or absent mucosal wave (usually asymmetric) that often affects phase closure (**Video Clip 33**). It is crucial to differentiate between an uncomplicated subepithelial cyst and an intracordal scar, as the latter is a more complex problem with worse prognosis for voice rehabilitation. With these factors in mind, the typical "pearls" used to distinguish polyps from cysts on stroboscopy have understandable limitations. Nevertheless, the utility of stroboscopy in appropriate diagnosis, patient counseling, and treatment intervention is vital to obtaining the best outcome.

References

1. Altman KW. Vocal fold masses. Otolaryngol Clin North Am 2007;40:1091–1108, viii
2. Jiang JJ, Diaz CE, Hanson DG. Finite element modeling of vocal fold vibration in normal phonation and hyperfunctional dysphonia: implications for the pathogenesis of vocal nodules. Ann Otol Rhinol Laryngol 1998;107:603–610
3. Altman KW, Atkinson C, Lazarus C. Current and emerging concepts in muscle tension dysphonia: a 30-month review. J Voice 2005;19:261–267
4. Kotby MN, Nassar AM, Seif EI, Helal EH, Saleh MM. Ultrastructural features of vocal fold nodules and polyps. Acta Otolaryngol 1988;105:477–482
5. Courey MS, Shohet JA, Scott MA, Ossoff RH. Immuno-histochemical characterization of benign laryngeal lesions. Ann Otol Rhinol Laryngol 1996;105:525–531
6. Hirano M. Surgical Anatomy and Physiology of the Vocal Folds. Chicago, IL: Mosby-Year Book; 1993:125–158
7. Ivey CM, Woo P, Altman KW, Shapshay SM. Office pulsed dye laser treatment for benign laryngeal vascular polyps: a preliminary study. Ann Otol Rhinol Laryngol 2008;117:353–358
8. Srirompotong S, Saeseow P, Vatanasapt P. Small vocal cord polyps: completely resolved with conservative treatment. Southeast Asian J Trop Med Public Health 2004;35:169–171
9. Johns MM. Update on the etiology, diagnosis, and treatment of vocal fold nodules, polyps, and cysts. Curr Opin Otolaryngol Head Neck Surg 2003;11:456–461
10. Sataloff RT, Spiegel JR, Hawkshaw MJ. Strobovideo-laryngoscopy: results and clinical value. Ann Otol Rhinol Laryngol 1991;100(9 Pt 1):725–727
11. Zhang Y, Jiang JJ. Chaotic vibrations of a vocal fold model with a unilateral polyp. J Acoust Soc Am 2004;115:1266–1269
12. Bouchayer M, Cornut G, Witzig E, Loire R, Roch JB, Bastian RW. Epidermoid cysts, sulci, and mucosal bridges of the true vocal cord: a report of 157 cases. Laryngoscope 1985;95(9 Pt 1):1087–1094
13. Shohet JA, Courey MS, Scott MA, Ossoff RH. Value of videostroboscopic parameters in differentiating true vocal fold cysts from polyps. Laryngoscope 1996;106(1 Pt 1):19–26
14. Loire R, Bouchayer M, Cornut G, Bastian RW. Pathology of benign vocal fold lesions. Ear Nose Throat J 1988;67:357–358, 360–362
15. Rosen CA, Lombard LE, Murry T. Acoustic, aerodynamic, and videostroboscopic features of bilateral vocal fold lesions. Ann Otol Rhinol Laryngol 2000;109:823–828

23

Laryngeal Inflammation

Natasha Mirza, Cesar Ruiz, and Katherine A. Kendall

Laryngitis, meaning inflammation of the larynx, is one of the most common conditions involving the larynx and occurs in both an acute and a chronic form. Acute laryngitis has an abrupt onset and is usually self-limited. The etiology of acute laryngitis includes exposure to noxious inhaled agents or infectious agents associated with upper respiratory tract infections. The infectious agents are most often viral but are sometimes bacterial (**Fig. 23.1**). When the etiology of acute laryngitis is infectious, white blood cells remove microorganisms during the healing process.

If a patient has symptoms of laryngitis for more than 3 weeks, the condition is classified as chronic laryngitis. Chronic laryngitis may be caused by environmental factors such as inhalation of cigarette smoke or polluted air (eg, gaseous chemicals), irritation from asthma inhalers, vocal misuse (eg, prolonged vocal use at abnormal loudness or pitch), or gastroesophageal reflux diseasse.[1-5] Rarely, laryngeal inflammation results from autoimmune conditions such as rheumatoid arthritis, relapsing polychondritis, Wegener's granulomatosis, or sarcoidosis (**Fig. 23.2**).

Laryngitis causes the patient to experience dysphonia or a hoarse voice. A hoarse voice is defined as one that demonstrates roughness, breathiness, and tension.[6] These symptoms can

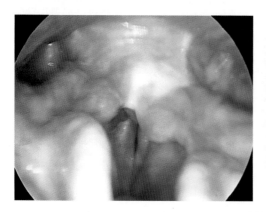

Fig. 23.1 Acute laryngitis. Note edema and erythema of the true vocal folds.

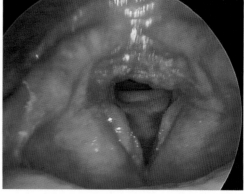

Fig. 23.2 Chronic laryngitis. Vocal folds are thickened and edematous with erythema.

result from a multitude of causes, however, and are not specific for acute or chronic laryngitis. Though usually self-limited, acute laryngeal inflammation leads to poor voice production secondary to the edema of the vocal fold tissues. Ng et al. found that fundamental frequency values were lower in patients with acute laryngitis than in patients with a normal voice.[6] The lowered pitch in patients with laryngitis is a result of irregular thickening of the tissues due to swelling along the entire length of the vocal fold.[7–9] Edema leads to an increase in vocal fold mass that results in a decrease in the frequency of vibration.

The thickening and edema of the vocal folds in acute laryngitis make the vocal fold cover stiff and more difficult to set into vibration. Phonation requires greater vocal fold adduction forces or tension and subsequent increases in subglottal pressure to overcome the increase in vocal fold stiffness. The phonation threshold pressure may increase to a degree that generating adequate phonation pressures in a normal fashion becomes difficult. Frank aphonia results when a patient cannot overcome the phonation threshold pressure required to set the vocal folds into motion. Increasing vocal fold adduction forces or tension further negatively impacts voice production, causing more injury to the vocal fold tissues and ultimately delaying recovery and a return to normal phonation.

◆ Pathophysiology

During the early stages of inflammation, the vascular endothelium becomes "leaky." This disruption of the blood vessels allows serum and other factors to leak into the lamina propria. The normal blood flow is altered at the site of injury. Other cells migrate to the site in response to locally released inflammatory factors. Clinically, acute inflammation results in vocal fold edema and erythema (**Figs. 23.1 and 23.2**).

Once acute inflammation occurs, three phases of vocal fold healing must be considered.[10] Recovery from an acute inflammatory injury begins as fibroblasts secrete new materials into the tissue injury site. Fibroblasts produce various extracellular matrix components including collagen, elastin, glycosaminoglycan, and proteoglycans. The appropriate combination of these components is important to maintain the viscoelastic shear property of the vocal folds. Any changes to the amount and configuration of any of these components results in decreased vocal fold pliability, thus altering vocal fold vibration. Hyaluronic acid, which is widely distributed in the superficial layer of the lamina propria, is essential to maintaining the viscosity of the vocal fold. Studies of this molecule have shown that it may be able to modulate scarless healing, implying that it has potential as a treatment designed to reduce scarring during the early recovery stages of vocal fold injury.[11,12]

Deposition of scar tissue is the second stage of healing, followed by wound contracture. As with wounds in other parts of the body, vocal fold scarring is seen as the end result of both acute and chronic inflammation. In cases of excessive collagen deposition, scarring causes a severe disturbance of vocal fold vibration resulting in considerable dysphonia. Sometimes, scarring is severe enough to cause outright fixation of the mucosa to deeper tissues. Once the vocal fold is scarred, the layered structure of the lamina propria is disrupted, and the mucosal vibratory properties are changed. Altered vocal fold vibration—depending on severity and extent—can cause a range of symptoms such as hoarseness, breathy voice, increased effort to speak, and voice fatigue.

◆ Examination

The diagnosis of laryngeal inflammation is based on a laryngoscopy. To fully characterize the exact nature of vocal fold injury secondary to inflammation, a more detailed evaluation is necessary with the help of a videostroboscopic exam. Videostroboscopy plays an essential role in the assessment of the elasticity, viscosity, volume, and tension of the vocal folds. For periodic vibration to occur, the mechanical properties of the vocal folds and the subglottic pressure must be in equilibrium. The superficial lamina propria, a loosely packed network of fibers that functions like a ball-bearing layer, allows the mucosa on top to be flexible and not tightly attached to the deeper tissues. For normal vibration to occur, the superficial lamina propria must be healthy.[13–16]

In inflammation, however, edema and cellular infiltration of the superficial lamina propria cause changes in the mechanical properties of the tissue that negatively affect vocal fold vibration. In general, videostroboscopic analysis of laryngitis reveals aperiodicity, vibratory asymmetry, decreased amplitude of vibration, and incomplete glottic closure with glottal gap and amplitude of vibration being most effected (**Video Clips 37 and 47**).

Glottic Configuration

The early stages of vocal fold inflammation are remarkable for edematous changes and thickening of the lamina propria. The inflammatory changes may compromise arytenoid approximation resulting in reduced vocal fold adduction. That, along with the irregular vocal fold margins, results in a glottic gap that allows air to escape, decreasing vocal loudness. Individuals who have a great demand for voice production will attempt to overcompensate by using the extrinsic laryngeal muscles to increase vocal fold adduction. This strategy usually results in an asymmetric approximation where only portions of the vocal folds make contact. The contact areas receive all the impact during phonation causing further localized tissue trauma and may result in the development of vocal nodules and polyps.[17]

Phase Characteristics and Vibration Amplitude

Inflammation of the vocal folds has been shown to increase the mean closed quotient, which is defined as the ratio of the closed phase to the pitch. The main perceptual correlate of an increase of the closed quotient is the need for increased pressure, in other words, a pressed voice. An increased closed quotient has been associated with a lower fundamental frequency, abnormal jitter and shimmer, decreased phonation time, abnormal harmonic to noise ratio, lower amplitude of vibration, and aperiodicity. Correlation analysis has demonstrated that these vocal parameters improved as the mean closed quotient decreased.[18]

Inflammation that is limited to the posterior part of the larynx may have the opposite effect (ie, an increase in the open quotient),

which is defined as the ratio of the open phase to the pitch. The open quotient is associated with increased breathiness and a decrease in vocal intensity.[19]

A unilateral or, more often bilateral, decrease of vibration amplitude is also noted with inflammation of the vocal folds secondary to the increase in mass and stiffness of the tissues.[20,21]

Mucosal Wave

In laryngitis, the propagation of the mucosal wave is reduced. Changes in the mucosal wave occur if the inflammation extends below the level of the vocal fold basement membrane, extending into the superficial lamina propria, leading to irregular swelling of the vocal folds and reducing the mobility of the overlying vocal fold cover. Ng et al. described the mucosal wave in laryngitis as appearing to have two distinct velocities of travel. The wave travels at one speed on the surface of the vocal fold, but, at a discrete point, it changes its speed of travel.[6] This finding was also described by Colton et al.[22] Possible mechanisms for this phenomena are the asymmetry of vocal folds, the desynchronization of vertical and horizontal vibration within and between the vocal folds, the coupling with other laryngeal oscillators in the subglottal and supraglottal airway, and the need to alter the airflow during phonation[22–25]

In summary, inflammation of the vocal folds causes irregular and/or reduced vibration that is further characterized on videostroboscopy by a decreased amplitude of vibration, a decrease in the mucosal wave, asymmetric vibration, and irregular glottic configuration with a lowering of the fundamental frequency. An understanding of how inflammatory pathophysiology affects vocal folds structures explains these findings. Two studies are cited here as clinical examples of how laryngeal inflammation from various causes impacts vibratory characteristics.

In a study of laryngeal tuberculosis by Agarwal and Bais, videostroboscopy revealed asymmetry of vocal fold vibration, a decrease in the amplitude of horizontal excursion of the vocal fold, a decreased mucosal wave, and aperiodic vibration on the affected side. In cases where generalized edema and an increase in thickness of the lamina propria of both vocal folds were found, the vibratory movements were symmetric but with decreased amplitude. If the inflammatory changes resulted in irregular scarring of the vocal folds, then the amplitude of vibration was absent or significantly reduced around the lesions.[26]

In a study of patients with chronic laryngitis secondary to asthma inhaler use, Mirza et al. found evidence of vascular dilation including varices and small areas of hemorrhage on laryngeal examination. The margins of the vocal folds also demonstrated areas of thickening and leukoplakia. Videostroboscopy demonstrated a decrease in vibration amplitude and a decrease in the mucosal wave.[5]

Reinke's Edema

Reinke's edema of the vocal folds is a special form of chronic hyperplastic laryngitis characterized by the collection of edema fluids directly under the vocal fold epithelium (**Fig. 23.3**). The stroma is hyalinized and thickened. The voice, which has a pressed quality, is harsh or breathy and has an exceptionally low pitch. On stroboscopy there is phase asymmetry because of impaired closure due to the irregular vocal fold margins and a mass effect (**Video Clip 36**). The shape of the glottic closure is irregular because of early contact of the irregular hyperplastic mucosa. The closed phase of the vibratory cycle is relatively long. The mucosal wave shows a decrease in amplitude.[27]

Leukoplakia and Pachydermia

Chronic irritation from long-standing inflammation can lead to leukoplakia and pachydermia consisting of hyperplasia of the epithelial layer of the vocal folds and greater hornification in the top layers of the epithelium. The ability of the vocal folds to vibrate is directly related to the thickness of the epithelium: the thicker and stiffer the epithelium, the more restricted the mobility of the vocal fold edges, resulting in a reduction of the ability of the vocal folds to vibrate. The voice is characterized by low pitch and a harsh or breathy quality (**Fig. 23.4**).[4]

Scarring

Scarring makes the vocal folds stiff. Stiff vocal folds need the generation of greater subglottal pressure to set them into vibration. Hence, patients with scarring in one or both vocal folds usually complain of increased effort with phonation and therefore voice fatigue. The scarred area is also slower to heal with each additional inflammatory insult. Scarring at the inferior (bottom) edge of the closing (striking) surface of the vocal folds is harder to detect. Usually the superior (top) edge of the closing surface can and will compensate. With increasing scar extent or severity, loss of vocal fold pliability increases, thus hampering additional phases of the vibratory cycle—and resulting in more severe voice symptoms (**Fig. 23.5**; **Video Clip 33**).[28]

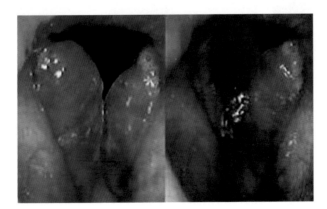

Fig. 23.3 Reinke's edema characterized by the collection of a thickened stromal fluid within the lamina propria. The vocal fold mass increases and the voice becomes lower in pitch.

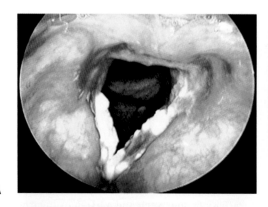

A

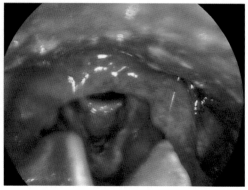

B

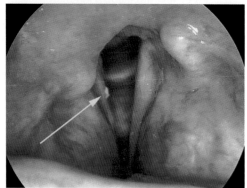

C

Fig. 23.4 (A) Leukoplakia of the vocal folds. The epithelium is thickened and keratinized. (B) Leukoplakia may be associated with erythema of the vocal folds. This lesion was biopsied, and histologic evaluation revealed carcinoma in situ. (C) The *arrow* points to a small area of leukoplakia that was identified adjacent to the resection margin of a region of carcinoma in situ. The lesion may represent recurrence at the margin of the resection.

Glottal Sulcus

The etiology of glottal sulcus is unknown but theoretically occurs at the site of a vocal fold injury or chronic inflammation. If this occurs over

the medial surface of the vocal fold, it results in a groove or infolding of mucosa (**Fig. 23.6**). In the area of the sulcus, the mucosa is tethered down to the underlying vocal ligament, giving it a retracted, tethered appearance. The mucosal cover may fibrose to the vocal ligament and results in a diminished or absent mucosal wave at the location of the sulcus. This decreased pliability restricts the Bernoulli and vocal fold

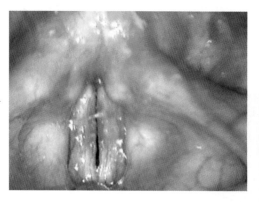

Fig. 23.5 Mild scarring of the vocal folds may be difficult to detect on examination with a constant light source. Videostroboscopy reveals a decrease in the amplitude of vibration, a decrease in the mucosal wave, and, in this case, a persistent glottic gap and irregular vocal fold margin.

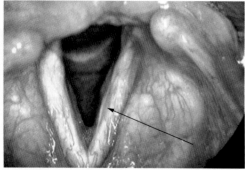

Fig. 23.6 Glottic sulcus may appear as a groove along the margin of the vocal fold as demonstrated at the tip of the *arrow* in this image.

myoelastic effects, whereby transglottic airflow medializes the leading edge of the vocal fold during vibration. The overall effect usually is a higher fundamental frequency with significantly reduced harmonics and harsher voice quality. There is also a defect in the medial surface of the true vocal fold along the sulcus that may produce a glottic gap. Videostroboscopy is an important tool used by the laryngologist to reveal linear depressions or areas of incomplete closure and areas of decreased mucosal wave corresponding with the sulcus.[29]

Reflux

Understanding the influence of laryngopharyngeal reflux on laryngeal inflammation and hence on the vibratory characteristics of the vocal folds is complicated due to inconsistencies in diagnosis. The gold standard for making a diagnosis of laryngopharyngeal reflux (LPR) disease is 24-hour dual-channel pH monitoring, wherein one sensor is placed in the esophagus and the other is placed just above the upper esophageal sphincter (UES). The incidence and duration of acidic conditions in the pharynx during a 24-hour period can thus be determined. Although 24-hour pH probe studies are considered to be very specific for the diagnosis of reflux, they are not considered to be sensitive and may fail to identify patients suffering from reflux episodes that occur less frequently than every 24 hours. In addition, the clinical reproducibility of the test has not been established. Furthermore, this technology is still not widely available, and many clinicians continue to make a diagnosis of LPR disease based on a combination of symptoms and examination findings along with the response to empiric treatment with proton pump inhibitors. Considerable controversy exists, however, on the reliability of using the signs of laryngeal inflammation, without pH study confirmation, to make a diagnosis of LPR disease.[4,30-38] Physical findings seen on laryngeal imaging that are commonly believed to be associated with LPR disease include increased interarytenoid or posterior glottic inflammation or erythema, hypertrophy of the posterior commissure (cobblestoning), vocal fold edema and erythema, vocal fold vascularity, and mucus accumulation (**Figs. 23.7 to 23.9**).

Complicating the issue of making a diagnosis of LPR disease on laryngeal imaging is the fact that there is poor reliability among clinicians regarding the ability to rate the visual criteria required to make a diagnosis of LPR disease. Branski et al. conducted a blinded study in

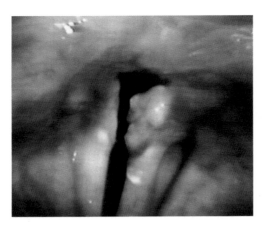

Fig. 23.7 This figure demonstrates some of the findings considered to be the result of gastroesophageal reflux disease: erythema of the mucosa over the arytenoid cartilages and the development of granulation tissue on the left arytenoid vocal process.

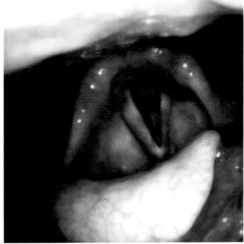

Fig. 23.8 One of the most common findings thought to be consistent with reflux disease: erythema of the mucosa overlying the arytenoid cartilages.

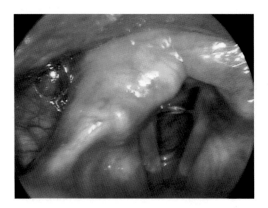

Fig. 23.9 This image demonstrates increased mucus collecting on the vocal folds and erythema of the true vocal folds in addition to erythema of the mucosa overlying the arytenoid cartilages. The arytenoid mucosa may also be edematous with evidence of edema of the tissues adjacent to the vocal process of the arytenoid cartilages. These findings are consistent with laryngeal inflammation that might be secondary to gastroesophageal reflux disease.

which five otolaryngologists reviewed the videostroboscopy studies from 100 consecutive patients presenting with voice complaints and rated signs of reflux disease. Interrater reliability was poor, in particular with respect to the degree of pachydermia, the overall severity of LPR findings, and the likelihood that LPR was contributing to the patient's symptoms. Raters were most likely to agree on the degree of involvement of the membranous vocal folds and were least likely to agree on the degree of involvement of the arytenoid cartilages. Only one rater was able to demonstrate consistent interrater reliability for the findings of reflux disease on examination.[39] The results from a study of 105 asymptomatic volunteers by Hicks et al. were somewhat better, with good intrarater agreement found between three raters for interarytenoid bar, arytenoid medial wall erythema, and cobblestoning. Like the previous study, there was "good" intrarater agreement for the finding of true vocal fold edema. However, a strong interrater agreement was not established for any of the signs rated in the study.[40]

Recently, in a study of differences in the detection of reflux-associated laryngeal signs based on imaging modality (flexible endoscope vs rigid endoscope, with or without distal chip technology), Eller et al. reported the interrater and intrarater reliability from five examiners who retrospectively evaluated both flexible and rigid exams from 34 patients. Subjects included in the study were consecutive patients presenting with voice complaints. The examiners rated the following signs: subglottic edema, ventricular obliteration, erythema, vocal fold edema, diffuse laryngeal edema, interarytenoid thickening, granuloma, thick mucus, and posterior erythema. Interrater reliability was generally higher (Cronbach $\alpha > 0.7$) when distal chip technology was used for imaging. Only the distal chip evaluation of subglottic edema and erythema had less than good intrarater reliability. Without the distal chip technology, intrarater agreement was less than 0.7 for all of the parameters except posterior erythema, which was reliable for both fiberoptic and rigid imaging. These findings might indicate that newer technologies have the potential to increase our ability to reliably evaluate these laryngeal signs. The same study, however, found that color evaluation (erythema) was more consistent when comparing flexible imaging without distal chip technology with rigid examinations than it was when comparing distal chip flexible scopes with rigid imaging.[41]

Even if good intrarater agreement could be developed, there remains a problem in that many of the signs considered indicative of LPR are, in fact, present in an asymptomatic population and are therefore not specific enough to make a diagnosis of reflux disease. In the Hicks study, 105 subjects without voice complaints were assessed. Individuals with a diagnosis of reflux disease were excluded from the study. Three evaluators blindly rated signs of reflux disease on videostroboscopy studies of the subject population. At least one tissue irritation finding was present on 86% of the asymptomatic study population. The most common findings were interarytenoid bar (70%), arytenoid medial wall erythema (29%), posterior pharyngeal wall cobblestoning (21%), interarytenoid bar erythema (15%), arytenoid medial wall granularity (13%), posterior cricoid wall edema (10%), arytenoid apex erythema (10%), and true vocal fold edema (10%). The findings of laryngeal irritation could not be correlated with a history of smoking or drinking alcohol or a diagnosis of asthma, thus excluding the possibility of secondary asymptomatic reflux as the reason for the examination findings.[40]

In another study from the same institution, the results of flexible fiberoptic examination of the larynx were compared with rigid videostroboscopy with respect to laryngeal inflammation signs in another group of asymptomatic volunteers. Unlike the study by Eller et al., this study determined that flexible laryngoscopy was more likely than rigid endoscopy to identify signs of laryngeal inflammation. The most common signs of laryngeal inflammation in this asymptomatic population were found to be abnormalities of the arytenoid complex such as erythema and edema of the arytenoid medial walls and apex (76%). Pseudosulcus, consistent with vocal fold edema, was found in 37% of the study population on flexible endoscopy.[13,41]

Despite the fact the laryngeal irritation signs are common in an asymptomatic population and there are significant reliability issues with the rating of these signs, many clinicians continue to believe that the improved image resolution of videostroboscopy makes it useful in the detection of subtle findings of chronic laryngeal irritation and that it can be used in the diagnosis of LPR disease. In a study at Baylor College of Medicine, 49 patients diagnosed with LPR disease by the combination of symptoms and physical examination findings were compared with 10 control subjects without a diagnosis of LPR disease. Photographs of the larynx from the LPR group were evaluated prior to treatment and again after 6 weeks of proton pump inhibitor therapy by three examiners. A rating scale was developed to determine a single severity value for the combined laryngeal irritation findings. Scores given to patients prior to treatment were significantly higher for irritation than those given to controls or to patients after treatment. Scores were based on a combination of ratings given for the following parameters: edema of the posterior supraglottis, edema of the vocal folds, edema of the subglottis, erythema of the posterior supraglottis, erythema of the vocal folds, and erythema of the subglottis. Findings that did not correlate with improvement after treatment include leukoplakia, nodules or prenodules, polyps, posterior pachydermia, web, or contact granuloma. Examiners did not

tend to agree, however, on absolute scoring of each region of the larynx. Despite the fact that use of a composite scoring system was able to distinguish general improvement in laryngeal inflammation, overall intrarater agreement was only moderate for this study. Only one rater was used to evaluate interrater agreement, which was found to be poor.[42]

At the time of the Baylor study, the idea of using a composite scoring system to rate laryngeal irritation signs in an attempt to improve our ability to identify patients with reflux disease and obviate the need for a pH study was not new. Belafsky et al. developed a scoring system (reflux finding score; RFS) using eight laryngeal signs thought to be associated with LPR and documented a difference in the scores from 40 patients with LPR disease confirmed by pH study compared with those from 40 normal controls. This study confirmed that patients with LPR disease have signs of laryngeal irritation (95% sensitivity); it does not, however, help to differentiate those individuals with laryngeal irritation due to reflux disease from those with laryngeal irritation due to other causes or as a normal variant because such patients were not included in the study.[43] In an independent evaluation of the RFS, Park et al. found that the RFS was positive in 80% of individuals with LPR disease confirmed by pH study but was negative in only 37.5% of patients demonstrating signs of laryngeal irritation but without LPR disease on pH study (sensitivity of 80.7% and specificity of 37.5%).[44]

In a more recent study using esophageal biopsy to establish the diagnosis of reflux disease, Pribuisiene et al. evaluated the sensitivity and specificity of their scoring system, the laryngoscopic reflux index (LRI). The study included 108 subjects. The authors excluded 19 patients from the study who presented with laryngeal inflammation but had negative esophageal biopsies, which is unfortunate because it invalidates their specificity calculations. This flaw in the study underscores the confusion regarding the usefulness of laryngeal signs in making the diagnosis of reflux disease and the importance of carefully evaluating each study that makes such claims. As in the study by Belafsky et al., the exclusion of patients with laryngeal reflux signs but no documented reflux by biopsy prevents an assessment of how often a false-positive diagnosis would be made based on the LRI alone. The authors compared the LRI from the biopsy-proven LPR subjects with those from 90 healthy controls and found a sensitivity of 96% and a specificity of 97% (falsely elevated due to patient selection factors) for the index. Although the previous studies found good interrater reliability for vocal fold erythema and edema, this study found it to be the least sensitive indicator of reflux disease.[43,45] This result is not surprising given that Hicks et al. and Qadeer et al. reported a 10% and 37% incidence of vocal fold edema in an asymptomatic population, respectively.[40,46]

It must be kept in mind that in many of the studies described, pH probe evaluations were not performed on the study population so the symptoms and laryngeal imaging findings could not be confirmed to correlate with measured acid exposure in the hypopharynx. Those studies that do correlate laryngeal signs with the results of a pH test demonstrate a poor correlation. The study by Park et al. demonstrated a 20% false-negative rate and an 63% false-positive rate in the use of laryngeal scoring compared with pH studies to determine if reflux is the etiology of patient complaints.[44] Other studies have found an even lesser degree of correlation between laryngeal findings and pH probe results. In a study of 42 patients with symptoms that were believed to be consistent with reflux disease, Noordzij et al. found only 69% to have LPR on dual-sensor pH probe study. There was no correlation between symptom severity and incidence of LPR. Signs of reflux disease were not significantly more severe in the patients with documented LPR. In fact, arytenoid edema was rated significantly worse in the group *without* documented LPR. None of the LPR signs correlated with LPR severity on pH study.[47] In the best-designed study to date, Pawar et al. conducted a prospective, randomized, placebo-controlled study of 76 patients with complaints of "post nasal drip" (considered to be a symptom of LPR disease) without evidence of nasal disease. All patients were tested with a dual-channel 24-hour pH study. The RFS was used to document laryngeal findings. Patients were then treated with either a twice-daily proton pump inhibitor or a twice-daily placebo for 3 months. The study evaluated the response of patient symptoms and RFS depending on the results of the treatment. At the outset of the study, the RFS failed to differentiate those with reflux documented on pH study (56%) from those without. Patients with and without documented reflux had a statistically significant improvement in their symptoms if treated with a proton pump inhibitor, possibly indicative of a significant placebo effect. Paradoxically, the RFS increased in the proton pump inhibitor group and decreased in the placebo group.[48]

Despite the difficulties in using laryngeal signs to make an accurate diagnosis of LPR disease, once a diagnosis of LPR disease has been made using a pH study, it may be possible to follow the response to therapy using an evaluation of laryngeal inflammation signs. Building on the results of the Baylor study, which documented improvement of laryngeal inflammation signs with the antireflux treatment, Qadeer et al. blindly evaluated the laryngeal signs on flexible laryngoscopy in 10 patients before and 1 year after successful fundoplication for the treatment of reflux disease. These patients had surgery because they did not improve on twice-daily proton pump inhibitor therapy. The most common preoperative findings in these patients included medial arytenoid wall erythema and edema (60%) and interarytenoid erythema (50%). Five of the patients had resolution of laryngeal irritation findings 6 months after the surgery, and another 3 patients had resolution of laryngeal irritation signs at 12 months after the surgery. The last two patients, who were additionally diagnosed with asthma and allergies, had improvement but not complete resolution of the laryngeal signs over the course of the study. Interestingly, the symptoms of sore or burning throat, hoarseness, and cough did not improve after surgery.[40,42,46]

In summary, although it is a common practice, the use of findings on laryngeal imaging must be done with caution to make the diagnosis of LPR disease. Even Belafsky indicated that although the irritation due to LPR usually occurs on the posterior larynx, this area makes up <5% of the entire larynx and stressed the importance of including other laryngeal irritants in the differential diagnosis in patients with significant inflammatory changes of the vocal folds.[49] Most of the emphasis regarding the signs of LPR on laryngeal imaging has been in the assessment of static signs rather than the impact of LPR on vocal fold vibratory characteristics. The degree of true vocal fold edema caused by LPR in individual cases will dictate the degree of abnormality seen on the evaluation of vocal fold vibratory characteristics. Vocal fold vibratory abnormalities caused by LPR will be consistent with the changes due to vocal fold inflammation from any cause. In a recent study, it was documented that pathologic reflux could lead to edema and hypertrophy of the laryngeal mucosa. These changes in turn interfered with phonation patterns. The most common finding was incomplete glottic closure. Other stroboscopic findings were irregularity of vocal fold vibration, asymmetry of vibration, and a reduced mucosal wave.[45]

◆ Conclusion

Laryngeal inflammation changes the composition and shape of the vibratory structures with a direct effect on vocal quality. Videostroboscopy and laryngeal image analysis are necessary to help in voice analysis and to provide in-depth information about the status of the vocal folds during periods of inflammation and chronic irritation. Stroboscopy has proved to be the best method to study the effects of inflammation and reflux on the vibratory patterns of the vocal folds and to monitor treatment. However, it is a valuable tool only in the presence of a thorough vocal history and physical examination.

References

1. Powitzky E. Extraesophageal reflux: the role in laryngeal disease. Curr Opin Otolaryngol Head Neck Surg 2002;10:485–491
2. Titze IR. On the mechanics of vocal-fold vibration. J Acoust Soc Am 1976;60:1366–1380
3. Behrman A. Global and local dimensions of vocal dynamics. J Acoust Soc Am 1999;105:432–443
4. Remacle M, Lawson G. Diagnosis and management of laryngopharyngeal reflux disease. Curr Opin Otolaryngol Head Neck Surg 2006;14:143–149
5. Mirza N, Kasper Schwartz S, Antin-Ozerkis D. Laryngeal findings in users of combination corticosteroid and bronchodilator therapy. Laryngoscope 2004;114:1566–1569
6. Ng ML, Gilbert HR, Lerman JW. Some aerodynamic and acoustic characteristics of acute laryngitis. J Voice 1997;11:356–363
7. Thompson L. Herpes simplex virus laryngitis. Ear Nose Throat J 2006;85:304
8. Jackson-Menaldi CA, Dzul AI, Holland RW. Allergies and vocal fold edema: a preliminary report. J Voice 1999;13:113–122
9. Spiegel JR, Hawkshaw M, Markiewicz A, Sataloff RT. Acute laryngitis. Ear Nose Throat J 2000;79:488
10. Branski RC, Verdolini K, Sandulache V, Rosen CA, Hebda PA. Vocal fold wound healing: a review for clinicians. J Voice 2006;20:432–442
11. Jiang J, Lin E, Hanson DG. Vocal fold physiology. Otolaryngol Clin North Am 2000;33:699–718
12. Ford CN, Inagi K, Khidr A, Bless DM, Gilchrist KW. Sulcus vocalis: a rational analytical approach to diagnosis and management. Ann Otol Rhinol Laryngol 1996;105:189–200
13. Milstein CF, Charbel S, Hicks DM, Abelson TI, Richter JE, Vaezi MF. Prevalence of laryngeal irritation signs associated with reflux in asymptomatic volunteers: impact of endoscopic technique (rigid vs. flexible laryngoscope). Laryngoscope 2005;115:2256–2261
14. Alberti PW. The diagnostic role of laryngeal stroboscopy. Otolaryngol Clin North Am 1978;11:347–354
15. Bless DM, Hirano M, Feder RJ. Videostroboscopic evaluation of the larynx. Ear Nose Throat J 1987;66:289–296
16. Cantarella G. Value of flexible videolaryngoscopy in the study of laryngeal morphology and functions. J Voice 1987;1:353–358
17. Postma GN, Koufman JA. Laryngitis. In: Bailey BJ, ed. Head and Neck Surgery—Otolaryngology, 2nd ed. Philadelphia, PA: Lippincott-Raven; 1998:731–739
18. Lim JY, Choi JN, Kim KM, Choi HS. Voice analysis of patients with diverse types of Reinke's edema and clinical use of electroglottographic measurements. Acta Otolaryngol 2006;126:62–69
19. Bouzid A, Ellouze N. Open quotient measurements based on multiscale product of speech signal wavelet transform. Research Letters in Signal Processing 2007;62521:10.1155/2007/6252
20. Schutte HK, Svec JG, Sram F. First results of clinical application of videokymography. Laryngoscope 1998;108(8 Pt 1):1206–1210
21. Schalén L. Acute laryngitis in adults: diagnosis, etiology, treatment. Acta Otolaryngol Suppl 1988;449:31
22. Colton RH, Woo P, Brewer DW, Griffin B, Casper J. Stroboscopic signs associated with benign lesions of the vocal folds. J Voice 1995;9:312–325
23. Mergell P, Herzel H, Titze IR. Irregular vocal-fold vibration—high-speed observation and modeling. J Acoust Soc Am 2000;108:2996–3002
24. Tigges M, Mergell P, Herzel H, Wittenberg T, Eysholdt U. Observation and modeling glottal biphonation. Acustica/Acta Acustica 1997;83:707–714
25. Neubauer J, Mergell P, Eysholdt U, Herzel H. Spatiotemporal analysis of irregular vocal fold oscillations: biphonation due to desynchronization of spatial modes. J Acoust Soc Am 2001;110:3179–3192
26. Agarwal P, Bais AS. A clinical and videostroboscopic evaluation of laryngeal tuberculosis. J Laryngol Otol 1998;112:45–48
27. Altman KW. Vocal fold masses. Otolaryngol Clin North Am 2007;40:1091–1108, viii
28. Hirano S. Current treatment of vocal fold scarring. Curr Opin Otolaryngol Head Neck Surg 2005;13:143–147
29. Lee ST, Niimi S. Vocal fold sulcus. J Laryngol Otol 1990;104:876–878

30. Kendall KA. Controversies in the diagnosis and management of laryngopharyngeal reflux disease. Curr Opin Otolaryngol Head Neck Surg 2006;14:113–115

31. Bove MJ, Rosen C. Diagnosis and management of laryngopharyngeal reflux disease. Curr Opin Otolaryngol Head Neck Surg 2006;14:116–123

32. Divi V, Benninger MS. Diagnosis and management of laryngopharyngeal reflux disease. Curr Opin Otolaryngol Head Neck Surg 2006;14:124–127

33. Galli J, Cammarota G, De Corso E, et al. Biliary laryngopharyngeal reflux: a new pathological entity. Curr Opin Otolaryngol Head Neck Surg 2006;14:128–132

34. Mahieu HF, Smit CF. Diagnosis and management of laryngopharyngeal reflux disease. Curr Opin Otolaryngol Head Neck Surg 2006;14:133–137

35. Pontes P, Tiago R. Diagnosis and management of laryngopharyngeal reflux disease. Curr Opin Otolaryngol Head Neck Surg 2006;14:138–142

36. Remacle M, Lawson G. Diagnosis and management of laryngopharyngeal reflux disease. Curr Opin Otolaryngol Head Neck Surg 2006;14:143–149

37. Katz PO. Gastroesophageal reflux disease—state of the art. Rev Gastroenterol Disord 2001;1:128–138

38. Modlin IM, Moss SF, Kidd M, Lye KD. Gastroesophageal reflux disease: then and now. J Clin Gastroenterol 2004;38:390–402

39. Branski RC, Bhattacharyya N, Shapiro J. The reliability of the assessment of endoscopic laryngeal findings associated with laryngopharyngeal reflux disease. Laryngoscope 2002;112:1019–1024

40. Hicks DM, Ours TM, Abelson TI, Vaezi MF, Richter JE. The prevalence of hypopharynx findings associated with gastroesophageal reflux in normal volunteers. J Voice 2002;16:564–579

41. Eller R, Ginsburg M, Lurie D, Heman-Ackah Y, Lyons K, Sataloff R. Flexible laryngoscopy: a comparison of fiber optic and distal chip technologies—part 2: laryngopharyngeal reflux. J Voice 2009;23:389–395

42. Beaver MES, Stasney CR, Weitzel E, et al. Diagnosis of laryngopharyngeal reflux disease with digital imaging. Otolaryngol Head Neck Surg 2003;128:103–108

43. Belafsky PC, Postma GN, Koufman JA. The validity and reliability of the reflux finding score (RFS). Laryngoscope 2001;111:1313–1317

44. Park KH, Choi SM, Kwon SUK, Yoon SW, Kim SU. Diagnosis of laryngopharyngeal reflux among globus patients. Otolaryngol Head Neck Surg 2006;134:81–85

45. Pribuisiene R, Uloza V, Kupcinskas L. Diagnostic sensitivity and specificity of laryngoscopic signs of reflux laryngitis. Medicina (Kaunas) 2008;44:280–287

46. Qadeer MA, Swoger J, Milstein C, et al. Correlation between symptoms and laryngeal signs in laryngopharyngeal reflux. Laryngoscope 2005;115:1947–1952

47. Noordzij JP, Khidr A, Desper E, Meek RB, Reibel JF, Levine PA. Correlation of pH probe-measured laryngopharyngeal reflux with symptoms and signs of reflux laryngitis. Laryngoscope 2002;112:2192–2195

48. Pawar S, Lim HJ, Gill M, et al. Treatment of postnasal drip with proton pump inhibitors: a prospective, randomized, placebo-controlled study. Am J Rhinol 2007;21:695–701

49. Belafsky PC, Postma GN, Amin MR, Koufman JA. Symptoms and findings of laryngopharyngeal reflux. Ear Nose Throat J 2002;81(9, Suppl 2)10–13

24

Laryngeal Paralysis and Paresis

Nazaneen N. Grant, Lucian Sulica, Ronda E. Alexander,
and Andrew Blitzer

◆ Pathophysiology of the Paralyzed Vocal Fold

The laryngoscopic appearance of vocal fold paralysis reflects the considerable variation in the underlying pathophysiology of the condition. Easily (and often) taken to represent a simple absence of innervation, vocal fold paralysis is in fact the product of a range of underlying neural dysfunction encompassing partial denervation, complete denervation, and variable degrees and patterns of reinnervation. An appreciation of this heterogeneity, coupled with the understanding that vocal fold paralysis is a dynamic condition that tends to evolve after onset, is at the core of interpreting the laryngoscopic examination.

A brief exposition of current knowledge regarding the relevant pathophysiology is in order, especially in contrast with long-held historical beliefs regarding the disorder. Traditionally, vocal fold paralysis has been conceptualized as an all-or-none phenomenon, with absence of motion resulting from a lack of neural input. However, both human and animal studies have shown that cases of vocal fold paralysis, unless the result of simple nerve section, differ in degree and extent of initial neural impairment. Moreover, the injury type itself is usually not uniform; most laryngeal neuropathies feature a mix of injury types among affected nerve fibers.[1,2] Further, laryngeal nerves appear to have a strong propensity for reinnervation.[2–4] Reinnervation appears to be the rule rather than the exception, occurring often even after deliberate recurrent nerve section, as was formerly done for spasmodic dysphonia.[5,6] A paralyzed vocal fold is thus only sometimes, and perhaps quite rarely, a denervated vocal fold.

In the larynx, regeneration of the recurrent nerve is more problematic than that of most peripheral nerves because it carries a mixed population of abductor and adductor fibers. In many—possibly most—cases, vocal fold reinnervation is dysfunctional and does not yield physiologic motion. This dysfunction extends beyond the classic definition of synkinesis, in which co-contraction of adductor and abductor muscle fibers produces no net vocal fold motion; such perfectly balanced antagonism is, after all, an extremely improbable outcome of a largely random process. Dysfunctional reinnervation may also result when nerve regrowth is appropriate but inadequate, which may result in decreased force of contraction, loss of motor unit specificity, and possibly also in changes in neural organization peripherally and centrally.[7] An altered afferent signal may also affect laryngeal behavior. The complex, highly specialized nature of the laryngeal neuromotor system leaves many ways in which reinnervation may miscarry.

These findings and observations have at least two important clinical implications. For most of the past century, the position of the paralyzed vocal fold was thought to reflect the site or type of lesion, a belief that has no physiologic basis and has been invalidated by careful clinical and laboratory work.[8–10] It should now be clear that the position of a given paralyzed vocal fold is most likely explained by its particular degree and pattern of innervation. Thus, time-honored terms like *paramedian* and *cadaveric* carry no topognostic significance and are not useful, except perhaps as purely descriptive conventions. Similarly, notions of discrete *adductor paralysis* and *abductor paralysis*, terms that still appear in academic journals with some frequency, also have no physiologic validity. There are no grounds for believing the adductor and abductor nerve fibers have different vulnerabilities or propensity for dysfunction.

Second, the natural propensity for reinnervation most likely accounts for the tendency for the voice—and the laryngoscopic examination—to improve over time in cases of vocal fold paralysis. Reinnervation, even when it does not restore motion, acts to restore or conserve muscle bulk and tone, increasing vocal fold mass and resistance to airflow, occasionally to the point that complete glottic closure during phonation is restored and conversational voice sounds normal, although the vocal fold itself remains immobile (**Fig. 24.1**). This explanation for the improvement commonly observed in cases of vocal fold paralysis over time is well supported by electrophysiologic evidence and should replace the time-honored notion of gradual contralateral compensation.[1,2] Gradual compensation, either as a spontaneous phenomenon or as the result of behavioral intervention, has not been convincingly documented in any study.

◆ Laryngoscopy of Vocal Fold Paralysis

Marked vocal fold hypomobility is the cardinal sign of paralysis. We deliberately avoid the term *immobility* because the vocal fold is rarely perfectly still, even if completely denervated. Simple in concept, hypomobility is sometimes surprisingly difficult to appreciate upon clinical examination. The examiner may be misled by small amounts of vocal fold motion caused by (1) an active interarytenoid muscle still partially innervated by the contralateral side, (2) an intact cricothyroid muscle, and/or (3) passive lateral displacement of the arytenoid cartilage of the paralyzed vocal fold by its pair during adduction. This last is known as the "jostle sign," described by Chevalier Jackson in the 1930s. When present, it offers evidence for poor ipsilateral muscle tone and against cricoarytenoid joint dysfunction. In ambiguous cases, asking the patient to alternate sustained vowel phonation and sniffing—the so-called /ē/-sniff maneuver—usually brings motion asymmetries into stark relief. This maneuver can also help reveal a rare

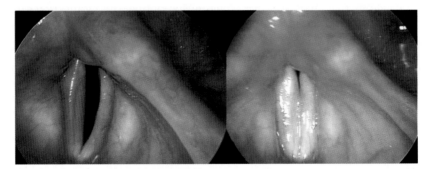

A   B

Fig. 24.1 Improvement in vocal fold paralysis: Comparison of best phonatory closure in a 76-year-old woman with left vocal fold paralysis after a carotid endarterectomy. **(A)** Image from an examination 1 month after injury. **(B)** Image from an examination 4 months after injury. In the interval, glottic closure has improved because reinnervation has restored muscle bulk and tone, although the left vocal fold itself remains immobile.

condition of inappropriate reinnervation resulting in adduction during sniffing or abduction during phonation. This is not to be confused with the entity called paradoxical fold motion, in which innervation is entirely intact and which has no relation to vocal fold paralysis.

Once vocal fold hypomobility has been identified, the larynx should be examined across a variety of activities, including respiration and phonation at a range of intensity and pitch. It is useful to consider these in a logical progression, from examination under continuous light during quiet respiration to examination under continuous light during phonatory tasks to examination under stroboscopic light.

Laryngoscopy at Quiet Respiration

The position of the arytenoid mound, composed of the arytenoid cartilage and overlying cuneiforms, is best assessed during quiet respiration. It may be upright and essentially symmetric with its pair or tipped into the airway to varying degrees; this displacement is frequently referred to as *prolapse* (**Fig. 24.2**; **Video Clip 30**). This represents a lack of muscular support of the cartilage and should not be mistaken for cricoarytenoid subluxation. The cricoarytenoid joint facets provide very little support for the arytenoid as they are broad and shallow to accommodate the multiple degrees of freedom in arytenoid movement. The arytenoid is stabilized principally by the intrinsic laryngeal muscles, much as a tent pole is supported by guy wires. When denervation

is profound, this support is lost. The predominant remaining pull is passive and anterior, due to the mass of the body of the vocal fold, including the vocal ligament and the thyroarytenoid muscle, and its attachment to the thyroid cartilage. Prolapse of the arytenoid mound displaces the vocal process, the anteromedial projection of the cartilage where the membranous vocal fold attaches, anteriorly and inferiorly. This three-dimensional displacement is easily overlooked as laryngoscopy yields the impression of predominately two-dimensional vocal fold motion.

As we have noted above, the position of the paralyzed vocal fold is not topognostic, and terms used to describe the position have not been shown to have a specific pathophysiologic correlate.

The vocal fold itself may appear to be of normal or decreased tone. The "slack" appearance in the latter condition typically results in a concave contour of the vibratory margin, often described as "bowing." Bowing may also be caused by underlying muscle atrophy from denervation. The two conditions—hypotonia and atrophy—are not synonymous, although they are both plainly related consequences of denervation and are in some respects similar on clinical examination. Hypotonia may appear immediately, as after nerve section, and is not associated with loss of vocal fold bulk (**Fig. 24.3A**; **Video Clip 27**). Atrophy takes some time to evolve—exactly how long is not established—and produces vocal fold thinning, retraction of the ventricular fold (which shares the same innervation), and enlargement of the

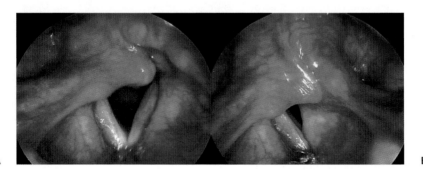

A   B

Fig. 24.2 Arytenoid prolapse: **(A)** In this case of idiopathic right vocal fold paralysis, the arytenoid cartilage is prolapsed into the glottis, lowering the vocal fold below the level of its partner. **(B)** In phonatory adduction, the prolapsed arytenoid interferes with the opposite cartilage and impedes closure. Rehabilitation without arytenoid repositioning surgery would very likely be suboptimal.

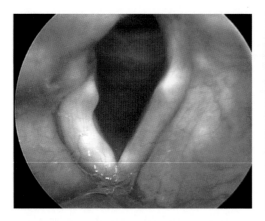

A

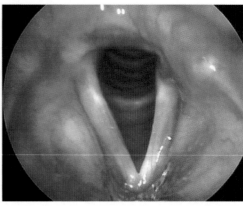

B

Fig. 24.3 Hypotonia versus atrophy. **(A)** The right vocal fold in this young woman with a metastasis at the jugular foramen is markedly hypotonic. **(B)** In contrast with the findings in **A**, the left vocal fold in this woman with long-standing idiopathic vocal fold paralysis is thin, and the ventricular fold has receded, exposing the ventricle. Both of these findings are the result of atrophy. It is common to find elements of both hypotonia and atrophy in cases of vocal fold paralysis.

ventricle (**Fig. 24.3B**; **Video Clip 29**). Paradoxically, ventricular fold retraction and ventricular enlargement may yield the impression that the vocal fold is larger, because more of its superior surface, sometimes extending well lateral to the superior arcuate line, is exposed to the examining eye. Careful examination will reveal the finding for what it is.

As hypotonia and atrophy are both incontrovertible signs of denervation, it is intuitively compelling to think that the longer from onset they are present, the poorer the prospects for recovery. This proposition has yet to be validated by experiment but already occasionally informs our clinical decision-making in vocal fold paralysis.

Valuable signs may also be observed away from the vocal fold proper. The presence of salivary pooling, typically in the piriform sinus on the side of the paralysis, speaks to the presence of a trio of deficits resulting from a lesion of the main trunk of the vagus—a so-called high vagal injury (**Fig. 24.4**; **Video Clip 48**). These are (1) hemilaryngeal hypoesthesia or anesthesia from involvement of the superior laryngeal nerve, (2) ipsilateral constrictor muscle hypofunction, and (3) cricopharyngeal muscle hyperfunction. Of these, the last is not always present due to bilateral innervation. Inferior constrictor hypofunction manifests as piriform sinus dilatation at rest or failure to contract during a pharyngeal squeeze maneuver. Together with glottic insufficiency, these deficits form a "perfect storm" for swallowing dysfunction by creating a hypopharyngeal reservoir of secretions that are neither well-propelled nor well-drained into the esophagus upon swallowing and that the larynx cannot sense. Upon reflection, it should be obvious that medialization alone will often not remedy this situation well, as it only addresses one component of the dysfunction; yet many

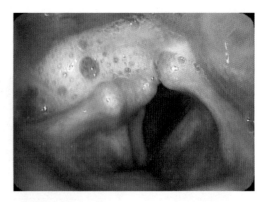

Fig. 24.4 "High vagal" injury: This examination of a 69-year-old man after surgery to remove a glomus jugulare tumor shows right vocal fold paralysis, ipsilateral salivary pooling, and dilatation of the right piriform sinus. The last two are hallmark signs of an injury involving the entire vagus rather than just the recurrent nerve. See also **Figs. 24.9 and 24.10**.

are often puzzled by continued aspiration after an adequate medialization laryngoplasty.

Laryngoscopy during Phonation

As the primary symptom of vocal fold paralysis is usually dysphonia, the importance of examination during phonation is self-evident. Clear visualization of the vocal folds may be impaired by supraglottic hyperfunction, most often manifested as contraction of the contralateral ventricular fold, a natural response to glottal insufficiency.[11] The ipsilateral ventricular fold, which shares innervation with the vocal fold proper, is usually quiescent under conditions of denervation (**Fig. 24.5**; **Video Clip 49**). "Unloading the larynx," or eliminating supraglottic hyperfunction by behavioral techniques, may be helpful to decrease supraglottic squeeze to clear the line of sight to the glottis proper.[11]

Dysphonia in vocal fold paralysis is principally, although not exclusively, the acoustic consequence of incomplete glottic closure and irregularities in vocal fold vibration resulting from differences in vocal fold tension and shape. Glottic insufficiency varies in both degree and configuration from case to case, and, as we have discussed above, may change in the same case over time. It is occasionally debated whether it is best evaluated by flexible or rigid laryngoscopy. Flexible transnasal laryngoscopy probably offers a more accurate impression of laryngeal function, as the tongue traction required for rigid peroral techniques introduces some artificial biomechanical factors that may be misleading. On the other hand, rigid examination, particularly when compared with fiberoptic rather than distal chip endoscopes, offers a far more precise image of the vibratory margin and may thus be the better tool for stroboscopic examination. Debate regarding the superiority of one or the other is somewhat academic, however, as there is absolutely nothing to prevent evaluation by both techniques when the clinician believes there is more information that can be obtained.

There exists no agreed-upon scale for the measurement of glottic insufficiency; most reports settle upon relative classifications such as mild, moderate, or severe. Given the variable angle and distance of the glottis from the examiner's endoscope and all of the variations in phonation (pitch and intensity foremost among them), an absolute measurement of glottic insufficiency that is reproducible from exam to exam is probably impossible. As a generalization, however, the larger the gap, the more profound the dysphonia, and the more aggressive will be the required rehabilitation procedure; medialization laryngoplasty is superior to injection augmentation in correcting large insufficiencies.

The configuration of glottic insufficiency in unilateral paralysis most commonly takes one of two shapes. It may be essentially spindle-shaped, involving principally the membranous

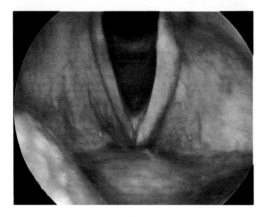

A

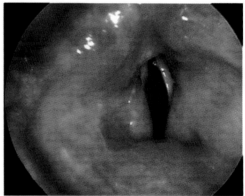

B

Fig. 24.5 (A) Vocal folds seen during quiet respiration in a case of left vocal fold paralysis after thyroid surgery. **(B)** Ventricular function in the same patient during phonation. Often, the ventricular fold of the unaffected side is engaged in effortful glottic closure in vocal fold paralysis, as in this case of left vocal fold paralysis after thyroid surgery. The resulting bulge can obscure the glottis in whole or in part.

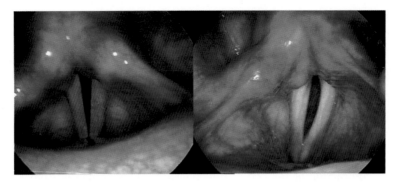

A   B

Fig. 24.6 Configuration of glottic insufficiency: **(A)** A case of left vocal fold paralysis after a thyroidectomy demonstrates a posterior gap. **(B)** A case of left vocal fold paralysis from a malignant mediastinal lymph-adenopathy in which closure at the vocal process is good. Compare also with the case in **Fig. 25.2**, which also demonstrates a large posterior gap.

portion of the vocal fold, or V-shaped, marked by a distance between the vocal processes of the arytenoid cartilage (**Fig. 24.6**). The latter is often called a *posterior glottic gap*; it is important to understand that the term does not refer to the absolute distance between the vocal process or to the size of the insufficiency but rather to its configuration. The presence of a posterior glottic gap argues in favor of an arytenoid stabilization procedure for rehabilitation because implant medialization alone, or injection augmentation for that matter, is notoriously inadequate for correction of this deficit.

A paralyzed vocal fold may not rest in the same plane as its partner. Such three-dimensional judgments are difficult to make in laryngoscopy, particularly when the vocal folds do not lie closely juxtaposed, which is the rule in vocal fold paralysis. Nevertheless, identification of a height mismatch is clinically relevant, as simple medial displacement of the paralyzed fold may not suffice for good apposition in phonation.

The real physiologic impact of hypotonia of the paralyzed vocal fold can only be accurately assessed during phonation. When challenged with subglottic air pressure, what may have appeared to be an only mildly bowed vocal fold during quiet respiration may be revealed to be far more flaccid. Obviously, this effect will be more pronounced the louder the volume solicited from the patient. Some patients reflexively tense the vocal fold to resist this subglottic pressure. Not only does this result

in a characteristic high-pitched voice known as a *paralytic falsetto*, but also it strongly suggests that the superior laryngeal nerve is intact to provide the cricothyroid muscle activation necessary for this response (**Fig. 24.7**; **Video Clip 25**).

Stroboscopy

Poor muscle tone and activity of the paralyzed vocal fold, besides contributing to glottic insufficiency, alters intrinsic tissue properties

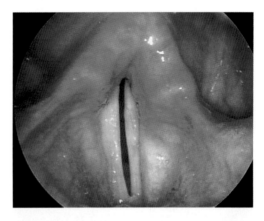

Fig. 24.7 Paralytic falsetto. This 69-year-old man with right vocal fold paralysis after cervical spine surgery uses his intact cricothyroid muscle to aid glottic resistance and improve projection. The pitch of the resulting voice is abnormally high, as would be expected.

to yield abnormalities in phonatory vibration when compared with the normal side. These, of course, are only discernible on stroboscopy. In general, decreased vocal fold tension yields increased amplitude of vibration, increased lateral displacement of vocal fold tissue during the vibratory cycle, and mucosal wave phase shifts or outright asymmetry in frequency of vibration. In the most severe cases, mucosal vibration will be frankly aperiodic. As stroboscopic examination depends on a stable frequency of vibration to time light flashes, such cases yield the illusion of nonsequential vibration, "skipping" video frames, and other irregularities.

The mucosal wave abnormalities are to be expected in vocal fold paralysis and, in and of themselves, are not particularly revealing. The real value of stroboscopy lies in more precise visualization of the configuration and degree of glottic insufficiency. Sharp delineation of the vibratory margin of the vocal fold during phonation is central to this task; only examination under stroboscopic light can reveal this adequately. Even in cases of borderline glottic insufficiency, stroboscopy may permit a more precise estimation of degree of glottic insufficiency by means of frame counting. The examiner begins review of a phonatory cycle on an image in which the glottis is unambiguously closed. Then, proceeding frame-by-frame until the cycle is completed, each image in which space is visible between the vocal folds is counted as "open." The total number of open frames is divided by the total number of frames in a cycle to yield the open quotient. This value varies at different pitches and volumes, but as a generalization, the normal open quotient is ~0.5 in modal phonation.

Examination after Rehabilitative Intervention

Dysphonia after rehabilitative surgery for vocal fold paralysis is not rare. It is typically due to technical factors, and surgical revision rates range from 5.4 to 14% to as high as 33% when all procedures to improve voice are considered.[12-14] Stroboscopy is particularly helpful in correctly assessing glottic closure as described earlier and prescribing corrective treatment. In injection augmentation, poor voice result is usually a matter of underinjection, overinjection, or misplacement of the injectate (**Fig. 24.8**; **Video Clip 50**). Most often, this last takes the form of diffusion into the superficial lamina propria, causing focal vibratory stiffness, best identified by stroboscopy.

The most common causes of suboptimal voice outcomes after medialization laryngoplasty include persistent posterior glottic gap, usually due to inappropriate omission of an arytenoid procedure, undermedialization,

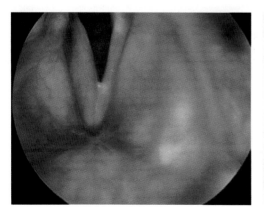

A

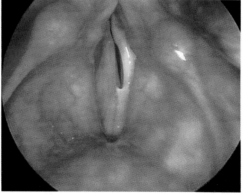

B

Fig. 24.8 Overinjection: This 51-year-old physician has had an injection medialization for right vocal fold paralysis after parathyroidectomy. He has a strained voice quality because of overinjection. (**A**) Vocal folds viewed during abduction. (**B**) The right vocal fold is convex and damps vibration of the left during phonation because of its bulk. It is quite stiff; its dun color represents edema.

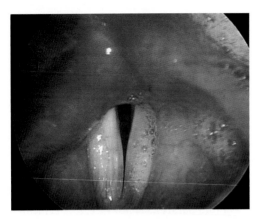

Fig. 24.9 Persistent posterior glottic gap: This 54-year-old woman with a left vocal fold paralysis after resection of a jugular foramen tumor underwent medialization laryngoplasty without an arytenoid adduction. As a result, there is a persistent gap at the vocal processes; closure overall is suboptimal. Note also the secretions overwhelming the larynx on the side of the paralysis typical of a high vagal injury.

or implant malposition, most often in too superior a position (**Fig. 24.9**; **Video Clip 51**). The first two of these are usually evident on careful examination. The last presents the impression of ventricular fold prominence that does not disappear with quiet respiration (**Fig. 24.10**; **Video Clip 52**).

◆ Laryngoscopy of Vocal Fold Paresis

Given the heterogeneity of the neural compromise underlying vocal fold paralysis, it should come as no surprise that paresis, or incomplete paralysis in which some or most gross vocal fold mobility is preserved, exists alongside paralysis as a clinical entity. While the existence of laryngeal paresis is beyond doubt, its incidence, presentation, and significance remain debated topics. Much difficulty stems from the fact that vocal fold paresis is often diagnosed by laryngoscopy, based on mild dynamic laryngeal asymmetries that are determined to be meaningful more by clinical expectations or hypotheses rather than by physiologic evidence. It is not much of an exaggeration to say that a determined observer may find signs of paresis in virtually every larynx. Separating innocent asymmetries from significant findings is the greatest challenge in the laryngoscopic characterization of vocal fold paresis.

As in paralysis, vocal fold hypomobility is probably the most common sign of motor paresis, although mobility is retained to a far greater extent in paresis. Rubin and colleagues have described the use of repetitive phonatory tasks during examination to fatigue inadequately innervated musculature to accentuate mild vocal fold hypomobility.[15] Glottic insufficiency during phonation may be difficult to discern because

A

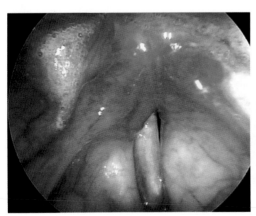

B

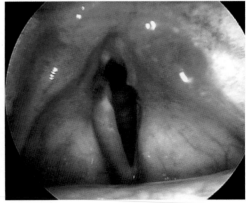

Fig. 24.10 (A) Superior implant malposition: This 27-year-old woman with a left vocal fold paralysis has a poor voice result because the implant rests above the vocal fold, medializing the ventricular fold.

The ventricular fold obscures the vocal fold, which is not well adducted. **(B)** This is not ventricular fold hyperfunction, as the ventricular fold remains full even in respiration, at right.

of its subtlety and also because of supraglottic hyperfunction, as discussed earlier. Asymmetries in vocal fold tension can be the result of both recurrent and superior laryngeal pareses and may manifest exclusively as asymmetry of mucosal wave motion, noticeable only on examination under stroboscopic light. It is worth repeating that not all such asymmetries are likely to be significant. The consistency of such findings across multiple pitches and intensities, and with patient complaints, is an important element in judging their relevance.

Virtually every author to address the subject of vocal fold paresis has remarked on the discrepancy of clinical observations and electromyographic findings.[15–18] Although electromyography is neither a perfect nor a complete means of neurologic assessment of the larynx, it comes far closer than does laryngoscopy to an objective diagnosis of neurologic impairment. In one series, around 1 in 4 patients had electromyographic findings not predicted by the endoscopic examiner; in another, the incidence of unexpected findings was still higher, about 40%.[17,19] Further, observations from blinded examinations of experimentally induced paresis demonstrate not only poor intrarater and interrater reliability but also extremely low diagnostic accuracy.[20] In this context, claims of diagnostic precision using laryngoscopy alone should be treated with great caution; laryngoscopy, whether under continuous or stroboscopic light, remains a tool of uncertain utility in vocal fold paresis.

◆ Conclusion

The laryngoscopic appearance of vocal fold paralysis reflects underlying pathophysiologic processes. A thorough understanding of these and their laryngoscopic correlates allows a precise, accurate, and insightful assessment of each case, which in turn informs and individualizes clinical care in the best interest of the patient.

References

1. Bielamowicz S, Stager SV. Diagnosis of unilateral recurrent laryngeal nerve paralysis: laryngeal electromyography, subjective rating scales, acoustic and aerodynamic measures. Laryngoscope 2006;116: 359–364

2. Blitzer A, Jahn AF, Keidar A. Semon's law revisited: an electromyographic analysis of laryngeal synkinesis. Ann Otol Rhinol Laryngol 1996;105:764–769

3. Woodson GE. Spontaneous laryngeal reinnervation after recurrent laryngeal or vagus nerve injury. Ann Otol Rhinol Laryngol 2007;116:57–65

4. Zealear DL, Hamdan AL, Rainey CL. Effects of denervation on posterior cricoarytenoid muscle physiology and histochemistry. Ann Otol Rhinol Laryngol 1994; 103:780–788

5. Aronson AE, De Santo LW. Adductor spastic dysphonia: three years after recurrent laryngeal nerve resection. Laryngoscope 1983;93:1–8

6. Netterville JL, Stone RE, Rainey C, Zealear DL, Ossoff RH. Recurrent laryngeal nerve avulsion for treatment of spastic dysphonia. Ann Otol Rhinol Laryngol 1991;100:10–14

7. Zealear DL, Billante CR. Neurophysiology of vocal fold paralysis. Otolaryngol Clin North Am 2004;37:1–23, v

8. Woodson GE. Configuration of the glottis in laryngeal paralysis. I: clinical study. Laryngoscope 1993;103(11 Pt 1):1227–1234

9. Woodson GE. Configuration of the glottis in laryngeal paralysis. II: animal experiments. Laryngoscope 1993;103(11 Pt 1):1235–1241

10. Koufman JA, Walker FO, Joharji GM. The cricothyroid muscle does not influence vocal fold position in laryngeal paralysis. Laryngoscope 1995;105(4 Pt 1): 368–372

11. Belafsky PC, Postma GN, Reulbach TR, Holland BW, Koufman JA. Muscle tension dysphonia as a sign of underlying glottal insufficiency. Otolaryngol Head Neck Surg 2002;127:448–451

12. Weinman EC, Maragos NE. Airway compromise in thyroplasty surgery. Laryngoscope 2000;110:1082–1085

13. Rosen CA. Complications of phonosurgery: results of a national survey. Laryngoscope 1998;108(11 Pt 1): 1697–1703

14. Anderson TD, Spiegel JR, Sataloff RT. Thyroplasty revisions: frequency and predictive factors. J Voice 2003;17:442–448

15. Rubin AD, Praneetvatakul V, Heman-Ackah Y, Moyer CA, Mandel S, Sataloff RT. Repetitive phonatory tasks for identifying vocal fold paresis. J Voice 2005; 19:679–686

16. Koufman JA, Postma GN, Cummins MM, Blalock PD. Vocal fold paresis. Otolaryngol Head Neck Surg 2000;122:537–541

17. Heman-Ackah YD, Barr A. Mild vocal fold paresis: understanding clinical presentation and electromyographic findings. J Voice 2006;20:269–281

18. Altman KW. Laryngeal asymmetry on indirect laryngoscopy in a symptomatic patient should be evaluated with electromyography. Arch Otolaryngol Head Neck Surg 2005;131:356–359

19. Koufman JA, Postma GN, Whang CS, et al. Diagnostic laryngeal electromyography: the Wake Forest experience 1995-1999. Otolaryngol Head Neck Surg 2001;124:603–606

20. Roy N, Barton M, Smith ME, Dromey C, Merrill R, Sauder C. An in vivo model of external superior laryngeal nerve paralysis: laryngoscopic findings. Laryngoscope 2009;119:1017–1032

25

Spasmodic Dysphonia and Muscle Tension Dysphonia

Gayle E. Woodson

Spasmodic dysphonia (SD) and muscle tension dysphonia (MTD) are voice disorders that disrupt speech and can sound very similar.[1,2] The clinical description of vocal quality in patients with adductor SD is "strained and strangled." Patients with MTD can also speak with a voice that is "strained and strangled," and even experienced and expert listeners find it difficult to differentiate between the sounds of these voice disorders. But the etiology and management of these problems is quite different. SD is a neurologic disorder.[3,4] MTD is believed to result from habitual misuse of the voice. What the two disorders do have in common is that the voice disorder is not due to a structural abnormality in the larynx, although MTD can lead to secondary lesions. Differentiation between SD and MTD can be accomplished by listening to the voice and examining the larynx with continuous light. Videostroboscopy does not usually play a role in this differentiation. However, in patients suspected of having MTD, videostroboscopy has a more important role. Presumed MTD patients who do not respond to voice therapy may actually have compensatory hyperfunction due to a mucosal or submucosal lesion that is not apparent on examination with continuous light.

For many years, SD was referred to as "spastic dysphonia." It was first described in 1871 by Traube, who reported that the sound of the voice was like that of a person trying to speak "whilst choking."[5] He believed that it was a psychiatric disorder. A psychiatric cause was accepted for many years, because no organic cause could be identified, and patients frequently reported that the onset of symptoms was during a time of stress. Because it is a debilitating disorder, most patients become discouraged, socially isolated, and even depressed. SD does not respond to any medical therapy, and speech therapy is only occasionally effective. However, in 1975, Dr. Herbert Dedo reported that surgically transecting the recurrent laryngeal nerve dramatically improved the voice in many patients with severe SD.[6] The efficacy of this surgical intervention provided strong evidence for an organic cause of the disease. Subsequently, injection of botulinum toxin into laryngeal muscles was shown to be effective in reducing the muscle spasm of SD, without totally denervating laryngeal muscles.[7–9] Psychological testing in patients before and after effective treatment of SD has documented improvement in mood and anxiety, indicating that the emotional disturbances observed in patients with SD are the result of the disorder rather than its cause.[10]

SD is now recognized to be a neurologic disorder. Specifically, it is a focal dystonia of the larynx, characterized by involuntary spasms of the intrinsic laryngeal muscles during speech. There are two basic forms of the disorder, adductor SD (AdSD) and abductor (AbSD). In AdSD, the most common form, the voice is strained due to spasmodic closure of the glottis.[11] In AbSD, the spasms abduct the vocal folds, opening the glottis, so that the voice is breathy.[12] Some patients have both adductor and abductor spasms. Speech is very effortful for patients with SD and they are clearly uncomfortable; however, there is no pain. It does not hurt to talk.

The muscle spasms in AdSD cause episodic and transient hyperclosure of the glottis, resulting in voice stoppage or pitch breaks. The occurrence of such voice breaks is the one feature that seems to be pathognomonic for AdSD, as these breaks have not been observed in patients with MTD. Adductor spasms are most prominent when the patient speaks words beginning with a vowel, such as "eggs" or "every." The frequency of voice breaks can be assessed by listening or quantified by measuring events in a sample of an acoustic recording of the voice. The frequency of voice breaks has been shown to decrease significantly in patients with symptomatic improvement from botulinum toxin treatment.[8,9] But the voice in patients with SD is not only disrupted by the direct effects of these muscle spasms. Patients adopt varying strategies to cope with the spasm, and these behaviors can significantly influence speech. For example, some patients with AdSD will whisper. Others may adopt vocal hyperfunction in an attempt to stabilize the voice. This is quite similar to the vocal behavior observed in patients with MTD, with false vocal fold closure, anterior-posterior squeezing of the glottis, and excess tension in cervical strap muscles. Less commonly, patients with AdSD learn to phonate on inspiration.

In AbSD, the voice is disrupted by sudden abductor spasms or delays in adduction at the onset of phonation, resulting in episodic or persistent breathy voice. These patients usually have breathiness during production of sustained vowels. The spasms are most prominent in words or syllables that begin with a voiceless consonant followed by a vowel. For example, "pay" begins with a voiceless consonant, "p," followed by a voiced vowel, "a." Pronunciation of this word requires abduction of the vocal folds during the "p," followed by rapid adduction of the vocal folds to produce the vowel. The vocal folds seem to "hang up" in the abducted position, so that the vowel is breathy, or even aphonic. As with AdSD patients, AbSD patients tend to adopt compensatory strategies that can be very similar to vocal behavior in MTSD.

The hyperfunctional voice in MTD is believed to involve excess activity in the extrinsic laryngeal muscles, including the cervical strap muscles.[1,2] There are no physiologic studies to support this assumption; however, physical examination in these patients usually reveals tight contraction and sometimes even tenderness in the cervical strap muscles. Additionally, it has been reported that many patients with MTD improve with speech therapy, specifically massage of the extrinsic laryngeal mucles.[13] There have been no controlled studies to rule out a placebo effect of massage. However, MTD is generally observed to be responsive to speech therapy. This response is a key clinical feature that can distinguish MTD from SD. But careful evaluation is usually effective in identifying patients with SD.

Clinicians should listen to patients perform a variety of vocal tasks. A standard assessment protocol has been recommended by the Research Planning Workshop on Spasmodic Dysphonia that convened at the National Institute on Deafness and Other Communication Disorders (NIDCD) in June 2005.[14] The voice should be assessed during conversational speech, sustained phonation, counting, whispering, and shouting, assessing vocal strain, detecting vocal tremor, and quantifying the frequency of voice breaks. Voice breaks and vocal strain should be absent during whispering and shouting, and the phonation is normal during laughter. **Table 25.1** lists 10 standardized sentences that the workshop recommended for use in evaluating patients with SD.[14] Ten of the sentences are more difficult for patients with AdSD, and 10 are more difficult for patient with AbSD. It is not necessary to use all 20 sentences, but the clinician

Table 25.1 Adductor and Abductor Sentences

List 1: Adductor Sentences

1. Tom wants to be in the army.
2. We eat eels every day.
3. He was angry about it all year.
4. I hurt my arm on the iron bar.
5. Are the olives large?
6. John argued ardently about honesty.
7. We mow our lawn all year.
8. Jane got an apple for Ollie.
9. A dog dug a new bone.
10. Everyone wants to be in the army.

List 2: Abductor Sentences

1. He is hiding behind the house.
2. Patty helped Kathy carve the turkey.
3. Harry is happy because he has a new horse.
4. During babyhood he had only half a head of hair.
5. Who says a mahogany highboy isn't heavy?
6. Boys were singing songs outside of our house.
7. The puppy bit the tape.
8. See, there's a horse across the street.
9. Sally fell asleep in the soft chair.
10. The policy was suggested in an essay on peace.

should ask the patient to speak as many of these sentences as necessary to clarify the diagnosis. Patients with SD should produce at least three breaks per sentence when using a normal voice but no breaks when speaking in a whisper. To differentiate between AdSD and AbSD, the patient should be asked to alternately speak sentences from the two groups. Group 1 sentences include words that begin with a vowel, as vowel onset is particularly prone to elicit adductor spasm. Group 2 sentences include words and syllables that begin with unvoiced consonants, immediately followed by a vowel. The transition from an unvoiced consonant to phonation elicits abductor spasm in AbSD patients, interfering with the glottic closure that is required for phonation. Thus, patients with AbSD should have more breathy breaks when speaking sentences from list 2 than when speaking sentences from list 1.

Patients with MTD perform very differently during this evaluation. Voice breaks are not observed in patients with MTD. The voice is continuously strained, without abrupt breaks. When reciting the standard sentences recommended by the NIDCD workshop, patients with MTD will have equal difficulty with sentences in groups 1 and 2. As mentioned above, patients with MTD frequently have tenderness in neck muscles and often report fatigue or even pain with continued speech. And unlike SD patients, MTD patients do not have an improved voice with shouting, singing, or pitch changes.

◆ Neurologic Evaluation

It must be noted that patients with some neurologic disorders may present with a voice that sounds similar to SD. In particular, Parkinson's disease can mimic SD. Patients with SD can sometimes have other associated dystonias, such as blepharospasm or writer's cramp. But any other associated signs and symptoms, such as dysarthria and dysphagia, are clues that the patient does not have SD but rather a more generalized neurologic disorder. Therefore, a careful neurologic examination is an important part of the evaluation.

◆ The Role of Laryngeal Endoscopy

Laryngeal examination is essential in the evaluation of any voice disorder. In SD, the larynx is structurally normal, but laryngeal motion is abnormal. In MTD, the etiology of the problem is not a structural abnormality, although there may be secondary changes due to vocal overuse, such as nodules, edema, or even polyps. MTD is caused by abnormal laryngeal behavior during speech. The voice assumes a characteristic "hyperfunctional" posture during speech.

Laryngeal behavior should be observed during a variety of phonatory and nonphonatory tasks. This can only be accomplished by flexible endoscopy, which permits observation of the larynx without interfering with its function during speech.[15] Either a fiberoptic endoscope or a flexible endoscope with a distal chip camera can be used. The enlarged image on a video monitor is superior for detecting mucosal pathology and assessing motion. A video recording of the examination can be replayed repeatedly and viewed in slow motion to provide detailed analysis of movement. It is also very useful to save the recording for comparison with future evaluations.

On passing the endoscope from the nasal cavity to the pharynx, function of the soft palate should be assessed. Patients with SD may have an associated tremor of the larynx and pharynx that also affects the palate. If so, this tremor can be observed during phonation of "ee." Observation of the palate is also important to exclude other neurologic impairments that could present with disrupted speech. The palate should elevate symmetrically and close snugly during swallow and phonation of "ee." Abnormal palate motion indicates that there is some other neurologic disorder, not SD. The endoscope should then be advanced into the hypopharynx to look for lesions and to assess function. Pooling of secretions in the hypopharynx indicates possible sensory or motor impairment.[16]

The larynx should be observed during breathing to confirm normal vocal fold motion with respiration. The vocal folds may appear motionless during quiet breathing, but the degree of motion varies with effort. Therefore, the patient should be instructed to sniff and cough to induce a greater range of motion. The vocal folds should abduct briskly during a sniff. Alternating sniffing with brief phonation is a good way to demonstrate the range of motion of the vocal folds. A voluntary cough is very useful to establish the potential range of motion in the larynx. There are three phases of laryngeal motion during a cough, whether spontaneous or voluntary. First the glottis opens widely for deep inspiration and then closes for the second stage, the compressive phase, with expiratory force against the closed glottis. In the third phase, the glottis suddenly opens widely while expiratory force continues, resulting in a sudden outrush of air.

Observation of laryngeal motion during speech is very important to detect hyperfunctional posturing and spasmodic activity and to differentiate between adductor and abductor spasms. Patients with SD often have an associated tremor of the larynx and sometimes the pharynx as well. As a rule, MTD patients do not have tremor. The larynx should be observed during sustained phonation as well as in recitation of selected sentences from the lists of recommended standard sentences. In AdSD, the vocal folds are continuously or episodically closed tightly, with spasmodic increases in adduction, particularly during speaking of sentences in list 1. In patients with AbSD, sudden vocal fold abduction and/or sluggish adduction is best observed during transition from voiceless consonant to vowel. These transitions are frequent in speaking of sentences in list 2. The abductor spasms may be difficult to detect due to vertical motion of the larynx and movement of the epiglottis. Detection is facilitated by playing the recorded examination back in slow motion. Spasms are usually asymmetric in AbSD. Abduction is usually much greater on one side than on the other. Determination of the dominant side is important in planning treatment with botulinum toxin or medialization surgery.[17]

Hyperfunctional behavior during speech is observed in some patients with SD as well as in all patients with MTD. Laryngeal manifestations of hyperfunction include anterior-posterior compression of the larynx and supraglottic constriction, with adduction of the false vocal folds and aryepiglottic muscles. In SD, hyperfunction is believed to be compensatory for the underlying spasm, and there may be great variation in laryngeal movement. In contrast, the hyperfunctional behavior in MTD is much more continuous and consistent. Hyperfunction and hoarseness in MTD patients do not vary with pitch or between sentences in the two standard sentence lists. Voice therapy probing can be conducted during the laryngeal examination, taking the patient through maneuvers to relax the larynx. Improvement during such probe therapy is strong evidence for MTD.

◆ Videostroboscopy

Stroboscopy is rarely useful in the diagnosis of SD, as the diagnosis is established on the basis of voice evaluation and laryngeal examination.

Moreover, the normal sound of the voice during shouting and laughter is strong evidence against any structural defect in the vocal fold. However, it is conceivable that a patient with SD could have a coexistent mucosal lesion of the larynx and that the diagnosis could be more elusive. In such a case, stroboscopic evaluation would be indicated. But it is often difficult to obtain a satisfactory stroboscopic examination of the larynx in a patient with SD. This is because stroboscopic illumination must be flashing very near the same frequency of the vibration of vocal fold mucosa. This is generally accomplished by acoustic analysis of the voice signal to extract the fundamental frequency. In severe SD, or in any patient with severe hoarseness, the acoustic signal of the voice is so irregular that a fundamental frequency cannot be identified. In many patients with SD, there are intervals of fairly stable vibration between vocal breaks, but these intervals are often too short to provide a stable signal.

Stroboscopic examination is more often of value in patients with MTD. Whereas there are definite clinical criteria that support a diagnosis of SD, the diagnosis of MTD is more dependent on the exclusion of other causes. Still, in most patients with MTD, the diagnosis is fairly certain after clinical evaluation, by listening to speech, assessing response to voice therapy, and by examining the larynx with continuous light to detect any gross lesions, such as polyps, nodules, or cysts. This examination can also detect the sequelae of hyperfunction, such as edema and erythema, or even vocal hemorrhage. In patients with documented hyperfuction, voice therapy is the first course of action, even when a gross lesion is detected. The observable pathology is quite often secondary to the overuse, or at least exacerbated by it. Reevaluation after a course of voice therapy is very informative.

In those cases with no observable pathology and no response to voice therapy, the possibility of a subtle structural problem, such as scar, sulcus, or an obscure cyst, should be considered, and stroboscopic examination would clearly be desirable. However, as with SD, stroboscopic evaluation can be difficult in the presence of significant dysphonia if the voice is too hoarse and too irregular to trigger the strobe.

One approach to obtaining a satisfactory stroboscopic evaluation of a patient with SD is to have the patient phonate on inspiration. This is a different motor act than normal speech, and in most SD patients, a stable vocal signal can be achieved. In fact, some patients with SD adopt inspiratory phonation as a compensatory strategy. The mucosal wave then flows in an opposite direction (rostral to caudal), but it is still possible to detect abnormalities of the vocal fold tissues that would impair vibration.

Another approach, which can be used in SD or MTD patients, or in any patient with severe dysphonia, is to drive the strobe light with a different signal than that of the patient's voice. The strobe light can be set to flash at a frequency near what the examiner perceives to be the frequency of the voice. The clinician can also mimic the sound of the patient's voice, with the microphone that drives the strobe timer on the examiner instead of the patient. If the vibration is so irregular that even these strategies fail, then the examination can be performed with the strobe flashing at an arbitrary frequency and then analyzed in stop action to capture individual images at different phases of the vibratory cycle. This is sometimes effective in identifying nonvibratory segments.

High-speed video is the best technique for imaging the vocal fold vibration in a patient with a severely irregular voice. It may also prove to be useful in detecting and studying the abnormal vocal fold movements of patients with SD. Currently high-speed video is not widely used because of the high cost of the technology at present.

◆ Conclusion

The diagnosis of SD and MTD is primarily based on clinical evaluation and standard laryngeal examination. Videostroboscopy is difficult to perform in patients with significant dysphonia because the frequency of vibration is too irregular to trigger the strobe. In cases of presumed MTD that do not respond to voice therapy, the possibility of structural pathology of the vocal fold must be considered, and stroboscopic examination is indicated. Alternate techniques of triggering the stroboscope can be helpful in these cases.

References

1. Morrison MD, Rammage LA, Belisle GM, Pullan CB, Nichol H. Muscular tension dysphonia. J Otolaryngol 1983;12:302–306

2. Morrison MD, Rammage LA. Muscle misuse voice disorders: description and classification. Acta Otolaryngol 1993;113:428–434

3. Shipp T, Izdebski K, Reed C, Morrissey P. Intrinsic laryngeal muscle activity in a spastic dysphonia patient. J Speech Hear Disord 1985;50:54–59

4. Nash EA, Ludlow CL. Laryngeal muscle activity during speech breaks in adductor spasmodic dysphonia. Laryngoscope 1996;106:484–489

5. Traube L. Zur Lehre von den Larynxaffectionnen heim Ileotypus. Berlin, Germany: Verlag Von August Hisschwald; 1871:674–678

6. Dedo HH. Recurrent laryngeal nerve section for spastic dysphonia. Ann Otol Rhinol Laryngol 1976;85(4 Pt 1)451–459

7. Miller RH, Woodson GE, Jankovic J. Botulinum toxin injection of the vocal fold for spasmodic dysphonia: a preliminary report. Arch Otolaryngol Head Neck Surg 1987;113:603–605

8. Blitzer A, Brin MF, Fahn S, Lovelace RE. Localized injections of botulinum toxin for the treatment of focal laryngeal dystonia (spastic dysphonia). Laryngoscope 1988;98:193–197

9. Ludlow CL, Naunton RF, Sedory SE, Schulz GM, Hallett M. Effects of botulinum toxin injections on speech in adductor spasmodic dysphonia. Neurology 1988;38:1220–1225

10. Murry T, Cannito MP, Woodson GE. Spasmodic dysphonia: emotional status and botulinum toxin treatment. Arch Otolaryngol Head Neck Surg 1994;120:310–316

11. Sapienza CM, Walton S, Murry T. Acoustic variations in adductor spasmodic dysphonia as a function of speech task. J Speech Lang Hear Res 1999;42:127–140

12. Edgar JD, Sapienza CM, Bidus K, Ludlow CL. Acoustic measures of symptoms in abductor spasmodic dysphonia. J Voice 2001;15:362–372

13. Roy N, Bless DM, Heisey D, Ford CN. Manual circumlaryngeal therapy for functional dysphonia: an evaluation of short- and long-term treatment outcomes. J Voice 1997;11:321–331

14. Ludlow CL, Adler CH, Berke GS, et al. Research priorities in spasmodic dysphonia. Otolaryngol Head Neck Surg 2008;139:495–505

15. Woodson GE, Murry T, Swenson M. Use of flexible laryngoscopy to classify patients with spasmodic dysphonia. J Voice 1991;5:85

16. Woodson GE. Management of neurologic disorders of the larynx. Ann Otol Rhinol Laryngol 2008;117:317–326

17. Woodson GE, Hochstetler H, Murry T. Botulinum toxin therapy for abductor spasmodic dysphonia. J Voice 2006;20:137–143

26

Laryngeal Leukoplakia and Neoplasm

Steven Bielamowicz and Lauren C. Cunningham

Vocal communication is an important element of human interaction. Voice is produced by the coordination of expiration and vocal fold closure. At the vocal folds, the gelatinous superficial lamina propria allows the overlying mucous membrane to vibrate fluidly while expired air flows over it, producing periodic acoustic energy, with the pharynx acting as a resonance chamber. We recognize this acoustic energy as the human voice. Lesions that begin on the mucous membrane of the vocal fold adversely affect vibration because the periodicity of the acoustic energy is disturbed.

Vocal cord vibration generates rhythmic waves of pressure in the air through the interaction of the vocal fold "cover" and the airstream. The "body-cover" theory of vocal fold vibration states that the underlying tissues, the deep connective tissue layer of the lamina propria, the vocal ligament, and the vocalis muscle, are relatively static, whereas the superficial lamina propria and the mucosa open and close to allow air to pass between the opposed mucosal surfaces. The mucosa moves in an oscillating fashion such that motion of one cord is the mirror image of the other. The mucosal wave originates at the inferomedial aspect of the vocal cord epidermis and propagates rostrally with expiratory airflow. As the rostral cord surfaces separate during the mucosal wave motion, exhaled air passes between the vocal folds. The negative pressure generated as air passes between the cords, as described by the Bernoulli effect, causes the inferior aspect of the vocal folds to pull together, followed by closure of the rostral aspect of the cords. Flow ceases until the build up of subglottic pressure overcomes the resistance of the closed vocal folds, and the cycle begins again.

Efficient vocal fold closure and the unique viscoelastic properties of the mucosal surfaces and superficial lamina propria are necessary for the formation of the mucosal wave. Lesions of the vocal folds may prevent symmetrical closure of the vocal folds or alter the viscoelastic properties of the tissues and interrupt the mucosal wave function. The result is a voice that is hoarse with a decrease in the vocal range. In this chapter, we analyze the histopathology of premalignant and early-stage malignant tumors of the vocal cords and the resultant abnormalities of vocal fold vibration as imaged with videostroboscopy.

◆ Histopathology

Laryngeal leukoplakia is defined as a white patch on the vocal cord and has been reported to have a malignant transformation potential

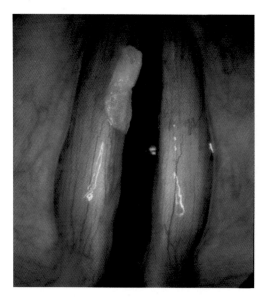

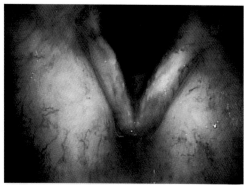

Fig. 26.2 Leukoplakia must be differentiated from candida infection of the vocal fold. This patient had received radiation therapy for laryngeal carcinoma 3 years previously. Although the exam is worrisome for recurrent carcinoma, these lesions resolved with antifungal therapy.

Fig. 26.1 A focal area of leukoplakia involving one vocal fold with variable thickness.

of 1 to 40% (**Fig. 26.1**).[1] Leukoplakia is the result of cellular changes in the overlying vocal fold epithelium and must be differentiated from candida infection of the vocal fold (**Fig. 26.2**). Leukoplakia may appear as a uniformly smooth superficial lesion affecting a portion of one or both vocal folds or as a thick, rough area of the vocal fold (**Fig. 26.3**). Some of these lesions extend across the anterior commissure (**Fig. 26.4**). Others involve a patch-like distribution across the vocal fold (**Fig. 26.5**). Rarely, leukoplakia may affect the supraglottic structures, the arytenoid body, and the interarytenoid region

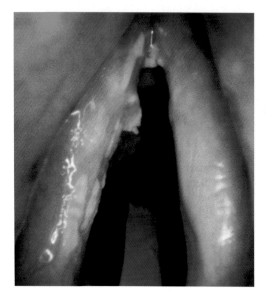

Fig. 26.3 Leukoplakia may appear as a patchy lesion with variable thickness as well as patchy white debris that is easily dislodged from the surface of the vocal fold as noted in the anterior commissure of this image.

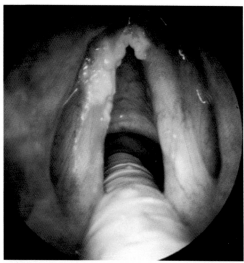

Fig. 26.4 Leukoplakia can extend across the anterior commissure.

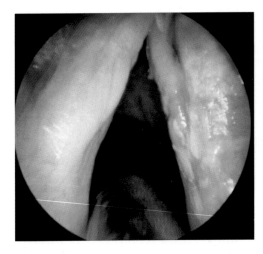

Fig. 26.5 The patchy nature of some leukoplakia lesions of the larynx can involve the true vocal fold as well as the ventricular fold.

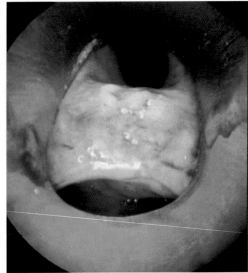

Fig. 26.6 A rare case of leukoplakia of the interarytenoid region. The vocal folds are in the upper portion of the image hidden by the laryngoscope.

(**Fig. 26.6**). Some leukoplakia is associated with erythema, and the term *erythroleukoplakia* is used (**Fig. 26.7**). Erythroleukoplakia is the most likely of these lesions to be malignant.[2,3]

Leukoplakia on the vocal cord represents a broad spectrum of pathology, with an array of corresponding malignant potential. Leukoplakia, without surrounding erythema, may represent a benign transformation called hyperkeratosis or parakeratosis. These lesions are confined to the vocal cord mucosa and have a thickened but ordered cellular maturation

from the basal layer to the surface and thus do not demonstrate any degree of dysplasia. On the other hand, a grossly similar leukoplakia of the vocal fold may demonstrate increasing disorder of the cellular maturation process from the basal layer to the surface and represent mild, moderate, or severe dysplasia, depending on the degree of abnormality. The risk of malignant transformation increases as the severity of dysplasia increases.[4] Lesions that are diagnosed as mild dysplasia are expected to transform in 2 to 12% of cases, and moderate dysplasia transforms in 7 to 27% of cases. Carcinoma in situ is diagnosed when the dysplastic changes are severe, yet the lesion does not penetrate the basement membrane. Invasive carcinoma occurs when the abnormal epithelial cells invade the tissues below the basement membrane (**Figs. 26.8 and 26.9**).

◆ **Videostroboscopic Evaluation of Leukoplakia**

The evaluation of patients with leukoplakia using videostroboscopy yields valuable information. The technique allows for the video-documentation of the geographic distribution

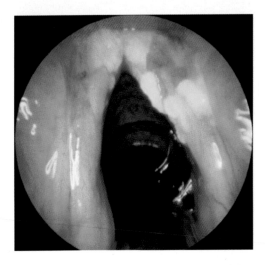

Fig. 26.7 This image reveals patchy erythroleukoplakia.

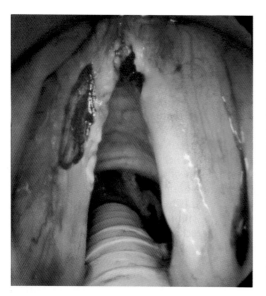 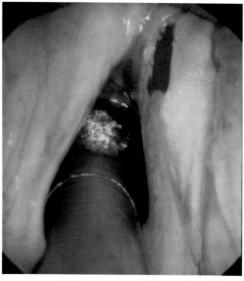

Fig. 26.8 An incisional biopsy of the lateral aspect of the left vocal fold was performed for an umbilicated lesion of the lateral aspect of the vocal fold after microinfusion. This biopsy revealed squamous cell carcinoma.

Fig. 26.9 This patient has been treated for isolated leukoplakia involving the free edge of the vocal fold with an excision of the lesion and preservation of the superficial layer of the lamina propria, in hopes of preserving vocal function. The pathologic examination revealed carcinoma in situ.

of leukoplakia over time. In many patients, the distribution of leukoplakia remains stable over time, and when the distribution of leukoplakia increases along the length of the vocal fold, malignant transformation should be considered. The use of videostroboscopy to evaluate and follow patients with leukoplakia is highly valuable. In patients with thin, superficial leukoplakia, the vocal fold vibration pattern may remain completely intact with a normal vibratory phase, amplitude, periodicity, and glottic closure. In this group of patients, malignancy is highly unlikely. In patients with isolated thick leukoplakia, the affected vocal fold may vibrate with normal vibration amplitude, periodicity, and phase; however, the glottic closure may be affected by the thick lesion. In addition, the area of thick leukoplakia will often demonstrate an adynamic segment within the vocal fold mucosa. Some of these isolated lesions may represent a benign lesion, whereas others may be malignant. Thus, these lesions may warrant surgical excision with a close resection margin and maximal preservation of the underlying superficial layer of the lamina propria.

In patients with bilateral leukoplakia and diffuse leukoplakia, the vibratory nature of the vocal fold is severely disturbed, and the periodic nature of vocal fold vibration is so abnormal that vocal fold vibration is absent as seen on videostroboscopy. The aperiodic nature of the fundamental frequency prevents the filter board within the videostroboscopic unit from providing light output that is asynchronous to the vocal fold vibration. Without adequate tracking of the sound source signal, videostroboscopy has minimal use. In these situations, the vibratory characteristics listed above cannot be evaluated. High-speed imaging may provide a significant improvement in the evaluation of these diffuse lesions and their effect on vocal fold vibration. In addition, patients with diffuse leukoplakia use significant supraglottic compression during voice production. The supraglottic compression is often so severe that visualization of the vibratory surfaces of the vocal fold during voice production is exceedingly limited. Similarly, in patients with inflammatory illness of the vocal fold, the vibration pattern is seen as restricted in amplitude along the full length of the vocal fold. This finding is seen in patients with unilateral erythroplakia.

When comparing hyperkeratosis, parakeratosis, and various degrees of dysplasia, videostroboscopy may not yield significant differences. These are all benign lesions that involve the vocal fold epithelium and do not extend into the superficial lamina propria. In theory, it may be possible to determine if there is deeper invasion by a vocal fold lesion when observing the degree to which the lesion alters vocal fold vibratory characteristics. From what is known about the biomechanics of vocal fold vibration, it is assumed that lesions that appear to vibrate on top of the superficial layer of the lamina propria, along with normal vibration of the surrounding tissues, imply minimal alteration of the vocal fold microstructure and are more likely to be benign. Similarly, lesions that involve the superficial layer of the lamina propria (invasive carcinoma) would be expected to reveal a greater degree of stroboscopic abnormality. In very superficially invasive lesions, the vibration abnormality is expected to be limited to the lesion itself. As the degree of invasion progresses, videostroboscopy might demonstrate a generalized loss of vocal cord vibration at the site of leukoplakia that extends to the surrounding vocal fold mucosa (**Video Clip 35**). Unfortunately, the expected changes in vibration with increasing degrees of tissue invasion are not clinically reliable. In a blinded study of premalignant and early-stage malignant changes of the vocal folds, Colden et al. demonstrated that the vibratory characteristics of the two groups of lesions are not consistently distinguishable by expert raters.[5]

As squamous cell carcinoma lesions advance in stage, vocal cord fixation or impaired movement of the vocal fold can be seen. Videostroboscopy shows changes not only of the vocal fold mucosa but also changes due to incomplete glottic closure associated with vocal paresis or paralysis. The loss of glottic closure is often associated with a contralateral ventricular fold hyperfunction as a compensation strategy.[6] This can limit the overall view of the mucosal wave during stroboscopic analysis. When the mucosal wave can be viewed in these patients, severe aperiodicity is common due to the restriction in the pliability of the vocal fold mucosa.

◆ Further Work-Up for Definitive Diagnosis

As the degree of dysplasia is thought to be the most reliable predictive factor for malignant transformation in laryngeal leukoplakia, a pathology evaluation must always be performed. A deep vocal fold biopsy provides a clear picture of the depth of the lesion but can result in scarring of the vocal fold mucosa and superficial lamina propria leading to vibration abnormalities at the biopsy site with devastating phonation results. Biopsies, therefore, should be performed using microlaryngeal techniques that maximally preserve normal structures.

The possibility of using a brush biopsy rather than a tissue biopsy to determine the risk of malignant transformation in leukoplakia has been studied. Woo quotes an 87% positive predictive value for brush biopsies using excisional or punch biopsy as a standard.[7] The ease of performing brush biopsy as an office procedure is more attractive to the patient and potentially allows the physician to closely monitor the progression of these lesions. The principal advantage of the brush biopsy is that this technique does not present any risk of injury to healthy tissues, thus functional changes due to biopsy are rare.

References

1. Bouquot JE, Gnepp DR. Laryngeal precancer: a review of the literature, commentary, and comparison with oral leukoplakia. Head Neck 1991;13:488–497
2. Qin GZ, Park JY, Chen SY, Lazarus P. A high prevalence of p53 mutations in pre-malignant oral erythroplakia. Int J Cancer 1999;80:345–348
3. Mashberg A, Meyers H. Anatomical site and size of 222 early asymptomatic oral squamous cell carcinomas: a continuing prospective study of oral cancer. II. Cancer 1976;37:2149–2157
4. Isenberg JS, Crozier DL, Dailey SH. Institutional and comprehensive review of laryngeal leukoplakia. Ann Otol Rhinol Laryngol 2008;117:74–79
5. Colden D, Zeitels SM, Hillman RE, Jarboe J, Bunting G, Spanou K. Stroboscopic assessment of vocal fold keratosis and glottic cancer. Ann Otol Rhinol Laryngol 2001;110:293–298
6. Bielamowicz S, Kapoor R, Schwartz J, Stager SV. Relationship among glottal area, static supraglottic compression, and laryngeal function studies in unilateral vocal fold paresis and paralysis. J Voice 2004;18:138–145
7. Woo P. Office-based laryngeal procedures. Otolaryngol Clin North Am 2006;39:111–133

VI

Pediatric Imaging

27

Imaging in Pediatric Patients

J. Scott McMurray

Children are increasingly presenting to clinicians for the evaluation of hoarseness. As young individuals, they pose their own set of difficulties. They often have no awareness, understanding, or interest in the reason for which they have been referred to the specialist. With this in mind, it is easy to understand why they may not be as cooperative as adults who seek an evaluation of their own accord. The evaluation of the hoarse child, however, is no less important than that of an adult. An accurate diagnosis is essential for appropriate management, which may prove to be lifesaving. Visualization of the laryngeal structures is the mainstay of accurate diagnosis.

The techniques used to visualize the adult larynx may also be used in children (**Fig. 27.1**). Smaller versions of fiberoptic and rigid endoscopes are available but often pale in clarity, resolution, and light delivery. As technological advances are made in endoscopy, advances are also made in the office evaluation of the pediatric larynx. It should be stated early, however, that operative endoscopy via a general anesthetic for an accurate diagnosis should be offered if sufficient visualization cannot be obtained in the clinic and if the endoscopist feels confident in his or her operative skills, support, and facility. A missed or delayed diagnosis from failure to adequately visualize the larynx is not acceptable.

The developing pediatric larynx also has a different appearance from the fully developed adult larynx. As the larynx descends into the neck of the adult, the supraglottic structures open up, exposing the true vocal folds for easier visualization. The infantile omega-shaped epiglottis and foreshortened aryepiglottic folds can at times obscure complete visualization of the child's glottis (**Fig. 27.2**). The true

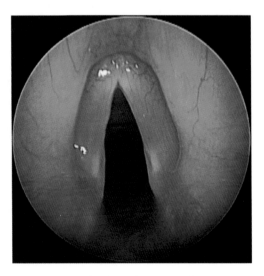

Fig. 27.1 Normal pediatric larynx seen during direct rigid endoscopy.

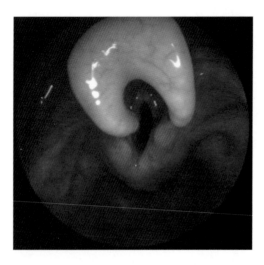

Fig. 27.2 The omega-shaped epiglottis and shortened aryepiglottic folds make visualization of the true vocal folds more difficult in this 18-month-old child.

vocal folds are also shorter in the child than in the adult. Not only are the vocal folds shorter, but also the ratio of the membranous vocal fold to the cartilaginous vocal process is nearly 1 to 1, much smaller than that in the adult (**Fig. 27.3**). The position and shape of the pediatric larynx dramatically differs from that of the adult.

As those who treat children know, the child is not the only patient in the room. The parents also must be involved and committed to the evaluation. An anxious parent will unknowingly and unwittingly transmit their anxiety to their child, making an occasionally difficult task nearly impossible. The key to a successful evaluation is to include both parent and child in the discussion of what will happen and what will be gained from the experience. With these issues properly addressed and with a calm and supportive parent, children are capable of cooperating with a thorough endoscopic evaluation.

Videotaping the laryngeal examination is extremely useful for many reasons. If the child is less than cooperative or if only glimpses of the larynx are obtained, documentation with videotape allows for replay, slow replay, and freeze-frame analysis of the larynx. Later comparisons of the laryngeal status are also important to track the progress of treatment. The usefulness of videotaping with frame-by-frame analysis cannot be emphasized enough. It allows the endoscopist to concentrate on obtaining the images during the endoscopy while affording replay for later review, reassessment, and for explanation of salient physical findings to the parent and child.

◆ Fiberoptic Endoscopy

The introduction of fiberoptic endoscopy has added tremendously in the evaluation of the aerodigestive tract in all age groups. With advancing technology, smaller fiberscopes are becoming available. This has allowed for the use of fiberscopes in even the youngest neonates for visualization of the functioning velopharynx, hypopharynx, and larynx. It is the rare case when a child cannot be evaluated by flexible endoscopy. Small, distal chip camera endoscopes, allowing for a more functional evaluation of the larynx, will likely someday completely replace the rigid angled telescope for laryngoscopy. This will especially hold true as optical quality improves (**Fig. 27.4**).

The choice of fiberoptic endoscope is based on its size, optical clarity, ability to couple with the video-recording source, and its durability. The endoscopist should trial each prospective endoscope with his or her own video system to be certain that the image is acceptable. Smaller endoscopes allow for more comfort for

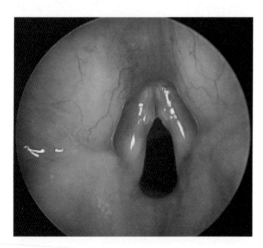

Fig. 27.3 These vocal nodules in the pediatric larynx extend across the total distance of the membranous fold. The ratio of the membranous fold to the vocal process is nearly 1 to 1.

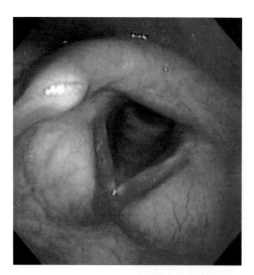

Fig. 27.4 Notice the clarity of this fiberoptic image in this office visualization of the larynx with a flexible, distal chip tip endoscope in a child.

the patient and therefore a longer and more agreeable evaluation, although their durability and optical quality at times are an issue.

Time, perhaps, is the most important component that leads to successful and thorough endoscopy. Time in explanation, time of preparation, and length of time of the examination will significantly enhance the evaluation. Children will be more acceptable to a procedure if they understand the reasons, the expectations, and the agreed upon limits prior to proceeding. Child-friendly terms, consistency, and trust are essential for successful endoscopy. As would be expected in an adult, if the patient does not trust the endoscopist or understand what to expect, cooperation will be minimal. Children should be approached with the same concern and compassion.

An accurate and complete description of the procedure should be given to the parents. If this can be done prior to the office visit, it is optimal. If the parent understands and "buys" into the procedure, it will be much easier to "sell" to the child. Children are masters at observing subtle cues from their parents to help them make decisions regarding their safety and well-being. An anxious parent may unwittingly transfer anxiety to his or her child.

Topical anesthesia and decongestion can be helpful in preparing the pediatric nose for the endoscope. Care should be taken in the very young, however, as significant but transient dysphagia and reflex apnea can occur. Lidocaine and oxymetazoline are the most common agents used in combination prior to the insertion of the flexible fiberscope. The flavor and sensation of atomized nasal sprays can also be disagreeable, however. This can usually be overcome with a lollipop of the child's choice prior to the spray. This can help mask the flavor as well as act as a reward for positive behavior.

If a child is unable to sit comfortably alone for flexible endoscopy, the parent may be enlisted to help with gentle restraint. With the parent seated in the endoscopy chair, the child can sit on the parent's lap. The parent can then give the child a gentle hug and control the hands and arms. An assistant can also help steady the head. The amount of physical restraint is kept light as long as the child does not move or reach for the fiberscope (**Fig. 27.5**). Demonstration of the action of the endoscope, capturing a head shot of the patient with the endoscopic camera and allowing the child to feel the fiberscope prior to insertion, can also be helpful to induce trust of the child.

Once the endoscopy has begun, stops along the way can be made to accommodate the child. With brief stops during insertion at the child's request, the child gains the understanding that he or she has some control during the endoscopy, and the procedure can then generally proceed with fewer interruptions. Once the endoscope is positioned, it should be left in place until the child can settle. When the movement of the scope ceases, discomfort and anxiety decreases and cooperation increases giving a better assessment.

Again, videotaping the examination allows for later explanation of the visualized structures to both the child and the parent. Frame-by-frame analysis can also be used when only brief glimpses of the desired anatomy are seen. Biofeedback can also be used and demonstrated with the videoendoscopy.

The advantage of the flexible endoscope is its nearly universal utility. It would be extremely unlikely that a child could not be examined by a fiberscope. It also allows for the functional evaluation of the nasal cavity, velopharynx, hypopharynx, larynx, and swallow, which cannot be done with the rigid endoscope. The

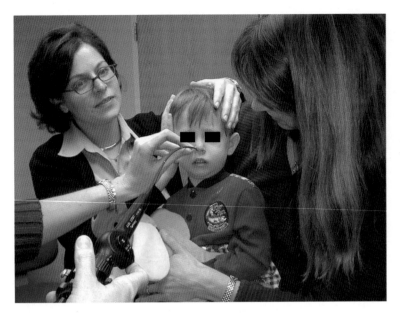

Fig. 27.5 This child is undergoing fiberoptic nasopharyngoscopy. The child is seated in the parent's lap who hugs him and controls his hands and arms. An assistant, a speech pathologist, steadies the head with gentle restraint.

disadvantage to the fiberscope lies in its relatively poor optics and at times inadequate light delivery for videostroboscopy.

◆ Rigid Endoscopy

Cooperative children, generally over the age of 5, can also be examined by the rigid endoscope. The advantages of the rigid angled endoscope are its clarity, quality, and brightness. Videostroboscopy has been found to be helpful in evaluating mucosal and submucosal lesions (**Fig. 27.6**). The typical 10-mm angled rigid endoscope can be used in most instances. Occasionally, the oropharyngeal inlet is narrowed by tonsillar hypertrophy. This can make insertion of the 10-mm endoscope difficult. Smaller angled telescopes are available and have been found to be useful. A 4-mm narrow-view angled endoscope with the light post on the viewing side has been helpful in children with large tonsils. The narrower or less blunt tip of the smaller endoscopes, however, can feel sharper in the posterior pharynx if the mucosa is touched, and so care must be taken to avoid contact with the pharyngeal walls. Superior light and optics, however, are provided by the rigid endoscopes.

The techniques and preparation for rigid indirect laryngoscopy in children are similar to those used in adults. A clear, age-appropriate explanation of the procedure is very helpful in obtaining patient compliance. Although it is up to the endoscopist's preference, fiberoptic endoscopy is often performed first to obtain an image of the larynx. If tolerated reasonably well, then rigid endoscopy can be introduced. This guarantees that some images of the larynx will be obtained yet it affords a chance to record images of the larynx with greater clarity, as well. Again, it should be emphasized that video recording during the endoscopy is extremely useful.

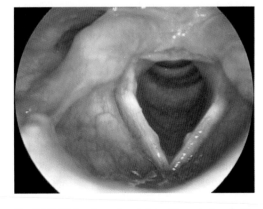

Fig. 27.6 Bilateral vocal nodules with posterior glottic edema and pachydermy consistent with laryngopharyngeal reflux observed via office rigid videoendoscopy.

◆ Operative Endoscopy

There are times during the evaluation of the pediatric larynx when office visualization does not yield an accurate diagnosis. Children may not be able to adequately comply with the fiberoptic exam in the office while awake. An incomplete examination due to anatomic issues, poor cooperation, or if the accuracy of the diagnosis is in question due to a failure in treatment are indications for further physical examination. In these instances, it may be necessary to take the child to the operating room for further evaluation. It may be that operative endoscopy, with a general anesthetic, is required to allow a thorough and more complete visual as well as tactile examination of the larynx (**Fig. 27.7**).

Although the techniques are similar to adult microlaryngology, in pediatric microlaryngology the instrumentation is smaller, airway management has different concerns, and the general anesthetic is often approached differently. This tool and approach, however, should be an integral part of the assessment of the pediatric larynx. Requirements for pediatric direct laryngoscopy include the appropriate instrumentation, support staff, and expertise to perform operative endoscopy. Comfort with the management of the pediatric airway is essential to the safe and accurate assessment of the pediatric larynx during general anesthesia. Beyond the expertise of the surgeon, a well-trained operating room staff and an anesthesiologist comfortable with the pediatric patient and airway are also required.

Telescopic examination or microscopic examination of the pediatric vocal folds may uncover pathology that was not otherwise recognized in the office. It has been shown by Dailey et al. that office endoscopy can miss or incorrectly diagnose 10 to 20% of adult laryngeal pathology.[1] Although this has not been studied in the pediatric larynx, it is likely that similar if not higher inaccuracies occur. An accurate assessment and diagnosis is required for proper treatment regimens.

There are many different techniques for operative endoscopy in the pediatric larynx. Spontaneous ventilation with direct assessment of the vocal folds by telescopes, whether zero-degree or angled, or by a microscope gives a magnified view of the vocal fold. Comfort with microlaryngeal surgical techniques is important for the evaluation of the pediatric larynx. Palpation of the vocal folds is then possible to assess for the presence of an intracordal cyst. Sulcus vocalis may also be recognized with palpation and manipulation of the vocal fold itself. Recognition of lesions other than vocal nodules is important, as these pathologic conditions may require vastly different therapies including surgery.

◆ Common Findings in Pediatric Laryngeal Imaging

Fortunately, the most common finding in a dysphonic child is vocal nodules. Vocal nodules are a thickening of the superficial layers of the vocal fold in discrete areas generally in the middle of the membranous vocal fold. Although attributed to vocal trauma, the exact etiology for vocal nodules is not known. Quiet children can have vocal nodules, whereas screamers may not. Vocal nodules also have different appearances. Soft tissue lesions that are often diagnosed as vocal nodules may have very different physical appearances. This also confirms our lack of understanding of the etiology of vocal nodules (**Figs. 27.8 to 27.15**).

It is important that the pediatric voice specialist be able to recognize different lesions of the vocal fold. It may be especially difficult to distinguish between a submucosal cyst and a vocal nodule in children (**Fig. 27.16**). This

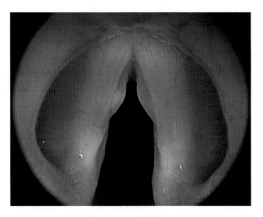

Fig. 27.7 These are symmetric vocal nodules at the midpoint of the membranous vocal fold. Again, the membranous to cartilaginous vocal fold ratio is 1 to 1.

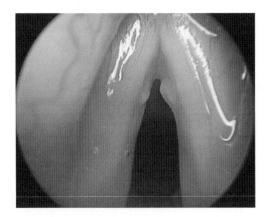

Fig. 27.8 Small asymmetric nodules and anterior vocal fold.

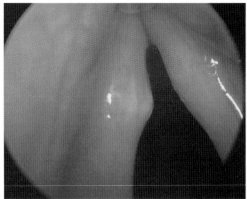

Fig. 27.9 Larger left vocal nodule with asymmetry when compared with the right vocal fold.

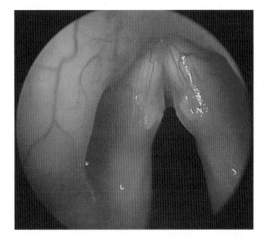

Fig. 27.10 Bilateral nodules with an angry thickened mucosal covering.

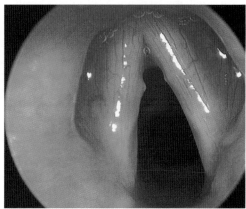

Fig. 27.11 Small but symptomatic nodules in the mid-membranous portion of the vocal folds.

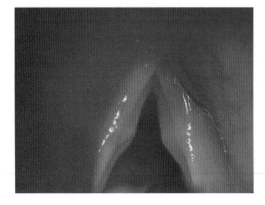

Fig. 27.12 Mildly asymmetric vocal fold nodules in a pediatric larynx.

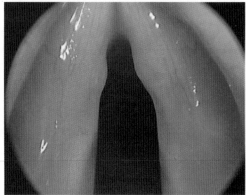

Fig. 27.13 Small symmetric nodules.

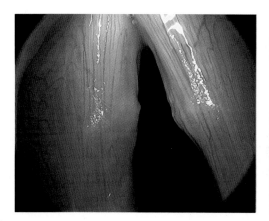

Fig. 27.14 Small nodules of different size and consistency.

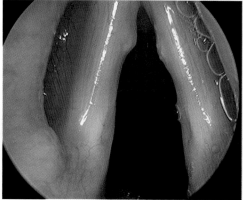

Fig. 27.15 These nodules have some asymmetry. There was no evidence of an intracordal cyst on closer examination.

differentiation is exceedingly important, however, as the primary treatment regiment is vastly different. Intracordal cysts may require surgical intervention or removal, whereas vocal nodules are often successfully treated with voice therapy alone (**Fig. 27.17**).

Sulcus vocalis is a pocket of mucosa that extends deep into the lamina propria. Sulcus vocalis lesions have been classified as superficial to very deep, with extension and occasionally scarring to the vocal ligament (**Fig. 27.18**). As it is in adults, the treatment of sulcus vocalis in children is controversial. Excision of this lesion without subsequent scarring is exceedingly difficult. Voice therapy alone, however, may not resolve the dysphonia. Despite the controversy in treatment modalities, an accurate diagnosis is helpful, as it may explain an inadequate or incomplete response to appropriate voice therapy.

Viral lesions from the human papilloma virus are the most common mass lesions on the pediatric larynx (**Fig. 27.19**). They may recur and cause significant voice disturbance

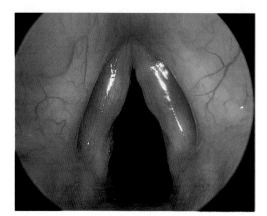

Fig. 27.16 The left vocal fold has an intracordal cyst. The only hint of the cyst is the yellow hue to the submucosal mass. The cyst was confirmed by exploration of the vocal fold. The right or contralateral side has a sulcus vocalis.

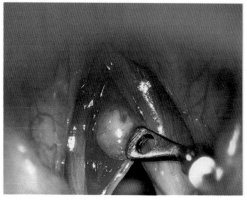

Fig. 27.17 An intracordal cyst is seen through an incision in the left vocal fold.

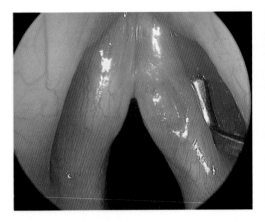

Fig. 27.18 On the right true vocal fold, the lesion seen is a pocket of mucosa, invaginating into the lamina propria, sulcus vocalis. The left vocal fold has an intracordal cyst.

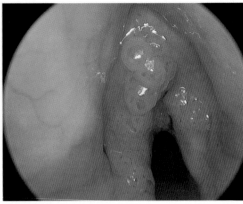

Fig. 27.19 Recurrent respiratory papilloma across the vocal folds and anterior commissure.

as well as respiratory embarrassment. Significant airway obstruction can result from growth of these viral lesions. Office endoscopy is usually diagnostic and may also be used to follow the course of the disease, but surgical intervention is often required for debulking the viral growths to prevent obstruction of the airway.

Congenital anomalies of the larynx may present in newborns or later in children. A few examples of congenital anomalies of the larynx include glottic web, laryngotracheal cleft, laryngomalacia, and supraglottic or saccular cysts (**Figs. 27.20 to 27.22**). Many of these are readily identifiable with office endoscopy, but some require direct laryngoscopy for confirmation.

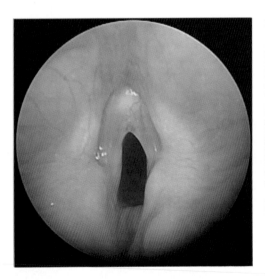

Fig. 27.20 A small laryngeal web is seen across the true vocal folds.

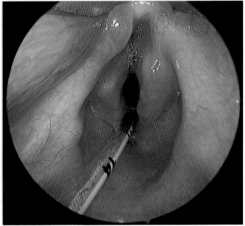

Fig. 27.21 This larynx has a large laryngotracheal cleft. There is a congenital cleft in the posterior glottis, between the arytenoids extending down through the cricoid cartilage. The tube seen is inserted into the esophagus, and the cleft is seen anterior to it.

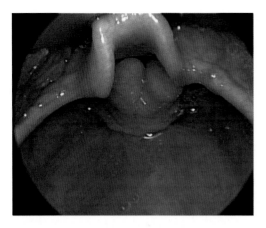

Fig. 27.22 The arytenoids are seen prolapsing into the glottis inlet in this patient with laryngomalacia. The shortening aryepiglottic folds were incised, and the prominent cuneiform cartilages were trimmed to treat this patient.

◆ Conclusion

Pediatric laryngeal pathology should be readily assessed with diagnostic endoscopy. Endoscopy may be performed in the office or in the operating room under general anesthesia. The tools and techniques are similar to those used for assessing adults. The approach, however, may be different. It is important to modify the approach to the child and the parent in the evaluation of the pediatric patient for successful diagnosis and treatment.

Reference

1. Dailey SH, Spanou K, Zeitels SM. The evaluation of benign glottic lesions: rigid telescopic stroboscopy versus suspension microlaryngoscopy. J Voice 2007;21: 112–118

VII

High-Speed Imaging

28

Laryngeal High-Speed Videoendoscopy

Dimitar Deliyski

The purpose of this chapter is to lay the foundation for broader understanding of one of the most promising laryngeal imaging techniques, high-speed videoendoscopy (HSV). This technique may have significant impact in helping us uncover new phenomena in the mechanism of voice production and to better understand laryngeal pathology along with its impact on voice quality. HSV is the most powerful tool for the examination of vocal fold vibration to date. It will provide further insights into the biomechanics of laryngeal sound production, as well as enable more accurate functional assessment of the pathophysiology of voice disorders leading to refinements in the diagnosis and management of vocal fold pathology. For the clinic, HSV is capable of providing unmatched functional and structural information about the larynx, which will ultimately improve clinical practice in speech-language pathology and otolaryngology.

Without claims of completeness, this chapter describes the origins and principles of the HSV technique, the technical considerations important for making HSV clinically useful, the advantages of HSV over videostroboscopy, the unsolved challenges to HSV delaying its wide clinical implementation, and the directions in which HSV is expected to improve our research and clinical abilities. Several clinical applications of HSV are reviewed.

◆ Origins and Principles of High-Speed Videoendoscopy

During phonation, the vocal folds usually open and close over 100 times per second and vibrate at velocities approaching 1 meter per second, making it impossible to view this activity with the unaided eye.[1] For centuries, scientists and clinicians have been trying to build instruments allowing visualization of this fast vibration. To present such fast vibration to the human eye, one has to "slow it down." There are three methods for slowing down fast motion.

The most obvious method to "slow down" vocal fold vibration is by optically photographing the fast-vibrating vocal folds at speeds several times faster than the frequency of vibration, then presenting those images to the human eye at significantly slower rates. This is the principle of high-speed imaging (**Fig. 28.1**). Until the late 19th century, little was known about the limits of visual perception, and building a high-speed imaging machine required technologies not available at the

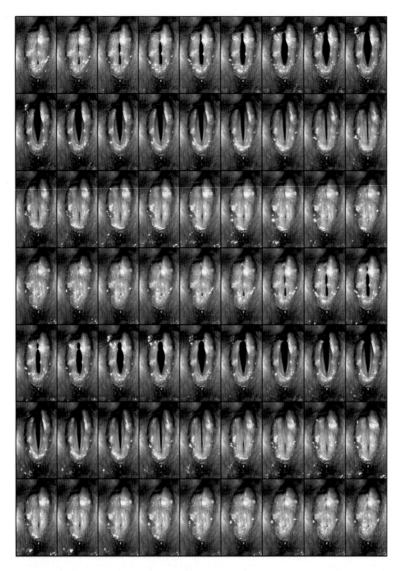

Fig. 28.1 Example of a sequence of color HSV images containing two glottal cycles. The frequency of vibration of the vocal folds (male subject) is 126 Hz and the HSV frame rate is 4000 fps, producing a sequence of ~32 images per glottal cycle (**Video Clip 53**).

time. Therefore, scientists and engineers had to search for alternative methods.

Another "indirect" approach to the evaluation of vocal fold vibration is by recording signals that result from the vibration and presenting them in a graphic format to the human eye. One can then infer conclusions about the characteristics of vocal fold vibration by analyzing the graphic images. The invention of the phonograph and the gramophone allowed for obtaining "visible graphic recordings" (ie, acoustic waveforms).[2] Consequently, the advances in acoustic voice analysis, in electroglottography (EGG) and photoglottography, and the ability to record signals for transglottal airflow and intraoral and subglottal pressure provided invaluable indirect information about the vibration of the vocal folds. The knowledge learned via these technologies helped to refine the models and theory of voice production and stimulated the building of instrumentation that improved clinical voice assessment.

The third approach for "slowing down" the vibration of the vocal folds is by taking advantage of the stroboscopic effect, which is possible due to the quasi-periodic nature of the vocal fold vibration. In the late 19th century, Oertel published the earliest application of stroboscopic principles for observing vocal fold vibration.[3] Later, combining indirect voice signals, acoustic or EGG, with a film or video camera, led to the invention of the most widely used instrument for laryngeal imaging today, the videostroboscopic system.[4] Chapter 11 provides full details about the principles and clinical application of videostroboscopy.

The first high-speed motion picture machine was built in the 1930s, leading immediately to several studies of vocal fold vibration.[5,6] These and other later studies have become some of the most important works in understanding laryngeal physiology.[5–8] But the technology for high-speed imaging was too impractical until the mid-1990s, when two types of high-speed imaging systems became commercially available, the videokymography (VKG) and the HSV systems.[9,10] VKG could scan a single line across the vocal folds at a speed of 7800 lines per second, and the HSV systems could scan a full image at speeds up to 2000 frames per second (fps). These first systems provided monochromatic images with poor resolution and image quality. The VKG was faster and less expensive than HSV but could scan only one section on the anterior-posterior plane of the vocal folds and lacked a mechanism for feedback about which line was being scanned. A new-generation VKG system has resolved many of these concerns.[11] In the meantime, bridging the technological gain in machine vision helped tremendously improve the HSV technology.[12] Today, high-speed cameras can record at frame rates up to 1,000,000 fps. They can record in color (**Fig. 28.1**), with high spatial resolution and excellent image quality, for longer durations.[13] Before overwhelming the reader by presenting technical parameters, it is important to explain: What makes HSV superior to videostroboscopy?

◆ Advantages of High-Speed Videoendoscopy over Videostroboscopy

Videostroboscopy

To elicit an effect of "slow motion," videostroboscopy relies on the assumption of the near-periodic nature of vocal fold vibration. **Figure 28.2A** reiterates an illustration of the principle of videostroboscopy from Chapter 11. In videostroboscopy, the resulting "slow-motion" glottal cycle is artificially assembled from images sampled from consecutive phases taken from different glottal cycles. The strobe light flashes are short (10 to 20 μsec), delivered only during the cycle phases for which images are taken.

It is important to realize that in the case of an aperiodic signal, the near-periodic assumptions do not hold. When the acoustic or EGG signal is aperiodic, the timing of strobe flashes does not correspond with the phases of the glottic cycle in the desired sequence. Even subtle variations in periodicity can produce completely distorted or unrealistic videostroboscopic sequences. Depending on the type of aperiodicity, the distortions may produce random-appearing vibrations, may change the balance between the timing of the opening and closing phases of the glottal cycle, may produce a reverse-appearing motion during a portion of the cycle or through the entire cycle, or may "lock" out of the closed phase, making it appear that the glottis never closes completely. All these effects can occur even in vocal fold vibration with very good overall periodicity, where the irregularity is so slight that it is not visually perceivable. At the same time, relatively pronounced aperiodic patterns may be able to synchronize well the strobe light, producing an illusory "regular" cycle. There are at least three reasons for these effects:

1. Videostroboscopy is a hybrid between an acoustic analysis system and an imaging system. The videostroboscopic effect relies on analysis of the acoustic or EGG waveform. We typically classify videostroboscopy under the category of laryngeal imaging systems. That is partially true, because the end

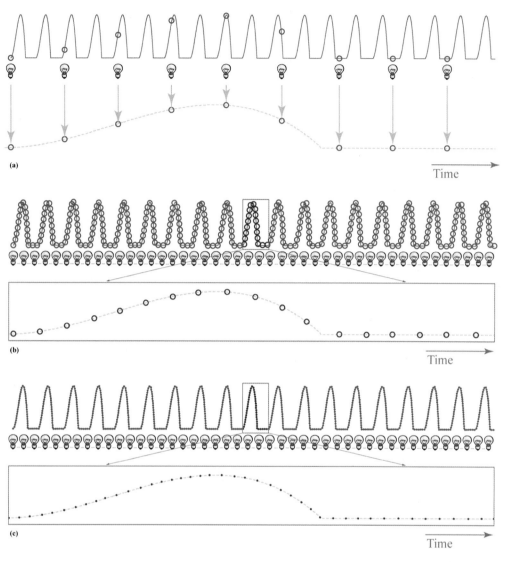

Fig. 28.2 Illustration of the principle of sampling in videostroboscopy **(A)** and in HSV **(B, C)**. **(A)** In videostroboscopy, the resulting "slow-motion" glottal cycle (below) is artificially assembled from images sampled from consecutive phases in different glottal cycles (above); whereas **(B)** in HSV, each cycle (below) is represented by images sampled within that very same cycle (above); that is, there is a "true" intracycle slow-motion viewing achieved by zooming, or warping the timescale. **(C)** When increasing the frame rate, HSV represents more accurately the details of the vibration within the glottal cycle.

product of a videostroboscopic exam is a series of images. However, which images are being presented depends on acoustic analysis. Therefore, from the point of view of the analysis of vocal fold vibration, videostroboscopy is an acoustic analysis technique, not a true imaging technique. The videostroboscopic vocal fold vibratory patterns are determined by the acoustic waveform, not by the actual biomechanical vibration. All limitations to acoustic voice analysis are present in videostroboscopy.[14]

2. For each video frame, videostroboscopy relies on pitch tracking through a laryngeal contact microphone or EGG to predict the phase of the upcoming glottal cycles. Thus, the acoustic or EGG signal during one 30-msec video frame is used to predict the frequency of the next phase of vibration that will be recorded in the upcoming video frame, assuming that the period will not change within the next 30 msec. Obviously, in the case of aperiodic vibration, or aperiodic acoustic or EGG waveforms, the videostroboscopic images will present in random or chaotic order and will not be representative of the actual vibration pattern.

3. It is also important to note that high aperiodicity of the acoustic or EGG signal does not always mean that the period of vibration is highly irregular. A visible irregular pattern of vocal fold vibration would always cause severe irregularities in the acoustic waveform, translating into perceptual effects of severe dysphonia or aphonia. However, period perturbations of the acoustic waveform do not necessarily mean that the period of vibration is visibly aperiodic. Most of the increased acoustic perturbation cases are not related to "visible" period irregularities of the vibration.[15] The variations of the acoustic period are not necessarily caused by variations in the period of the glottal cycle. The glottal cycle period may be stable overall, but the cycle-to-cycle variations of local (intracycle) vibratory features, such as glottal width, symmetry, open quotient, mucosal wave, mucus bridges, and/or loss of contact, may be producing acoustic period perturbations. Videostroboscopy interprets these acoustic period perturbations as vibratory period instability, leading to an overdiagnosis of aperiodicity.[15,16]

In summary, aperiodic vibration, or aperiodic acoustic waveforms cause the strobe light to become asynchronized with the actual phase of vocal fold movements preventing visualization in "slow motion." As a result, videostroboscopy cannot be used on persons whose voice disorder has caused their vocal fold movement, or acoustic waveform, to become aperiodic. Thus, many patients, mainly those exhibiting dysphonia, cannot benefit from the technology of videostroboscopy even though it is considered the current gold standard for laryngeal imaging.

Videostroboscopy is a technique that revolutionized clinical management of voice disorders and laryngeal pathology. However, it is applicable only on sustained phonation tasks for individuals with stable phonatory characteristics. Accurate and reliable assessment cannot be achieved for individuals with pronounced dysphonia. Videostroboscopy is not applicable for evaluating transient vocal fold vibratory behaviors, such as, phonatory breaks, laryngeal spasms, and the onset and offset of phonation. It cannot be used for tasks involving vocal attack, coughing, throat clearing, laughing, and other activities including rapid laryngeal maneuvers.

High-Speed Videoendoscopy

In contrast with videostroboscopy, HSV is the only technique that captures the true intracycle vibratory behavior through a true series of full-frame images of the vocal folds. Therefore, HSV, by default, overcomes the above limitations of videostroboscopy, providing for the possibility of a more reliable and accurate objective quantification of the vocal fold vibratory behavior regardless of whether this behavior is periodic or aperiodic.

Figure 28.2B illustrates the principle of HSV sampling in comparison with stroboscopic sampling (**Fig. 28.2A**). In HSV, each resulting glottal cycle is represented by several images sampled within that very same cycle (ie, there is a "true" intracycle slow-motion viewing achieved by zooming the timescale). The lighting is constant, not intermittent as in stroboscopy. HSV is recording constantly, and no information can be missing between the frames. HSV data contains all frames, not just selected ones. Therefore, HSV supersedes videostroboscopy. We have demonstrated that videostroboscopy can be produced from HSV using simulated stroboscopy with audio (SSA).[13] The advantage of SSA is that it uses the actual vibration, not an indirect acoustic signal, to establish the glottal cycle phases in producing the stroboscopic effect, thus it does not suffer the tracking errors typical for videostroboscopy.

In addition, HSV is a superset of VKG, because it contains all the VKG lines from the anterior to the posterior, whereas VKG contains only one line.[13] Therefore, kymography can be produced from HSV by selecting a particular line across the anterior-posterior axis, a process termed digital kymography (DKG).

These properties make HSV uniquely suitable for either spatial and/or dynamic representation of the same content (ie, as a movie) or kymographically. Not only does HSV record the true glottal cycle: It records a series of many glottal cycles, allowing for the study of cycle-to-cycle variation in the local (intracycle) vibratory features over time.

Assessment of Vibratory Features of Sustained Phonation

The purpose of videostroboscopy is the assessment of vocal fold vibratory features in sustained phonation. In a stroboscopic exam, the voice assessment protocol includes vibratory features such as periodicity, symmetry, mucosal wave, open quotient, glottal closure, and mucus aggregation. HSV can be used to elicit all features of the stroboscopic protocol. However, due to the higher temporal resolution and tracking reliability of the HSV technique, some of the features appear differently, and new important aspects of these features can be observed.

Symmetry

Vibratory symmetry of the glottal cycle can be regarded in several ways. In a videostroboscopic evaluation, asymmetry is judged in the left-right dimension evidenced by amplitude and phase differences between the left and right vocal folds. A recent systematic categorization of asymmetry differentiated four aspects of left-right asymmetry: amplitude, phase and frequency differences, and axis shifts.[17] Another important aspect of asymmetry is the anterior-posterior phase asymmetry,

which is often manifested through the hourglass or zipper effects during vocal fold closure.[18] Anterior-posterior phase asymmetry is defined as the anterior and posterior portion of one vocal fold reaching maximal glottal opening at different times within the glottal cycle. Left-right phase asymmetry is defined as the two vocal folds reaching maximal glottal opening at different times within the glottal cycle. Left-right amplitude asymmetry is defined as the two vocal folds having different maximal amplitudes of glottal opening within the glottal cycle. Left-right frequency asymmetry is defined as the two vocal folds vibrating at different frequencies. Axis shifts are defined as the spatial location of the opening of the vocal folds within the glottal cycle shifting to the left or to the right from the location of last contact. HSV allows for the objective visualization of all five aspects of asymmetry, whereas videostroboscopy can be used only for two, left-right amplitude and phase asymmetry.[18,19] In videostroboscopy, these two features are usually judged together because it is difficult to perceptually separate them, and their visualization is limited only to periodic vibration and acoustic waveforms.

Period and Glottal Width Irregularity

Regularity, or periodicity, of vocal fold vibration can be defined as the exact repetition of a spatial-temporal pattern. Thus, irregularity and aperiodicity refer to any change of this pattern over time. The most common visually judged features of vocal fold vibratory regularity are glottal period regularity and glottal width regularity, which reflect the two aspects of the spatial-temporal pattern.[15,19] Both HSV and videostroboscopy can be used for assessing period and glottal width regularity. However, the reliability of videostroboscopy suffers significantly in the presence of irregularity due to tracking problems, whereas HSV can visualize any irregular vibratory pattern. In videostroboscopy, the determination of irregularity is essentially based on the acoustic or EGG signal's properties, not on the actual vibration properties. In addition to the ability to precisely record irregular patterns, HSV allows for presenting these patterns in a spatial-temporal domain using DKG, making them more comprehensible.

Mucosal Wave

Mucosal wave is one feature that is generally thought to be a good global indicator of vibratory behavior. Mucosal wave is the propagation of the epithelium and superficial layer of the lamina propria from the inferior to the superior surface of the vocal folds during phonation. The presence, magnitude, and symmetry of the mucosal wave are indicators of tension and pliability of the underlying vocal fold tissue and are essential to the production of good voice quality.[20] Due to the anatomic configuration of the vocal folds and the superficial viewpoint of rigid endoscopy relative to them, the mucosal wave is viewed through two different aspects. The first viewing aspect is the lateral propagation of the mucosal wave between the vocal folds, where the mucosal wave is seen as the differential between the lower and the upper margins of the vocal folds during closing. This view begins with the closing phase, from the moment of adduction of the lower margins of the vocal folds through the end of the adduction of the entire folds. The second viewing aspect is the propagation of the mucosal wave on the upper surface of the vocal folds. This view begins during the closing phase from the upper margins of the vocal folds. While the vocal folds are adducting to close the glottis, the mucosal wave is traveling in the opposite direction, toward the exterior margins of the vocal folds. Both HSV and videostroboscopy allow visualization of the two mucosal wave aspects. However, HSV provides more objective visualization, especially through the use of DKG. Due to its high velocity of propagation, the mucosal wave is the feature most sensitive to the frame rate of the HSV system.[20] Our investigations show that for achieving full viewing of the mucosal wave features, the frame rate has to be at least 16 times higher than the frequency of vibration. That is, for a man with a fundamental frequency (F_0) of 125 Hz, the frame rate has to be at least 2000 fps, for a woman with $F_0 = 300$ Hz, it has to be at least 4800 fps, and for a woman producing falsetto with $F_0 = 1000$ Hz, it has to be at least 16,000 fps to track the detail of mucosal wave propagation.

Open Quotient

Open quotient is the amount of time the vocal folds are in the opening and closing phase, versus the duration of the entire vibratory cycle.[19,21] HSV allows for measuring open quotient because it provides the true intracycle information for each glottal cycle.

Contact and Loss of Contact

Glottal closure is the pattern of vocal fold contact at the closed phase of vibration. It is generally categorized as closed, hourglass, anterior gap, posterior gap, or irregular. This feature can be viewed through both HSV and videostroboscopy. However, it is very important to report whether the realization of contact and loss of contact are changing from one cycle to the next. Only HSV can provide this information due to its inherent true cycle-to-cycle visualization.

Mucus and Mucus Bridges

Vocal fold mucus aggregation is common in persons with voice disorders. It is known that an increase in vocal fold mass, from mucus, will change vocal fold vibratory behavior. Mucus has been noted as the causal factor of rough vocal quality. The presence, type, thickness, location, and pooling of mucus aggregation are important indicators of how mucus is impacting vocal quality.[22] Mucus can be evaluated with both HSV and videostroboscopic techniques, and videostroboscopy is generally more sensitive due to its better spatial resolution and image quality. However, another feature important for voice quality, the cycle-to-cycle variation of mucus bridges forming between the vocal folds during loss of contact, can be studied only through HSV.

As indicated, many vibratory features can be studied by either videostroboscopy or HSV. However, most of the features appear different from videostroboscopy when viewed using HSV.[15,16,18,20,22,23] Voice clinicians, including speech-language pathologists and laryngologists, have been highly trained to use videostroboscopy. When using HSV, they may attempt interpreting vibratory features relative to the norms used in the clinic with videostroboscopy. Thus, there is a risk that a new and very different technique may not be found useful, unless a smooth transition is realized. An important first step in such transition is to generate HSV-specific clinical norms. This topic is covered later in the section "High-Speed Videoendoscopy in the Clinical Speech-Language Pathology Practice."

Analysis of Aperiodic Phenomena

HSV is uniquely suited for studying aperiodic vibration and other fast movements. This is an area in which videostroboscopy has no utility. Videostroboscopy cannot be used on persons whose voice disorder has caused vibration with perturbed periodicity. Not only can HSV visualize such vibration, but also it allows measuring the degree of perturbation. HSV is applicable for evaluating most transient vocal fold vibratory behaviors.

Phonatory Breaks, Laryngeal Spasms, Onset and Offset of Phonation

HSV is the only imaging technique that can effectively record and visualize transient phonatory events. A better understanding of the nature and occurrence of these events is a very important area of voice research with strong implications for clinical practice, from the functional evaluation and diagnosis of various voice disorders through treatment planning and intervention.

Phonatory breaks are transient instabilities or short interruptions of the phonatory process. They are a typical phenomenon associated with several voice disorders. We have seen them also sometimes in vocally normal populations, especially within the first 100 msec after phonatory onset. HSV allows for precisely tracking the phonatory breaks, visualizing them, and assessing their temporal pattern and duration.

Laryngeal spasms can result in vocal fold abduction or adduction. They are thought to occur in neurologically based voice disorders and are most typical in spasmodic dysphonia. HSV allows for precisely tracking, categorizing, and measuring laryngeal spasms.

The characteristics of phonation onset and offset of phonation may be indicative of a specific type of voice disorder. Little is known in this area. The evaluation of vocal offset can provide invaluable information about vocal fold pliability by judging how quickly and orderly the end of phonation occurs. The evaluation of vocal onset can provide objective information about the maneuvers the patient performs in reaching the optimal phonatory threshold to begin phonation or about asymmetries due to left-right differences in mass and tension, which may not be visible during stable sustained phonation. HSV places this information at our fingertips, and it is only a matter of conducting sufficient research to create better protocols for objective voice evaluation.

Vocal Attack Time

The speed with which the vocal folds adduct to the midline is considered an important variable in the etiology of some voice disorders and may also be a meaningful indicator of central or peripheral neural dysfunction. Measuring vocal attack time has been addressed by Moore and by Werner-Kukuk and von Leden.[5,8] HSV allows for precisely recording the voice onset for different types of glottal attacks and measuring useful physiologic characteristics. Recently, we have used HSV to successfully validate a vocal attack time measurement, which is discussed in more detail later in the section "High-Speed Videoendoscopy as a Research Tool for Voice Science."[24]

Coughing, Throat Clearing, Laughing, and Other Activities Involving Rapid Laryngeal Maneuvers

Coughing and throat clearing are considered to be potentially harmful to the vocal folds from the point of view of vocal hygiene. Clinicians typically recommend "safer" mucus clearing behaviors, such as "soft" cough and clear. But little is known about the biomechanics of these processes and how are they actually harmful to the tissue. HSV allows for precise visualization, registration, and measurement of the physical attributes of these behaviors. Our ongoing research effort in this area may provide clinically useful data. On a separate note, laughing, clearing, and other similar quickly varying laryngeal tasks are clinically useful as media for eliciting phonation in aphonic patients. HSV can be used for visualizing the vocal fold vibration during the short phonatory segments elicited though such clinical techniques.

Alaryngeal Speech

Developing instrumental or perceptual techniques for the evaluation of alaryngeal voice has always been a significant challenge. These voices do not qualify for acoustic voice analysis, present difficulties in using perceptual scales, and cannot be documented via EGG or videostroboscopy.[14] HSV has been successfully used for visualization of the vibratory characteristics of the substitute voice generator and for automatic image segmentation of the neoglottis.[25] The ability of HSV to visualize and measure vibration after laryngectomy is important for evaluating the success of voice restoration.

Objective Automated Analysis

After everything said about HSV, it is important to make a clarification. HSV is a lot more than a slow-motion movie. Videostroboscopy is a technique designed primarily for slow-motion visualization of the fast vocal fold vibration during sustained phonation in real time, which is very limited in terms of objective measurement of the vibration. HSV is fundamentally different in that respect. The visualization is very accurate, presented in warped (delayed) time. Every characteristic of the visualized vibration is potentially measurable, because it is inherently accurately represented in the recording. HSV can be described as a data "cube," which has two spatial coordinates, x (left-right) and y (posterior-anterior), and one temporal coordinate, t (time). All three dimensions are described by the intensity of each pixel. It is a solid "cube": there is no missing information along any of the dimensions. Therefore, it is essential to demonstrate what is clinically relevant to develop the appropriate analytic technique for measuring it.

Several automatic and semiautomatic HSV-derived measurements have been reported in the literature.[26] They have been classified as follows:

- *Measures related to frequency of vibration:* fundamental frequency; period perturbation quotient; coefficient of variation of F_0; voice breaks; vocal tremor (F_0-modulation) frequency and magnitude.
- *Measures associated with glottal symmetry:* left-to-right phase, amplitude, and frequency symmetry quotients; axis shifts; posterior-to-anterior symmetry concurrence (showing whether some parts along the vocal fold have different symmetry parameters than others).
- *Measures related to glottal width and area characteristics:* open and closed quotient; glottal area perturbation quotient; coefficient of variation of glottal area; soft phonation index; vocal tremor (glottal area modulation) frequency and magnitude.
- *Measures reflecting unilateral dynamic characteristics:* activity/displacement of the left or the right vocal fold, and ratio of left versus right vocal fold.
- *Measures related to mucosal wave properties:* mucosal wave presence; symmetry quotient; relative area to glottal open area; sharpness pattern.
- *Measures related to vertical movement during phonation:* left-to-right vertical symmetry, computed through the image intensity.
- *Measures assessing modal types:* vibration-based voice typing (similar to types 1, 2, and 3 per Titze); automatic classification of bifurcation patterns (eg, periodic, biphonia, diplophonia, vocal fry, aphonia, vocal onset, vocal offset, etc.); subharmonic level (ie, which is the most active subharmonic of F_0 [first, second, etc.]).[14]
- *Semiautomatic measures reported objectively:* manually placed posterior and anterior commissure markers; manually tagged transient events; visually classified patterns of vibration.[17]

Some of these objective measures have been compared with visual perceptual ratings: period and glottal width irregularity, left-right phase and amplitude asymmetry, axis shifts during closure, and open quotient.[15,18,21] The findings suggest that usually objective measures differ from visual subjective ratings, underscoring the limits of human perception and the importance of developing robust automated measurement techniques. New objective HSV measures are being developed through the phonovibrography method.[27] Objective measures that have been reported using VKG—amplitude symmetry, speed quotient, and phase symmetry index—are highly applicable to HSV.[28] Whereas several research teams are actively developing HSV-based objective measures, the clinical efficacy of these measures is still under investigation. There are no established standards or commercially available software products at this time.

Relationships between Vibration and Acoustics

Due to the high temporal resolution of HSV, it is possible for the first time to precisely align the HSV images with acoustics and other voice signals (**Fig. 28.3**), such as EGG, transglottal airflow, intraoral and subglottal pressure, and accelerometry. This is exciting for two reasons. First, voice science can better understand the relationships between vocal fold vibration and the resulting voice, leading to important refinements of the models of voice production. Additionally, combining HSV measures of vocal fold vibration with concurrent acoustic and EGG measures may provide complementary, high-precision measures that can improve the clinical practice. Scientific investigations of these relationships are under way. Several examples are presented later in the section "High-Speed Videoendoscopy as a Research Tool for Voice Science."

◆ Technical and Methodological Considerations Using High-Speed Videoendoscopy

This section is intended to provide a practical understanding of the HSV technology. There are two aspects, technical and methodological. The technical part is concerned with acquiring high-quality HSV data. That is, making sure that all vibratory information of interest was recorded correctly, with sufficient spatial and temporal image quality. The methodological aspect is concerned with the efficacy of presenting the relevant information to the clinician or researcher. That is, finding ways of complementing the playback of the HSV movie by other, more intuitive facilitative playbacks and objective measures that can reveal the relevant content, which is often hidden to the human eye through the HSV movie playback.

Important Technical Characteristics of High-Speed Videoendoscopy

An HSV system typically consists of the following elements: a digital high-speed camera (monochrome or color); a 70-degree or 90-degree rigid laryngeal endoscope; an endoscopic lens adapter; a powerful light source (usually 300 W constant xenon); a trigger button; a computer controlling the camera via specialized software for image acquisition and real-time video feedback; a computer monitor; and a wheeled equipment cart. The camera may be connected to the computer either via a specialized hardware card or via a standard Ethernet or FireWire interface. In some cameras, the digital processing circuitry is in a separate box installed on the cart, which allows for a lighter camera head attached to the endoscope. Heavier cameras, 2 lb and above, may be weight-balanced using a camera crane. The synchronous recording of additional signals is available with more advanced configurations. Such systems include additional hardware and software. Our HSV system, designed at the Voice and Speech Laboratory, University of South Carolina (Columbia, SC) (**Fig. 28.3**), includes the following additional elements: an 8-channel data acquisition card; a head-mount condenser microphone; a microphone preamplifier; an EGG device; a frequency divider; data acquisition software; and a second monitor to separate the HSV image from the channel data feedback.

Sensitivity

The digital high-speed cameras are photon-integrating devices. The complementary metal-oxide semiconductor (CMOS) photo sensor of the camera is divided into pixels (individual

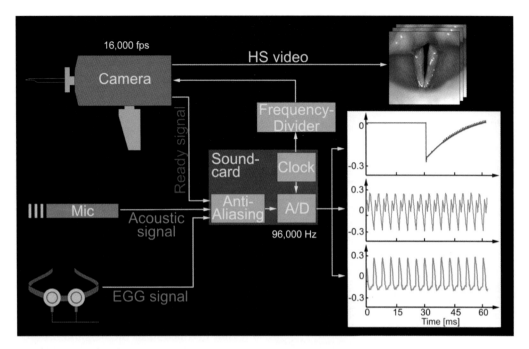

Fig. 28.3 A block-circuit of the HSV system designed at the Voice and Speech Laboratory, University of South Carolina, which allows aligning precisely the HSV images with acoustic, EGG, and other voice signals. A Phantom v7.3 high-speed camera (Vision Research, Inc.) is clocked by the sampling rate of an 8-channel M-Audio Delta 1010LT data acquisition card (Avid Technology, Inc.) after 1:6 frequency division. The camera "Ready" signal makes it possible to achieve accuracy of synchronization of 11 μsec. This architecture permits exactly attributing the six acoustic or EGG samples corresponding with each frame.

photo cells), each usually 10 μm × 10 μm in size, or larger, up to 22 μm by 22 μm. For the duration of one frame of the recording, each pixel "counts" the number of photons being reflected from the surface of the anatomic structures that "fall" on the surface of that sensor. The stronger the intensity of light reflection and/or the longer the integration time, the higher is the number recorded for that pixel (ie, the brighter that pixel will be in the recorded movie). The amount of light that the tissue can absorb safely is limited. Thus, the sensitivity of the sensor's pixels and the duration of each frame's integration time are important parameters for eliciting an image. The most sensitive high-speed cameras today have monochrome sensitivity of 6400 ISO per 1280 × 800 pixels sensor (Vision Research, Inc., Wayne, NJ) and 6400 ISO per 1000 × 1000 pixels sensor (Photron Inc., San Diego, CA), which provides similar sensitivity per pixel. The

sensitivity of the color versions of these cameras is 1600 ISO.

Integration Time

The high-speed camera integrates the light reflected from the tissue surface for a given time corresponding with one frame. Each recorded sample is an image, termed *frame*, constructed of many pixels. For example, if the HSV frame rate is 2000 fps, each second of time is divided into 2000 recording sessions following every 500 μsec. The integration of each frame takes most of the 500-μsec period, given that the only time the integration is not active is during the "reset" time for each frame, which is negligible (~2 μsec). This is the most fundamental difference between stroboscopy and HSV. In videostroboscopy, the strobe flashes are intermittent. If they cannot be precisely timed, the resulting reconstructed glottal cycle image sequence is incorrect. HSV is recording everything and no information is missing between the frames (**Fig. 28.2**).

Frame Rate

Although HSV technology provides true sampling of vibration, the selection of an appropriate frame rate is very important for the accurate recording of some of the relevant vibratory features. **Figure 28.2C** illustrates the effect of increasing the HSV frame rate on the accuracy of representing the vibration details within the glottal cycle compared with lower frame rates (**Fig. 28.2B**). The frame rate determines the integration time (ie, the time between frames). If the integration time is too long and the velocity of the features being filmed is too high, the fast-moving features are averaged through the integration period, and they appear blurred, out of focus, or may even become invisible. The faster the motion, the shorter the integration time has to be, thus the frame rate has to be higher. Based on our data, the fastest vocal fold vibratory features are the mucosal wave propagation and the movement of the vocal fold edges during the closing phase. Based on visual testing, we established a rule of thumb that the frame rate has to be at least 16 times higher than the frequency of the glottal cycle (in periodic sustained phonation same as F_0). That is, each cycle has to be presented by at least 16 images (**Fig. 28.1**). Therefore, in clinical settings, the optimal frame rate is ~8000 fps, allowing for the evaluation of voicing tasks not exceeding F_0 of 500 Hz. That frame rate would cover most clinical tasks for men and women, such as habitual pitch and loudness phonation, onset and offset, high and low pitch in modal register, and breathy and pressed phonation. In some special tasks, such as falsetto register or pitch glides, even the rate of 8000 fps may be insufficient and some features may be underrepresented. Obviously, the commonly used frame rate of 2000 fps is inadequate and would misrepresent the vibratory features of persons with a F_0 above 125 Hz (ie, most women would appear to lack a mucosal wave).[20] Several older studies have suggested that increased pitch relates to a reduced mucosal wave, probably a conclusion partially resulting from inferior technology at the time.

Color

Traditionally, HSV systems have been monochromatic (black and white). The Voice and Speech Laboratory integrated the first known color HSV system back in 2003.[13] Since then, we have learned about the advantages and caveats of color. Color is clinically important for correctly identifying anatomic structures and especially for identifying lesions and structural tissue changes. However, to achieve color, the sensitivity of the camera is reduced ~4 times, because the light has to be channeled into three color filters (for red, green, and blue), and additional light loss is caused by filtering-out the infrared and ultraviolet components, light absorption, and reflection. That translates into a 4-times reduction of the maximum frame rate of the HSV system for the same image quality relative to monochrome. Additionally, color significantly reduces the effective spatial resolution of the camera due to the Bayer mosaic color filtering used in single-chip color sensors. Consequently, for the very same model camera, the color and monochrome versions at the same pixel resolution have a significantly lower effective resolution of the color camera because the image is obtained through interpolation. Thus, the edges of the vocal folds represented using the monochrome camera are more accurate. Color HSV systems have advantages when viewing the vocal fold, but monochrome images allow for more accurate measurement of the vibratory characteristics.

Lighting

HSV technology requires a lot of light due to the CMOS photon integration principles. Thus, increasing the amount of light can improve HSV image quality and frame rates. The type of light source used with most HSV systems today is 300 W constant xenon light. There is, however, a safety concern that further increasing the amount of light used with HSV can cause tissue damage. Additionally, it is considered possible that long exposures to a 300 W constant xenon light can cause tissue damage.

No reports of such damage have been filed to date, but as a precaution it is recommended that the amount of time the vocal folds are exposed to light during an HSV exam be reduced to less than 20 seconds.

Spatial (Pixel) Resolution

Our experience shows that spatial resolution above 300 × 300 pixels is adequate for quality images and for automated analysis. The spatial resolution of modern high-speed cameras allows for much higher resolution, including high-definition resolution of 1920 × 1080 pixels, and up to 2048 × 2048 pixels (Vision Research, Inc.).

Effective Dynamic Range

Dynamic range is a measure of brightness resolution of the sensor (ie, the ratio between the largest possible to the smallest possible light that the camera can register). That ratio is related to the sensitivity of the camera in a combination with the quantization levels (bits per pixel). For example, 8 bits per pixel provide for a maximum dynamic range of 256 (48 dB), whereas 12-bit quantization supports a maximum dynamic range of 4096 (72 dB) per pixel. Whether this is an effective dynamic range depends on the amount of noise in the lower bits (the smaller intensity values). If noise is present, the effective dynamic range is reduced relative to the maximum dynamic range. A high effective dynamic range allows one to "brighten" a dark image or to "darken" a very bright image without causing a distortion or loss of information. That is very important for achieving high image quality and for accurate image analysis.

Weight

The achievement of ultrahigh speeds requires that all hardware, including the memory, be physically located inside the body of the camera. Thus, the fastest high-speed cameras are too heavy to be held by hand during the exam. The camera used in the Voice and Speech Laboratory system, Phantom v7.3 (Vision Research Inc.), weighs 7 lb. To compensate for the weight, we attached the device to a camera crane (model CamCrane 200; Glidecam Industries, Inc, Kingston, MA). The camera weight is balanced, to appear weightless to the operator, while allowing the most degrees of freedom for motion by using a ballhead. Other than creating weightlessness, the crane was found to reduce significantly the endoscopic motion and tilt, thus introducing a comfortable system to operate. Based on that experience, we recommend using a camera crane regardless of the weight of the camera.

Color and spatial resolution are very important factors when identifying lesions, vascularities, and tissue changes and for accurately representing the glottal edges. Spatial resolution is also important as it allows for the wide view angle necessary to examine the full anterior-posterior view of the vocal folds and their surrounding anatomic structures. The frame rate is essential for accurately displaying the mucosal wave and providing sharp glottal edges, especially when viewing high-pitched samples. Long recording duration is necessary to register multiple phonatory tasks in a continuous recording (ie, comfortable, high and low pitch, glides, loudness levels, repetitive phonation, and forced inhalation), adduction and abduction of vocal folds, and phonatory onset and offset. An increased dynamic range allows for improved viewing quality and increased accuracy of the automated image analyses. Due to insufficient clinical experiments with HSV, the necessary requirements for these factors have not yet been standardized.

Of all factors that influence HSV, the color, temporal resolution, and dynamic range are the ones limited by the sensitivity of the camera sensor. The spatial resolution, temporal resolution, and dynamic range are in a reciprocal relationship as they share the same hardware bandwidth and memory resources. The sample duration and spatial resolution depend on the memory available, while the view angle depends on the spatial resolution and the optics installed. Therefore, improvements in HSV technology depend on three factors: sensitivity of the camera sensor, hardware speed, and memory size. The most important and the most challenging factor is the sensitivity, due to the limitations of CMOS technology and the lack of demand for high sensitivity from the traditional market sectors using high-speed cameras.[13]

An ongoing collaborative effort between the Voice and Speech Laboratory, University of

South Carolina, and the Center for Laryngeal Surgery and Voice Rehabilitation, Massachusetts General Hospital (Boston, MA), led recently to the following breakthrough advances in HSV technology:

1. Color HSV allowing for high-quality 42-bit rigid videoendoscopy at the speed of 6000 fps at a spatial resolution of 400 × 480 pixels and for 24-bit rigid color HSV at 10,000 fps and 320 × 320 pixels resolution.
2. Ultrahigh-speed monochrome HSV allowing for high-quality 12-bit rigid videoendoscopy at the speed of 16,000 fps at a spatial resolution of 320 × 320 pixels and for 8-bit rigid HSV at 48,000 fps and 128 × 200 pixels resolution.
3. High-precision temporal synchronization of monochrome HSV at 16,000 fps with multiple channels of other data allowing for accuracy of synchronization around 11 μsec at a sampling rate of 96,000 Hz per data channel.
4. High-definition HSV allowing for optically zoomed, high-quality, 12-bit monochrome imaging of the vibrating vocal fold tissues at the speed of 4000 fps and spatial resolution of 600 × 800 pixels.
5. Flexible HSV allowing for the use of a regular nasal fiberscope at the speed of up to 6000 fps and spatial resolution of 320 × 320 pixels.

These examples are presented to the reader to provide a notion of what is considered to be the state of the art in year 2009. Although these HSV system integrations are experimental and not currently commercially packaged for clinical use, it is likely that in another 5 years from now, HSV systems with similar and better parameters will be available to the clinic at a nonprohibitive cost. More importantly, and in the meantime, the research on the clinical efficacy of HSV needs to accelerate to "catch up" with the advance of technology.

Methodology: High-Speed Videoendoscopy Offers Much More than a Slow-Motion Movie

The improvement of the HSV camera technology is essential for the accurate recording of the biomechanical information of vocal fold movement. The biggest advantage of HSV is the true visual presentation of movement of an anatomic structure that humans, especially the skilled clinicians, understand best.[13] Advanced image processing techniques will complement the visual data automated analyses and measurements.

That is, the presentation of the HSV content to the clinician can be made either visually or through measurements. Thus, the methodology for voice evaluation via HSV can be achieved via visual perceptual ratings and via automatic or manual objective measures. These are two mutually complementary approaches. In the rich HSV content, some of the vibratory information is difficult for the human eye to perceive but can be measured automatically, whereas other features are difficult to formalize as an algorithm but are intuitive to the human brain. Therefore, it is most likely that the HSV clinical voice evaluation protocol of the future will be a combination of visual ratings and objective measures.

Facilitative Playbacks

As noted earlier in the section "Advantages of High-Speed Videoendoscopy over Videostroboscopy," HSV is a lot more than a slow-motion movie. There are many creative ways of presenting the HSV content in an intuitive form by preserving some of the spatial information so the clinician can follow the anatomy while the features of interest are emphasized for easy comprehension. This approach facilitates visual perception, improves the accuracy of quantification, and increases the reliability of visual rating. Special tools for enhanced visualization have been created, termed *facilitative playbacks*.[13,27] The following are some of the facilitative playbacks that have been successfully used thus far for research and clinical purposes: digital kymography playback, mucosal wave playback, mucosal wave kymography playback, and phonovibrogram.

Digital Kymography Playback. The normal sequence of viewing HSV recordings, termed *HSV playback*, is by sequentially presenting image frames with spatial coordinates *x* and *y* along the time axis *t*. DKG playback corresponds viewing DKG image frames with coordinates *x* and *t* in a sequence presented along

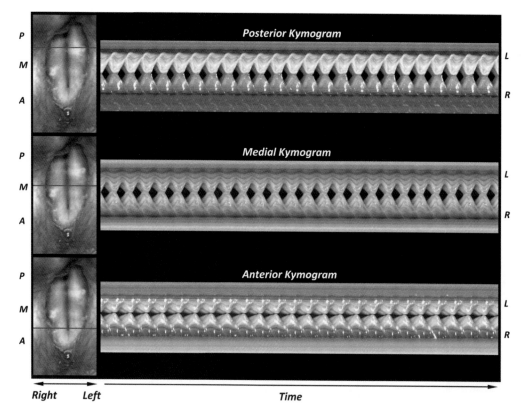

P M A — **Posterior Kymogram** — **L R**

P M A — **Medial Kymogram** — **L R**

P M A — **Anterior Kymogram** — **L R**

Right   Left   Time

Fig. 28.4 Example of a DKG playback of sustained phonation. DKG playback is a movie playing from posterior to anterior. The figure provides three snapshots taken in the posterior, medial, and anterior areas, respectively. The image on the left shows an average image of the vocal folds with the line being scanned across the glottis. On the right, the corresponding kymographic image is shown. The actual DKG playback movie used in this example is provided as **Video Clip 54** in the DVD accompanying this book.

the posterior-anterior axis *y*. In DKG playback, the DKG frames are viewed as a movie sequence that plays from the posterior toward the anterior.[13] The DKG playback can be regarded as a step up from multiplane kymography.[29] **Figure 28.4** provides three snapshots from a DKG playback of sustained phonation taken in the posterior, medial, and anterior areas along the posterior-anterior axis. **Figure 28.5** shows two snapshots from a DKG playback of a phonatory offset, taken in the posterior and medial areas. The DKG playback was found useful for demonstrating the change of the dynamic characteristics while viewing damaged tissues, such as lesions, scars, and discolored areas. Dynamic changes due to stiffness of the tissue, shown as a movie, may also help to reveal the nature of lesions (ie, cysts vs polyps). It is essential

to point out the importance of endoscopic motion compensation in ascertaining time alignment of the anatomic structures for valid DKG representations.[30]

Mucosal Wave Playback. The mucosal wave (MW) playback is produced by modifying the HSV image sequence into a series of frames, in which the pixel intensity encodes the motion of the upper and lower margins of the vocal folds and the mucosal edges. As illustrated in **Fig. 28.6**, in the MW playback, the color indicates the direction of motion (ie, the opening edges are encoded in green and the closing edges in red).[13] The frame selected for the example in **Fig. 28.6** demonstrates the effectiveness of the MW playback in emphasizing the

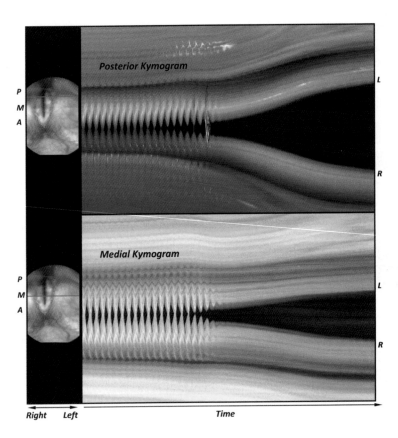

Fig. 28.5 Example of a DKG playback of a phonatory offset. The figure provides two snapshots taken in the posterior and medial areas, respectively. The image on the left shows an average image of the vocal folds with the line being scanned across the glottis. On the right, the corresponding kymographic image is shown. The DKG playback movie used in this example is provided as **Video Clip 55** in the DVD accompanying this book.

fact that during the beginning of the closing phase, when the lower margins are closing, the upper margins of the vocal folds may still be opening. The width of the differential between the upper and lower margins is a measure of the extent of the lateral phase of the mucosal wave.

Mucosal Wave Kymography Playback. Mucosal wave kymography (MKG) playback corresponds to viewing kymographic frames of mucosal wave along the posterior-anterior axis *y* (**Fig. 28.7**). Thus, MKG playback is a kymographic playback of the mucosal wave movie content. The MW and MKG playbacks have a substantial clinical potential as facilitative visual techniques as they allow for the assessment of the fine detail of the mucosal wave including the propagation of the mucosal edges during the opening and closing glottal phases.[13,18,20]

Phonovibrogram. Phonovibrogram (PVG) is a two-dimensional diagram of the vocal fold vibration. It is obtained by segmenting the edges of the vibrating vocal folds and transforming the obtained contour data into a two-dimensional image without loss of information.[27] Within a PVG image, the segmented contours of the moving vocal folds are unambiguously transformed into a set of geometric objects. PVG images can be regarded as fingerprints of vocal fold vibration and enable a direct and intuitive assessment of vocal fold vibration. The interpretational power and the quantitative analysis of PVG have been demonstrated on persons with voice disorders and vocally normal individuals.[27]

Objective Measures

Human perception is imperfect when evaluating visual content, especially content such as

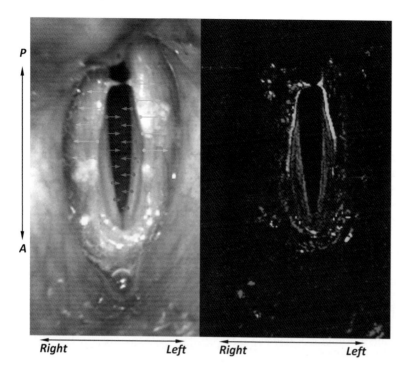

Right   Left   Right   Left

Fig. 28.6 Example frame of an MW playback taken at the beginning of the closing phase during sustained phonation. In the MW playback, the color indicates the direction of motion (ie, the opening edges are encoded in green and the closing edges in red). This example demonstrates the effectiveness of the MW playback in emphasizing the fact that in the begin- ning of the closing phase, when the lower margins are closing, the upper margins of the vocal folds may still be opening. The width of the differential between the upper and lower margins is a measure of the extent of the lateral phase of the mucosal wave. The MW play- back movie used in this example is provided as **Video Clip 56** in the DVD accompanying this book.

that of HSV where a vibration pattern is repeated over and over and variations may be insignificant relative to the overall pattern. For example, it is impossible for the human brain to compare the pattern of a glottal cycle with a pattern 10 cycles later after seeing the cycles in between. Objective, unbiased measures are important for overcoming the limitations of

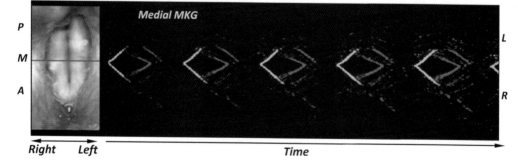

Right   Left   Time

Fig. 28.7 A medial position frame of an MKG playback of sustained phonation. This type of display allows for the temporal representation of the dynamics of the mucosal edges during glottal opening and closing in consecutive glottal cycles. The color shows the phase of motion (opening is green, closing is red). The mucosal wave extent appears as a double-edged or thicker red curve during the closing phase. The MKG playback movie used in this example is provided as **Video Clip 57** in the DVD accompanying this book.

human perceptions, as well as for documenting and comparing quantitatively the HSV content. The earlier section "Advantages of High-Speed Videoendoscopy over Videostroboscopy" already covered in detail the possible HSV measures that have relevance to voice assessment. To make these measurements automatically, researchers first have to build valid, reliable, and accurate segmentation and registration algorithms. Segmentation is a process of detecting and extracting the features of interest that are later subjected to measurement. In the context of HSV, there are three types of segmentation: temporal, image (spatial), and kymographic (spatial-temporal) segmentation.

Temporal Segmentation

Because HSV contains rich temporal and spatial information, it takes a very long time to view the HSV playback, and it is impractical to use DKG and other facilitative playbacks on lengthy HSV samples. Luckily, more than 95% of the vibratory information available through HSV is dynamically redundant due to the repetition of a pattern. Therefore, during sustained phonation, viewing shorter segments inclusive of just a couple of glottal cycles can be representative for the relevant information in the HSV sample. The process of automatically analyzing the temporal redundancy and selecting short segments representative of the whole HSV sample is termed *temporal segmentation*.[13,31] Temporal segmentation allows for navigating through the enormously large HSV content by mapping the specific areas of interest. After the segments are selected, they are either subjected to motion compensation to produce facilitative playbacks or subjected to image or kymographic segmentation to produce objective measurements.[30]

Image and Kymographic Segmentation

Image segmentation is a process of partitioning a digital image into multiple segments (sets of pixels). The goal of image segmentation is to simplify and/or change the representation of an image into something that is more meaningful and easier to analyze. HSV image segmentation is used to locate the vocal fold edges and to approximate them with lines and curves, which then can be numerically analyzed. Typically, HSV image segmentation is applied on each HSV frame (ie, in spatial domain). There is a variety of HSV segmentation algorithms in the published literature, and the algorithms are based on different methods: thresholding, region growing, active contours (snakes), level sets, and so forth. Segmentation has been applied also on VKG using snakes.[28] This type of spatial-temporal segmentation is termed *kymographic segmentation*. It is an approach applicable to HSV with significant potential. Based on our research, kymographic segmentation offers faster and more reliable and accurate HSV segmentation than the spatial image segmentation.[32] The added benefit of using kymographic segmentation is the inherent temporal registration (ie, the process of tracking the movement of the segmented vocal fold edges over time), a feature not available through spatial-domain image segmentation.

◆ Unsolved Problems with Laryngeal High-Speed Videoendoscopy

Despite its obvious advantages, HSV has not yet gained widespread clinical adoption because of remaining technical, methodological, and practical issues and an associated lack of information regarding the validity and clinical relevance of HSV. These limitations are highly interrelated.[13] Improvements of technology and methodology are usually driven by the clinical demand. However, the research needed to demonstrate the clinical relevance of HSV, which is necessary for guiding the development of the appropriate methodology, is still in an early stage. Given that there are no established requirements, standardized clinical protocols, and clearly demonstrated benefits, there are no sufficient incentives among clinicians to implement this new, costly technology.

Clinicians and researchers usually consider the cost of HSV systems as being the most prohibitive factor for the clinical implementation of HSV. But this is only partially true. The cost of HSV technology is comparable with that of stroboscopy. Clinicians are accustomed to using and interpreting videostroboscopy, and they view HSV as a technique supplemental to videostroboscopy; a technique offering further detail about the glottal cycle or about irregular patterns. As we already pointed out, the same vibratory features may appear different on HSV than they do on videostroboscopy. Thus, the new information gained by the clinician from HSV may not be complementary, because it is not comparable. It is understandable why the clinician may feel discouraged. Adding to the cost of the equipment, the time spent for training, performing the procedure, and maintenance—without a health insurance billing/coding procedure in place for financial reimbursement—is indeed discouraging. Thus, the most prohibitive factor is not necessarily the cost of the HSV equipment, but rather the fact that there are more factors contributing to a greater cost, which is not yet justified through clinical evidence. As soon as the clinical value of HSV and its superiority over stroboscopy is demonstrated through research, HSV will supplant videostroboscopy in the clinic.

Many technical and methodological challenges still need to be addressed and studied. Effective techniques for the visualization and measurement of the features of the mucosal wave, vibratory regularity and symmetry, the vocal fold edge, glottal closure, vibratory amplitude, and the open quotient should become available. New methods for assessment of nonstationary laryngeal dynamics, such as onsets, offsets, and breaks, should be developed. Although camera technology capable of meeting the technical characteristics for clinical application is available, a lot of practical issues have yet to be addressed, such as the weight of the cameras and the creation of special optical lenses better serving HSV, and further increase in sensitivity, memory size, and storage would be very beneficial. More unanswered questions affect the practicality of HSV: Does the bright constant xenon light pose any risks to the patients? How to store the huge amount of data? Appropriate image compression techniques are essential. How to quickly view the lengthy HSV recordings? For example, 10 seconds of HSV data recorded at a speed of 10,000 fps would require 2 hours 46 minutes to view the whole recording at a speed of 10 fps. That is impractical, and the need for effective automatic temporal and image segmentation and facilitative playbacks and objective measurements is obvious. Currently, there are no commercial software tools for such analyses, and the commercial HSV integrated systems are still a step away from the necessary speed and image quality. More clinical research is necessary. Until the practicality, validity, reliability, and clinical relevance of HSV are formally studied, voice specialists will not be willing to change their methods for evaluating the vibratory behaviors of the vocal folds.

◆ High-Speed Videoendoscopy as a Research Tool for Voice Science

Historically, high-speed imaging has been used mainly as a research tool. Since the 1930s, different high-speed techniques helped in building our current understanding of voice production.[5-8] A summary of the state of the art in high-speed digital imaging as of the end of the 20th century has been written by Kiritani.[33]

The most recent and significant advancement of the HSV technology allowed for capturing unprecedented details about the biomechanics of laryngeal sound production. The HSV technology is already helping to guide innovations in surgical voice restoration and to develop the next generation of clinical tools for improving the functional evaluation of voice disorders.[13,19,34] Before and above the potential of HSV as a clinical tool remains the role of HSV as a powerful technique for refining our understanding of voice production.

The purpose of this section is to update the reader about currently ongoing voice research using HSV including examples. There are several laboratories worldwide conducting HSV-based research to answer basic voice science questions. Our purpose is not to conduct a systematic review but rather provide a few examples stemming from our own experience, which will demonstrate the power of HSV in addressing current basic questions. The following is a summary of five different basic voice science studies with significant potential to impact clinical practice. These studies are not directly related and are currently at various stages of their completion. All five studies, however, have one thing in common: HSV is used as an intermediate technique, or as a "physiologic marker," for validating concepts using other, indirect measurement techniques.

Improved HSV technology became essential in investigating the interrelations between the biomechanical aspects of vocal fold vibration (ie, the vocal fold physiology) and other biofeedback signals that have traditionally been used for the evaluation of vocal function. Such traditional biofeedback signals include the acoustic voice waveform (sound pressure), EGG, transglottal airflow, intraoral/subglottal pressure, and accelerometry. These indirect signals have been the basis for objective measures of laryngeal function. The relationship between these measures and vocal fold physiology has been largely assumed, depending on the current theoretical paradigm. However, little direct evidence about the correlation of these signals and measures to the actual biomechanical vibration of the vocal folds has been reported to date.

Measure of Vocal Attack Time

It this study, we hypothesized that the time lag between the rise of the sound pressure (SP) and EGG signals, measured at the onset of phonation, provides a useful index of vocal attack time, which is an important variable in the etiology of some voice disorders and may also be a meaningful indicator of central or peripheral neural dysfunction.[24] HSV was used for the experimental validation of this measure, whereby the SP and EGG signals were recorded synchronously with HSV. DKG images were subsequently generated from the HSV and used to manually measure the time from the beginning of vocal fold oscillation to the first vocal fold contact. The study demonstrated that, after appropriate signal processing, the intersignal time delay provides a potentially useful measure that varies with vocal attack characteristics. HSV-based techniques were essential for providing a physiologic understanding and quantitative validation of the proposed measure.

Relationship between the Glottal Flow and Glottal Area Waveforms

A very important but little studied aspect of human voice production is the relationship between the vocal fold vibration and the transglottal airflow. To analyze this relationship, in this study we combined HSV of the glottis for determining the glottal area waveform (GAW) with inverse filtering of the acoustic signal for estimating the glottal flow waveform (GFW).[31] The HSV system, recording at 16,000 fps, and the audio recording hardware were synchronized with an accuracy of 11 μsec. We developed an image segmentation algorithm for automatic extraction of the GAW from the HSV images based on region growing. The HSV samples and the corresponding acoustic signals were obtained from 14 vocally normal individuals for different voicing conditions (ie, various registers, adductory adjustment, longitudinal tension, or nonstationary phonatory behavior). The revealed waveform shapes and slopes of the vocal fold vibration and the transglottal flow were in agreement and changed correspondingly with the different phonatory conditions. However, the delay between the glottal area and flow signals varied in a very wide range, sometimes exceeding the glottal cycle length. This contradicts current models estimating delay based on vocal-tract length and speed of sound. Thus, further research is warranted.

Signature-Based Measurement of the Delay between Voice Signals

Relating intracycle landmarks of vocal fold vibration to corresponding features of indirect voice signals is a question of high importance for basic science and clinical practice, as shown in the previous study. The recent refinement of HSV allowed for accurate synchronization of HSV image data with acoustics and other signals. Synchronization is a necessary prerequisite for aligning these signals with high temporal precision. However, a remaining problem is the inherent delay between the signals measured at the laryngeal level versus those measured inside or outside the vocal tract. Traditionally, these delays have been estimated based on distance and speed of sound. Recent findings cautioned us that actual delays may be significantly different, usually greater than estimated. Therefore, delays should be measured rather than estimated.

The purpose of this study was to develop a technique for accurate and reliable measurement of the delay between different types of voice signals.[35] The technique relies on the premise that although different types of signals have inherently dissimilar waveforms due to differences in phase and spectral characteristics, they carry a common signature encoded in the fluctuations of their fundamental frequency. The method comprises a 3-stage high-precision autocorrelation-based frequency signature decoder applied on two synchronously recorded voice signals, followed by statistical procedures for eliciting the actual delay. The validity, accuracy, and reliability of the technique were tested on a data set of 720 two-channel samples with various delay between the channels. The results demonstrate the proposed technique warrants the required accuracy and reliability necessary for intracycle landmark alignment. The new technique is currently being applied for signature-based delay measurement on HSV images versus other signals.

Complementing High-Speed Videoendoscopy with Electroglottography

The purpose this study was to assess the utility of combining HSV with EGG indices of glottal and vocal fold function.[36] Because EGG is sensitive to changes in vocal fold contact area during phonation, it can be a valuable tool for both voice researchers and clinicians. Clinical observation and the application of various physical and mathematical models have been used to identify important EGG signal landmarks and to relate changes in signal morphology to specific aspects of laryngeal physiology. The continued refinement and applicability of HSV allows the synchronization of the EGG signal with endoscopic images of the vocal folds. It is the purpose of this study to investigate variations of specific EGG features and relate

them to HSV-observed changes in vibratory behavior.

In this ongoing study, 14 vocally normal speakers were recorded using synchronous HSV (16,000 fps) with EGG (96,000 Hz) with an accuracy of 11 μsec as they produced the vowel /i/ sustained in eight different modes of phonation: habitual, high and low pitch, breathy and pressed phonation, glottal fry, tremor, and falsetto. Based on current EGG models, 10 signal features were identified and grouped into four categories: cycle-phase–related features, temporal features, noise-related features, and configuration-related features. The resulting data were compiled to compare differences related to the phonatory mode and the sex of the subject. Using custom-designed software with a specialized graphic user interface, the EGG signals were precisely aligned with multislice digital kymography derived from HSV (**Fig. 28.8**), and color-encoded marks were manually placed at five characteristic EGG landmarks. The classified EGG features were then related to specific vocal fold vibratory characteristics using the custom-built software. The software allowed dynamically allocating vocal fold contact on the HSV images and DKG for any lateral line and precisely matching the HSV contact features to the EGG landmarks.

Relations among High-Speed Videoendoscopy Image Analyses and Aerodynamic, Electroglottography, and Acoustic Measures

The purpose of this ongoing study is to create a cross-classification scheme between noninvasive integrative measures (glottal flow, oral pressure, sound pressure, accelerometer, and EGG) and specific physiologic moments of glottal dynamics (derived from HSV), as well as to use computer phonatory models to provide similarities to the cross-classification scheme created with the human data. A modified Rothenberg mask is used to record flexible nasal HSV at 4000 fps with the other 5 data channels. The goal is to use HSV as a tool for the experimental validation and refinement of current theoretical models of voice production.

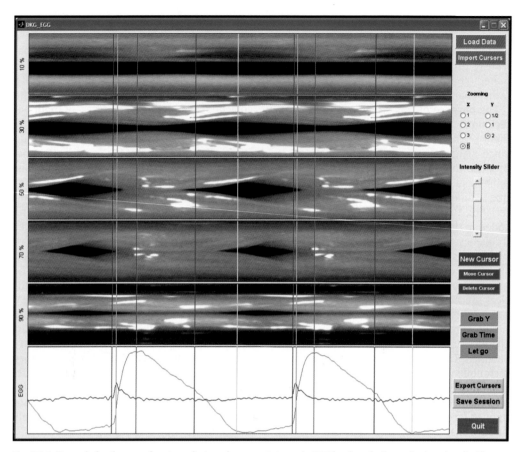

Fig. 28.8 Example for the use of custom-designed software with a specialized graphic user interface for precisely aligning EGG signals with multislice digital kymography derived from HSV. Five color-encoded marks are manually placed at the corresponding intracycle EGG landmarks for each glottal cycle. The position of each landmark is then compared with the phase of vocal fold vibration at each of the five posterior-to-anterior positions.

◆ High-Speed Videoendoscopy in the Clinical Speech-Language Pathology Practice

The speech-language pathology practice can benefit tremendously from HSV by refining the current protocol for voice evaluation. The vibratory features of sustained phonation currently rated using videostroboscopy can become more accurate and reliable if measured using HSV-based technology, and new features of aperiodic vibration will become clinically applicable, such as voice breaks, laryngeal spasms, vocal attack time, and onset and offset of phonation.

Several clinical research teams have addressed the clinical comparison of videostroboscopy and HSV.[13,15,16,18,20,22,23] One thing is similar in the results of all these experimental studies; that is, most of the analyzed vocal fold vibratory features (ie, periodicity, mucosal wave, symmetry, open quotient, glottal closure, and mucus aggregation) appeared different on HSV relative to videostroboscopy. For several features, there was a difference in sensitivity and specificity between the two imaging modalities. Videostroboscopy often had lower intrarater and interrater reliability.

The earlier section "Advantages of High-Speed Videoendoscopy over Videostroboscopy" already elucidated the inherent reasons for differences between videostroboscopy and HSV, based on the principles of these techniques. Because voice clinicians have been trained to use videostroboscopy, they may attempt interpreting vibratory features relative to the norms used in the clinic with videostroboscopy. Thus, there is a risk of overdiagnosing or misdiagnosing when HSV features are compared with the norms developed for videostroboscopy.

Normative Data for High-Speed Videoendoscopy

One main limitation to the clinical use of HSV is the lack of norms. An important first step in establishing the clinical utility of HSV is to generate HSV-specific clinical norms. The ability of the clinician to differentiate normal physiology from pathology using HSV images depends on valid norms. The following is a summary of findings achieved through recent research comparing videostroboscopy with HSV for commonly used clinical vibratory features.[13]

Phase Symmetry

Investigations of left-to-right phase symmetry revealed more instances of asymmetry than symmetry across a variety of HSV facilitative playbacks.[18] In comparison, there was an even larger prevalence of asymmetrical ratings for posterior-to-anterior phase symmetry. An increased percentage of cases were rated as symmetrical during pressed versus comfortable phonation at habitual pitch and loudness, which could reveal physiologic differences between the two types of phonation.

Period and Glottal Width Irregularity

Through the visual rating of vocal fold vibratory period and glottal width regularity using stroboscopy and HSV-based facilitative playbacks, a greater number of glottal width irregularities than period irregularities were noted.[15] A similar difference was realized through manually achieved objective measures. If the relative lack of period irregularities is further substantiated, this finding would change our understanding of indirect measures of frequency perturbation.

Additionally, approximately twice as many cases of glottal width irregularity were noted for pressed versus habitual phonation. This finding supports the notion of pressed phonation relying on a less typical and possibly less stable vibratory pattern. The increased irregularities noted from the kymographic playbacks stress the importance of kymography in the voice evaluation arsenal. The differences between visual ratings and objective measures demonstrate the importance of quantification to evaluation of vocal fold vibratory irregularities.

Mucosal Wave

There are three conclusions from this study: atypical mucosal wave was abundant for normophonic speakers; variations in ratings were observed across visual playback techniques; and the HSV frame rate influenced visibility of mucosal wave.[20] The results reinforce the idea that the magnitude and symmetry of the mucosal wave in normophonic speakers can be atypical. Thus, caution should be used when determining the abnormality of mucosal wave variations during clinical visualization procedures, especially when applying the norms from stroboscopy to HSV. The variation of ratings across the HSV and HSV-derived playbacks demonstrates the strength of using different views providing a balance between specificity and sensitivity. This suggests that it may be beneficial to use HSV and HSV-derived playbacks together to maximize the visualization of the mucosal wave. An important conclusion of this investigation is the finding that the temporal resolution of 2000 fps (used in many commercial systems) is insufficient to record the intracycle information necessary to assess features of mucosal wave when the frequency of vocal fold vibration is higher. This conclusion is based on findings of reduced mucosal wave from the habitual phonation of females with F_0 above 200 Hz. It is known that the mucosal wave is reduced at high pitch. However, a follow-up comparison of high-pitched phonation recorded at 2000 fps and 10,000 fps showed that the reason for a reduced mucosal wave in females was the temporal resolution of HSV. Future studies should address the differences in information provided via full view and kymographic techniques and the normality of variations in extent and symmetry of mucosal wave magnitude.

Open Quotient

The majority of normophonic speakers exhibited open quotients between 40% and 60% for both modal and pressed phonation when rated and measured from laryngeal videoendoscopic recordings.[21] When variations occur, it is most likely that a trend toward an increased open quotient is noted for modal phonation. Conversely, variations typically take the form of a decreased open quotient for pressed phonation. Discrepancies between perceptual and objective measures of open quotient reveal the ability of future quantitative analysis techniques to strengthen both research and clinical applications of open quotient measures. Future investigations should compare these findings with those from a variety of pathologies and further study the relationship between direct evaluation of the open quotient and information gained through indirect techniques.

High-Speed Videoendoscopy Data from Patients with Voice Disorders

Several ongoing studies provide preliminary data using HSV and videostroboscopy in patients with voice disorders. Specifically, the vibratory features of phase symmetry, period and glottal width irregularity, and mucosal wave have been investigated. For phase symmetry and period and glottal width irregularity, the preliminary findings suggest that stroboscopy is more sensitive but less specific in identifying asymmetry and aperiodicity. Similar to studies in vocally normal individuals, HSV detected fewer instances of moderate to severe aperiodicity, or asymmetry, when compared with stroboscopy. HSV, MW, and MKG playbacks differentiated hypofunctional and hyperfunctional voice disorders at a statistically significant level, whereas stroboscopy did not. The general conclusion is that using the videostroboscopy norms for HSV-based features would lead to a classification of the large majority of persons with voice disorders as vocally normal.

◆ High-Speed Videoendoscopy in the Clinical Otolaryngology Practice

HSV can lead to substantial refinements in the clinical practice of laryngology. The HSV technology is already helping to guide innovations in surgical methods and bioimplants for repairing damaged vocal fold superficial lamina propria, a major factor in many voice disorders.[34] These efforts to restore the delicate biomechanical properties of the superficial lamina propria need the type of increased accuracy that HSV can potentially provide to assist with precisely defining/mapping specific damaged areas and to target them for repair. HSV is also important for accurately assessing the impact of such interventions on the fine temporal details of vocal fold vibration. HSV provides more accurate descriptions of the underlying pathophysiology of disordered voice production than is possible with stroboscopy. Such increases in accuracy will lead to important refinements in the assessment and diagnosis of vocal pathology.

Recently, HSV was used to gain better insights into the voice production mechanisms of patients who have undergone endoscopic phonosurgical treatment of early glottic cancer.[19] The investigation was accomplished using a system described earlier in this chapter that can acquire digital color images of vocal fold vibration using HSV with time-synchronized recordings of the acoustic voice signal during phonation. This enabled direct correlations between acoustic parameters and measures of glottal closure and vibratory symmetry extracted from the high-speed digital recordings using custom-designed image-processing algorithms. This approach allows for the application of automated digital image and signal processing methods to reveal critical relationships between vocal fold vibratory function and the resulting acoustic characteristics of the voice. Such investigations are not possible with videostroboscopy. This information should substantially assist surgeons in identifying biomechanical phonatory mucosal deficits and the effectiveness of implant reconstruction efforts.

HSV has also substantial potential in applications not involving the vocal folds, such as voice restoration after laryngectomy, or mapping and assessing the success of upper airway reconstruction.

In conclusion, HSV is a fast-emerging technique with great potential in clinical voice evaluation and phonosurgery, as well as a powerful tool for basic voice science. HSV has numerous advantages over videostroboscopy. Ultimately, HSV will supplant videostroboscopy in the daily clinical practice. The high-speed camera technology is reaching the level necessary to support such a transition. However, there is a lack of sufficient research supporting HSV with clinical evidence. Consequently, the methodology for effective visualization and measurement of HSV is lagging behind the existing technology. More clinical evidence-based research using HSV is warranted. Likely within the next couple of years, the current videostroboscopy-based clinical protocols will migrate to HSV leading to more comprehensive protocols including new physiologic features. Videostroboscopy will continue to be used for specific applications requiring very high spatial resolution and image quality.

Acknowledgments This chapter made multiple references to the author's ongoing or completed research related to HSV. That research is/has been funded by NIH research grants from the National Institute on Deafness and Other Communication Disorders (R01 DC007640 and T32 DC00038), by the Institute for Laryngology and Voice Restoration, and by an R&PS grant (11560-KA01) from the South Carolina Research Foundation. This is research conducted in collaboration with the following researchers and clinicians: Robert E. Hillman, Ph.D.; Steven M. Zeitels, M.D.; Robert F. Orlikoff, Ph.D.; Pencho P. Petrushev, Ph.D.; Heather Shaw Bonilha, Ph.D.; Raphael R. Schwarz, Ph.D.; Terri Treman Gerlach, Ph.D.; Ron J. Baken, Ph.D.; Ben C. Watson, Ph.D.; Song Wang, Ph.D.; Ronald C. Scherer, Ph.D.; Fariborz Alipour, Ph.D.; Bonnie Martin-Harris, Ph.D.; Tomasz P. Zielinski, Ph.D.; Darrell A. Klotz, M.D.; N. Neil Howell, M.D.; Daryush D. Mehta, S.M.; Maria E. Golla, M.S.P.; Habib J. Moukalled, M.S.; Cara Sauder, M.A.; Lori Ellen Sutton, M.A.; and Susan C. Hanks, M.S.

References

1. Schuster M, Lohscheller J, Kummer P, Eysholdt U, Hoppe U. Laser projection in high-speed glottography for high-precision measurements of laryngeal dimensions and dynamics. Eur Arch Otorhinolaryngol 2005;262:477–481

2. Scripture EW. Elements of Experimental Phonetics. New York, NY: Charles Scribner's Sons; 1902

3. Oertel MJ. Das Laryngo-Stroboskop und die Laryngo-Stroboskpische Untersuchung. Archiv für Laryngologie und Rhinologie (Berlin) 1895;3:1–16

4. Nagashima H, Tuda K, Marui M. Larynx stroboscope for photography. U.S. Patent No. 4,232,685; 1980

5. Moore P. Motion picture studies of the vocal folds and vocal attack. J Speech Disord 1938;3:235–238

6. Farnsworth DW. High-speed motion pictures of the human vocal cords. Bell Lab Record. 1940;18:203–208

7. Moore GP, White FD, Von Leden H. Ultra high speed photography in laryngeal physiology. J Speech Hear Disord 1962;27:165–171

8. Werner-Kukuk E, von Leden H. Vocal initiation. High speed cinematographic studies on normal subjects. Folia Phoniatr (Basel) 1970;22:107–116

9. Švec JG, Šram F, Schutte HK. Videokymography: a new high-speed method for the examination of vocal-fold vibrations. Ototinolaryngologie a Foniatrie. 1999;48:155–162

10. Kay Elemetrics Corp. High-Speed Video Model 9700: Instruction Manual. Lincoln Park, NJ: Kay Elemetrics Corp.; 1999

11. Qiu Q, Schutte HK. Real-time kymographic imaging for visualizing human vocal-fold vibratory function. Rev Sci Instrum 2007;78:024302

12. Masi CG. Video for voice. Vision Systems Design 2009;5:37–41

13. Deliyski DD, Petrushev PP, Bonilha HS, Gerlach TT, Martin-Harris B, Hillman RE. Clinical implementation of laryngeal high-speed videoendoscopy: challenges and evolution. Folia Phoniatr Logop 2008;60:33–44

14. Titze IR. Workshop on Acoustic Voice Analysis: Summary Statement. Iowa City, IA: National Center for Voice and Speech; 1995

15. Bonilha HS, Deliyski DD. Period and glottal width irregularities in vocally normal speakers. J Voice 2008;22:699–708

16. Kendall KA. High-speed laryngeal imaging compared with videostroboscopy in healthy subjects. Arch Otolaryngol Head Neck Surg 2009;135:274–281

17. Švec JG, Šram F, Schutte HK. Videokymography in voice disorders: what to look for? Ann Otol Rhinol Laryngol 2007;116:172–180

18. Bonilha HS, Deliyski DD, Gerlach TT. Phase asymmetries in normophonic speakers: visual judgments and objective findings. Am J Speech Lang Pathol 2008;17:367–376

19. Mehta DD, Deliyski DD, Zeitels SM, Quatieri TF, Hillman RE. Voice production mechanisms following phonosurgical treatment of early glottic cancer. Ann Otol Rhinol Laryngol 2010;119:1–9

20. Shaw HS, Deliyski DD. Mucosal wave: a normophonic study across visualization techniques. J Voice 2008;22:23–33

21. Shaw H, Deliyski D. Symmetry and Open Quotient: Normative High-Speed Videoendoscopy Findings.

Presented at: 34th Symposium of the Voice Foundation: Care of the Professional Voice; June 2005; Philadelphia, PA

22. Bonilha HS, Aikman A, Hines K, Deliyski DD. Vocal fold mucus aggregation in vocally normal speakers. Logoped Phoniatr Vocol 2008;33:136–142

23. Patel R, Dailey S, Bless D. Comparison of high-speed digital imaging with stroboscopy for laryngeal imaging of glottal disorders. Ann Otol Rhinol Laryngol 2008;117:413–424

24. Orlikoff RF, Deliyski DD, Baken RJ, Watson BC. Validation of a glottographic measure of vocal attack. J Voice 2009;23:164–168

25. Lohscheller J, Döllinger M, Schuster M, Schwarz R, Eysholdt U, Hoppe U. Quantitative investigation of the vibration pattern of the substitute voice generator. IEEE Trans Biomed Eng 2004;51:1394–1400

26. Deliyski D, Petrushev P. Methods for objective assessment of high-speed videoendoscopy. Proceedings: 6th Int Conf Advances in Quantitative Laryngology Voice and Speech Research AQL, Hamburg, Germany. Universitätsklinikum Hamburg-Eppendorf 2003;6:1–16

27. Lohscheller J, Eysholdt U, Toy H, Döllinger M. Phonovibrography: mapping high-speed movies of vocal fold vibrations into 2-D diagrams for visualizing and analyzing the underlying laryngeal dynamics. IEEE Trans Med Imaging 2008;27:300–309

28. Manfredi C, Bocchi L, Bianchi L, Migali N, Cantarella G. Objective vocal fold vibration assessment from videokymographic images. Biomed Signal Process Control 2006;1:129–136

29. Tigges M, Wittenberg T, Mergell P, Eysholdt U. Imaging of vocal fold vibration by digital multi-plane kymography. Comput Med Imaging Graph 1999;23:323–330

30. Deliyski DD. Endoscope motion compensation for laryngeal high-speed videoendoscopy. J Voice 2005;19:485–496

31. Schwarz R, Deliyski D. Experimental analysis of the relationship between the glottal flow and glottal area waveforms. J Acoust Soc Am 2008;123:3740

32. Moukalled HJ, Deliyski DD, Schwarz RR, Wang S. Segmentation of laryngeal high-speed videoendoscopy in temporal domain using paired active contours. In: Manfredi C, ed. Proceedings of the 6th International Workshop on Models and Analysis of Vocal Emissions for Biomedical Applications MAVEBA. Florence, Italy: Firenze University Press; 2009:137–140

33. Kiritani S. High-speed digital image recording for observing vocal fold vibration. In: Kent RD, Ball MJ, eds. Voice Quality Measurement. San Diego, CA: Singular Publishing Group; 2000:269–283

34. Zeitels SM, Burns JA, Lopez-Guerra G, Anderson RR, Hillman RE. Photoangiolytic laser treatment of early glottic cancer: a new management strategy. Ann Otol Rhinol Laryngol Suppl 2008;199:3–24

35. Deliyski D, Schwarz R. Signature-based measurement of the delay between voice signals. Presented at: 38th Symposium of the Voice Foundation: Care of the Professional Voice; June 2009; Philadelphia, PA

36. Golla ME, Deliyski DD, Orlikoff RF, Moukalled HJ. Objective comparison of the electroglottogram to synchronous high-speed images of vocal-fold contact during vibration. In: Manfredi C, ed. Proceedings of the 6th International Workshop on Models and Analysis of Vocal Emissions for Biomedical Applications MAVEBA. Florence, Italy: Firenze University Press; 2009:141–144

29

Clinical Applications for High-Speed Laryngeal Imaging

Katherine A. Kendall

The introduction of high-speed imaging of the larynx into clinical practice has expanded our ability to image vocal fold vibration to include situations that cannot be successfully evaluated using videostroboscopy. High-speed laryngeal imaging uses a high-speed camera to capture real-time images at a minimal rate of 2000 frames per second. This frequency of image capture is fast enough to obtain multiple images from a single cycle of vibration (usually 175 to 250 cycles per second) and when played back can be viewed as an *actual* slow-motion movie of vocal fold vibration. Because high-speed laryngeal imaging does not require the measurement of a stable vibratory frequency to adjust the rate of image acquisition, it can be used successfully in situations where the frequency of vibration is changing rapidly, such as during the onset and offset of voicing and in patients with aperiodic voices, tremor, or laryngeal spasms. Thus, high-speed digital imaging offers benefits over standard videostroboscopy in the diagnosis and analysis of patients with irregular vocal fold motion.

High-speed imaging of the larynx has been performed since the 1930s but remained impractical for clinical use because of cumbersome equipment and high costs. The recent development of advanced, cost-effective, and commercially available high-speed imaging systems has made it practical to use this technology in a clinical setting. It has the potential to advance the functional assessment of the pathophysiology of voice disorders, ultimately improving the ability to diagnose and manage vocal fold pathology.

◆ Indications for High-Speed Laryngeal Imaging

Hoarseness, the clinical complaint usually investigated with laryngeal imaging, is the result of abnormalities in vocal fold vibratory function and is an indication for high-speed laryngeal imaging. Laryngeal pathology that results in hoarseness is commonly associated with an unstable frequency of vibration, leading to difficulties in using videostroboscopy for analysis of vibratory characteristics in these patients. High-speed laryngeal imaging can be used in patients in whom the strobe is unable to find a stable frequency. Characteristics of vibration usually assessed with videostroboscopy (amplitude of vibration, mucosal wave, periodicity, phase characteristics, glottic configuration, symmetry, and the presence of adynamic segments) can all be evaluated with high-speed laryngeal imaging.

Because the rate of image capture with high-speed laryngeal imaging is stable, the number of images captured per vibratory cycle depends on the frequency of vocal fold vibration. More images are captured per cycle at low vibration frequencies and fewer images are captured at higher frequencies of vibration. For example, at the low end of the fundamental frequency range, 150 Hz, between 13 and 14 images are captured per vibratory cycle when the capture rate is 2000 per second. At the higher end of the range, 250 Hz, only 8 images per cycle can be captured. In female singers, the rate of image capture may be insufficient to analyze vocal abnormalities that occur at the high end of their singing register.

◆ Supportive Research

In a research setting, high-speed laryngeal imaging has been used to learn more about normal vocal fold vibratory behaviors. The digitization of the imaging enhances the ability to accurately quantify many characteristics of vibrating vocal folds not possible with the analog imaging of videostroboscopy. Tissue characteristics as well as the influence of other forces such as aerodynamics, muscle tension, and vocal fold length have been studied.[1-3] High-speed laryngeal imaging has also allowed the evaluation of normal laryngeal functioning in situations of rapid pitch change, such as during the onset and offset of voicing and during a glissando (**Video Clip 58**). The technology can be adapted to make objective measures of normal vibration that correlate with acoustic measures.[1] This type of analysis has advanced our understanding of normal vibratory physiology and is critical to the development of successful surgical and medical techniques used to restore normal vocal fold vibratory function to patients suffering from hoarseness.

High-speed laryngeal imaging analysis of the glottal area and the amplitude of vibration for each vocal fold has been applied to the evaluation of patients with unilateral vocal fold paralysis both before and after medialization.[4,5] Another area where high-speed laryngeal imaging has great potential for clinical application is in the assessment of vocal tremor and in the differentiation of spasmodic dysphonia from muscle tension dysphonia (**Video Clips 20 and 59**). Due to the acoustic characteristics of tremor and breaks in phonation, videostroboscopy cannot capture the vibratory pattern in these patients (**Video Clips 60 and 61**). High-speed laryngeal imaging is being applied to assist with quantification of vocal tremor, which has been very difficult with videostroboscopy.[6] As more information is gathered regarding normal function and function in patients with these disorders, better treatment modalities may be developed.

Further research of vocal fold vibration using high-speed laryngeal imaging is under way to evaluate how various dynamics of the vocal folds as seen with high-speed imaging can be interpreted and which features of vocal fold oscillations are important. The reader is referred to Chapter 28 for a more in-depth review of the science and current research pertaining to high-speed laryngeal imaging.

◆ High-Speed Laryngeal Imaging Technique

Clinically Available Equipment

The Kay Pentax High-Speed Video System is available in combination with a Digital Stroboscopy System. Because both technologies are incorporated into a single workstation, it is easy to switch back and forth between the two imaging modalities during a patient evaluation. The rigid endoscope used for stroboscopy can be easily attached to the high-speed camera for high-speed laryngeal imaging.

Exam

High-speed digital imaging techniques use conventional rigid endoscopes to record images of the larynx with a full view of the superior laryngeal surface (**Fig. 29.1**). Due to the amount of data generated from that number of images, recording time is usually limited to ~8 seconds. This, however, has been found to be a sufficient amount of time to evaluate most phonatory behaviors. The recorded

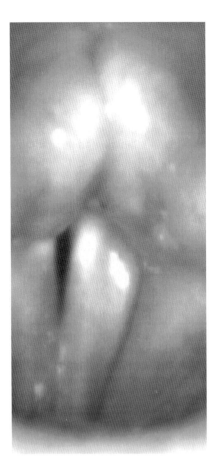

Fig. 29.1 The larynx as viewed with high-speed imaging.

images can be played back in slow motion for analysis. At a recording rate of 2000 fps, 8 to 20 images per vibratory cycle are recorded depending on the frequency of vibration. Keep in mind that videostroboscopy, on the other hand, is unable to record events that are shorter than four to five cycles in duration with four to eight cycles occurring per single image captured.

Patient positioning for high-speed imaging is the same as for videostroboscopy. The focal length of the high-speed camera is relatively narrow, and it is helpful to try to prefocus the camera using a template while positioning the scope end about 2 inches from the template. The camera is inserted into the pharynx transorally, in the same manner as is done for videostroboscopy, and the images can be viewed on a monitor. Using a foot pedal con-

trol, the examiner can save the last 8 seconds of recording for future playback and analysis. The playback speed can be adjusted as needed.

In general, the development of an examination protocol is recommended. This ensures that the final recording is optimal for a full evaluation of all vibratory parameters. Because the onset and offset of voicing is one parameter that can only be evaluated with high-speed laryngeal imaging, it should be included in the examination protocol. In developing the imaging protocol, it must be kept in mind that with high-speed laryngeal imaging, 2000 frames are recorded for each second of vibration and review of the images is done at a rate of 9 frames per second. Therefore, ~2.5 minutes are needed to review 1 second of voicing, and up to 30 minutes is needed to review the entire 8 seconds of voicing recorded in the study. Most clinicians do not have 30 minutes to review each study and generally will look at much smaller segments of the study to make assessments.

An attempt should be made to record voicing at or near the patient's fundamental frequency; however, this is not always an easy task. Often, to bring the larynx into view for recording, the patient is asked to voice at a frequency above the fundamental, effectively elevating the larynx for viewing. It is therefore important to establish the fundamental frequency prior to the onset of recording and then to attempt viewing of the larynx at that frequency. In general, a range of 20 Hz above or below the average fundamental frequency is accepted as representative of the fundamental frequency. Because some vibratory abnormalities occur only at certain frequencies and because vibratory characteristics are affected by the frequency of vibration, it is important that recording at a high pitch and then at a lower pitch also be performed. The remainder of the examination can be tailored to the patient's specific complaints.

Study Interpretation

There remains a paucity of published normative data regarding vocal fold vibratory characteristics as documented by high-speed laryngeal imaging. As a result, our ability to identify pathologic vocal fold function using high-speed laryngeal imaging is limited to a degree by our inability to distinguish it from normal function. To establish the range of normal function as documented with high-speed laryngeal imaging, we performed high-speed recordings in 50 healthy individuals without voice problems and compared the high-speed recordings with videostroboscopy performed in the same subjects.[7] Three blinded raters then reviewed the studies and judged the following characteristics of vibration: glottal configuration, vibratory symmetry, phase closure, mucosal wave propagation, amplitude of vibration, and periodicity of vibration. The data from high-speed studies was then compared with data from the videostroboscopic studies performed in the same subject population. Intrarater and interrater reliability was calculated for both imaging modalities.

Although each judge who participated in this study had extensive clinical experience with making clinical judgments of laryngeal imaging studies, there was a substantial amount of disagreement within and between judges. Previous studies of videostroboscopy judgments with high interrater agreement generally depend on the use of specific segments of the study to establish interrater agreement.[5,8,9] When clinicians are free to make assessments from any part of the study, there may be differences in interpretation based on variables including loudness, pitch, effort level, and modal register of the subject.[10,11] Recent studies regarding reliability of clinicians evaluating imaging from a large patient population report reliabilities similar to those found in this study.[5,12]

Because each clinician who participated in this study likely chose a slightly different part of the imaging study for making their judgments of vibratory characteristics, their findings varied. Recording made near the subject's fundamental frequency was done to minimize this variability but could not eliminate it. This finding highlights the importance of communication between clinicians regarding the findings of laryngeal imaging and the importance of using the clinical picture to help interpret the results. There is also a need to continue the development of quantitative methods of measurement using imaging studies.[11,13] Strict imaging protocols with respect to frequency, phonation mode, and loudness may help to minimize variability. However, any test that requires significant patient participation and cooperation will likely exhibit some variability based on patient factors that cannot be completely eliminated.

Overall, the comparison of videostroboscopy ratings with ratings from high-speed imaging studies did not reveal any statistically significant difference between the two modalities for any of the measures *except* for the assessment of *periodicity*. Aperiodic vibratory characteristics were noted in 26% of the videostroboscopy studies and in only 2.6% of the high-speed studies ($p = 0.0006$). Aperiodic vibrations were more easily identified with videostroboscopy because when there was aperiodic vocal fold vibration, the strobe failed to track, causing the images to jump from place to place in the vibratory cycle. In addition, changes in frequency of vibration may not be as easily identified with high-speed imaging because the observed difference from cycle to cycle may be subtle and requires the examiner to review many cycles to assess. Using the kymography function, aperiodic vibrations are easily identified with high-speed imaging. The kymograph displays the movement of the vocal fold edges at a point along the anterior-posterior axis of the vocal folds. The point can be chosen by the examiner. The computer then creates a vertical display of the movement at that point over time. Several cycles of vibration can be seen simultaneously, and changes in vibration frequency can be easily identified. The kymograph function is also helpful with the evaluation of symmetry of vibration between the two vocal folds.[14,15] Segments of aperiodic vibration in 26% of a normal population indicates that previous estimates of the percentage of patients likely to benefit from high-speed laryngeal imaging may be low.

In addition to high rates of aperiodicity, *asymmetry* of vibration was found in 25% of the population, regardless of imaging modality. Periods of vibratory aperiodicity and periods of asymmetry seen in our normal subjects indicate that these findings may not represent a vocal fold vibratory abnormality when documented in patients.

When the normal range of *glottal configuration* is considered, significant variability was found within this normal subject population (**Table 29.1**). Every type of glottal configuration

Table 29.1 Glottal Configuration

Modality	Complete Closure(%)	Posterior Gap(%)	Anterior Gap(%)	Hourglass(%)	Incomplete (%)
Videostroboscopy	56	27	9	6	1
High-speed imaging	48	35	8	6	3

was identified although the closed configuration predominated, being found in 52% of the subjects studied. The next most common configuration was a posterior glottic gap, identified in 31% of the study population. Previous studies of glottal configuration in normal females have found a posterior glottic opening in 30% while voicing at the subject fundamental frequency.[8,16] In addition, a posterior glottic opening was seen more frequently in younger females than in older females in our study group, and this finding is also consistent with the results of other studies.[17] We also found more variability in the ratings of glottic configuration in the females when compared with the males in the study.

Differences between imaging modalities and between raters for glottic configuration indicate variability of the parameter in a given subject. For example, one subject was rated as having incomplete closure on the high-speed imaging study by both speech-language pathology raters. The otolaryngology rater evaluated the high-speed study twice, but rated the glottic configuration as closed on both of those assessments. The otolaryngologist also rated the videostroboscopy study in this individual and rated the glottic configuration as demonstrating an anterior glottic opening. Re-review of the studies revealed that the videostroboscopy clip was slightly over 2 minutes long. There was evidence of anterior-posterior and lateral-medial hyperfunction throughout the study. An anterior gap was identified for most of the study, and this was confirmed by one of the other raters. The high-speed study was variable and could have been judged as complete closure, anterior gap, or incomplete closure depending on where the judgments were made. There were 11,196 frames in the clip. The study starts with an anterior gap and then changes to complete closure, and this is inconsistent. The subject then takes a breath and starts

voicing again with the anterior gap. Five hundred eighty-nine frames later, there is complete closure (with much anterior-posterior squeeze, so there may have been a gap that was not visible). Then, 522 frames later, there is definitely an anterior gap. And 119 frames later, the closure is incomplete for 2804 frames, and then goes back to an anterior gap. Once again, 483 frames later, the glottic configuration changes to complete closure, and the clip then goes back to an anterior gap until done. This type of variability within a single examination underscores the caution clinicians must use during examination interpretation.

The *amplitude of vocal fold vibration* and *mucosal wave propagation* was rated for both imaging modalities on a 100-point scale with 41 designated as "normal" for both parameters. The majority of the ratings for both mucosal wave and amplitude fell within 5 points of "normal," irrespective of image modality, and there was no significant difference in the ratings based on image modality (**Figs. 29.2 and 29.3**). As expected, the ratings of vibration amplitude and mucosal wave were clustered around the designated "normal," however, the range of ratings was skewed toward an increased amplitude of vibration with some of the "normal subjects" demonstrating vocal fold vibration amplitudes rated to be as high as 28 points above the "normal" mark. In other words, diminished amplitude of vibration and mucosal wave likely represent pathology as the normal population is skewed toward larger values for these two parameters.

The distribution of the *percent open phase* ratings in our normal subject population demonstrated two distinct patterns when comparing the two image modalities (**Fig. 29.4**). The videostroboscopy ratings were based on the "montage" function of the strobe system that selects 10 images from a single virtual composite "cycle" of vibration and displays

Vibration Amplitude

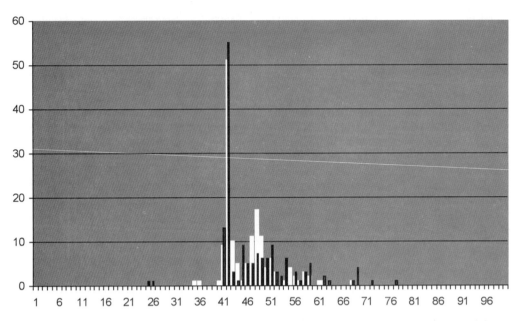

Fig. 29.2 Amplitude of vibration. The white bars indicate the ratings from videostroboscopy studies, and the black bars represent the ratings from high-speed studies.

Mucosal Wave

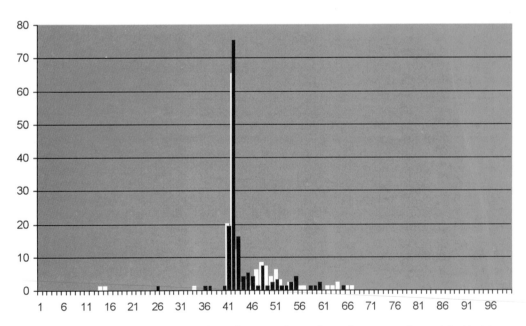

Fig. 29.3 Mucosal wave. The white bars indicate the ratings from videostroboscopy studies, and the black bars represent the ratings from high-speed studies.

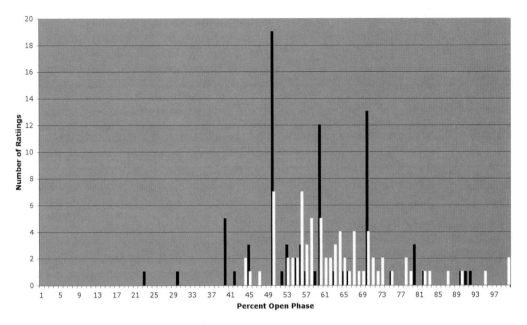

Fig. 29.4 Percent open phase. The black bars indicate the ratings from videostroboscopy studies, and the white bars represent the ratings from high-speed studies.

them on the screen. The rater then counts the number of images with open vocal folds. This method results in estimates of the percent open phase that are multiples of 10. Consequently, the percent open phase data from videostroboscopy falls into distinct groups. Almost 7% of the studies were rated to have a 40% open phase, 25% of the studies were rated to have a 50% open phase, 16% of the studies were rated to have a 60% open phase, and 17% were rated to have a 70% open phase. Another 23% were given ratings that fell in between these integers and are the result of the rater sampling from several points in the study and averaging the percent open phase from several montages. The other 13% were given open phase ratings above or below these values. On the other hand, because high-speed imaging of the larynx has a fixed rate of image capture, the number of images per cycle varies. The measurement of the number of frames with open vocal folds per cycle results in data of a more continuous nature due to the potential smaller increments of measurement. The mean value of the percent open phase as measured from high-speed imaging was 62.3% and ranged from 44 to 100%.

Report Creation

Our patient evaluation begins with videostroboscopy and is followed with high-speed imaging. We currently include both the high-speed and videostroboscopy findings in our final report. At present, there is no mechanism to bill separately for the high-speed portion of the study, so it is integrated into our overall "laryngeal imaging" procedure. This is not difficult to do because the addition of high-speed imaging to the protocol simply requires a change of camera after the videostroboscopy is complete and a few more seconds of recording. Certainly, not every patient needs further evaluation with high-speed imaging after videostroboscopy. However, at this time, we perform high-speed imaging on every patient undergoing laryngeal imaging and have been gratified by the additional information that is gained, even in patients in whom the videostroboscopy exam was optimal for evaluation.

◆ High-Speed Laryngeal Imaging Limitations

Currently, high-speed laryngeal imaging remains complementary to videostroboscopy in a clinical setting. Because only a relatively few vibratory cycles are reviewed with a high-speed imaging study, intermittent pathology may be missed. Using the technology in concert with videostroboscopy, however, provides a more complete assessment of vibratory function over a longer recording period. In addition, it provides assessment of vibratory function in real time and allows imaging during voicing onset and offset. With the kymography function, the high-speed imaging system can be used to assess changes in periodicity and symmetry over time and help with further analysis of intermittent vibratory irregularities, provided that they occur during the 8 seconds recorded during high-speed imaging.

The images recorded with older high-speed imaging systems are in black and white. If an assessment of tissue color is desired with these systems, then videostroboscopy is required. We have found that it has been helpful at times, however, to visualize pathology of the vocal folds in the black-and-white allowing a better assessment of the limits of the pathology that was obscured by color changes on videostroboscopy. In particular, cases of vocal cyst viewed with high-speed imaging are easily distinguished from polypoid changes, which may be difficult to differentiate with videostroboscopy.

It must be kept in mind that the stable frequency of image capture with high-speed imaging means that fewer images per cycle are recorded at high frequencies. Frequencies greater than 500 Hz will be difficult to assess with high-speed imaging because less than four images per cycle will be recorded. A soprano complaining of difficulty with the high end of her singing range is an example of this situation.

◆ Clinical Application Examples of High-Speed Imaging

We have found several instances where additional clinical information was gained with high-speed imaging of the larynx in patients with good tracking on videostroboscopy. These patients might not initially be considered for high-speed imaging because the videostroboscopy appeared easy to interpret. However, when the high-speed imaging study was reviewed, unexpected findings were appreciated.

◆ *Early postoperative recovery:* Previous studies using videostroboscopy to assess the return of the mucosal wave in patients after surgery of the vocal fold report that the mucosal wave generally begins to return 3 weeks after surgery. With high-speed imaging, we have found cases of mucosal wave recovery as early as 1 week after surgery. Videostroboscopy performed at that time revealed stiffness in the area of surgery, likely due to poor tracking in the healing vocal fold segment because it vibrated at a different frequency from the rest of the normal vocal fold (**Video Clip 62**). On high-speed imaging, however, clear vibrations were identified in the healing segment (**Video Clip 63**). Based on this finding, we have been able to allow these patients to advance more rapidly with voice rehabilitation.

◆ *Behavior assessment:* Although no further information regarding the type and degree of pathology is obtained in patients with vocal fold nodules on high-speed imaging, significant information regarding behavioral pathology can be recorded. By recording voicing onset, we have found several cases of what appears to be extreme muscle tension and supraglottic squeezing at voicing onset that was not appreciated with videostroboscopy (**Video Clips 36 and 64**). In addition, although no objective measures can be made, subjectively there appears to be an increase in the force with which the vocal folds contact during voicing. When viewed with high-speed imaging, the vocal folds of these patients appear to be slamming together (**Video Clips 65 and 66**). These observations may provide clues into the pathophysiology of nodule formation. Following these patients with serial high-speed imaging studies may provide a mechanism by which to monitor the progress of therapy. Eventually, the technology could be used to assess patients prior to surgery to determine if they have successfully eliminated the muscle tension behavior, thereby increasing the likelihood of successful outcomes with surgery.

- *Nodule/polyp versus cyst:* Occasionally, it is difficult to distinguish various types of vocal fold pathology along the vocal fold margin. In particular, it is important to determine if a cyst is present. This type of lesion does not respond to voice therapy and requires surgical excision for cure. Often, however, there is significant surrounding secondary pathology such as edema and erythema that obscure the margins of the cyst, making it difficult to distinguish from a nodule or polyp. We have found that by viewing this type of pathology with high-speed imaging in black-and-white, the margins of the lesions appear more distinct and that the diagnosis of a cyst can be made more definitively. As a result, the patient is spared prolonged voice therapy prior to surgical treatment.
- *Aperiodicity versus stiffness:* Using videostroboscopy, a part of a vocal fold may appear adynamic when, in actuality, it is vibrating but at a frequency that is irregular and/or different from the measured frequency of voicing. Because the strobe is not tracking the frequency of vibration of that part of the vocal fold, it appears stiff. With high-speed imaging, however, it is possible to see the vibrations in that segment. (See the previous discussion regarding early postoperative recovery.)

◆ Future Developments in High-Speed Laryngeal Imaging

The continued use of high-speed laryngeal imaging will likely elucidate more clinical situations in which it is helpful, and this will encourage manufacturers to refine the technology. The addition of color to high-speed imaging has already occurred with most of the commercially available systems. Linking the images to an audio recording of the patient's voice and further refinements in image resolution would provide additional clinical information to the study. The digitization of the imaging enhances the ability to accurately quantify many characteristics of vibrating vocal folds, and future systems are likely to offer the ability to quantitatively assess vocal fold vibration.[18,19]

In conclusion, high-speed imaging of the larynx offers many benefits over standard videostroboscopy in the analysis of patients with voice disorders, particularly those with irregular vocal fold motion. As the technology advances and the knowledge base with this form of laryngeal analysis expands, our ability to evaluate and treat patients will improve.

References

1. Sundberg J. Vocal fold vibration patterns and modes of phonation. Folia Phoniatr Logop 1995;47:218–228
2. Berry DA, Montequin DW, Tayama N. High-speed digital imaging of the medial surface of the vocal folds. J Acoust Soc Am 2001;110(5 Pt 1):2539–2547
3. Döllinger M, Braunschweig T, Lohscheller J, Eysholdt U, Hoppe U. Normal voice production: computation of driving parameters from endoscopic digital high speed images. Methods Inf Med 2003;42:271–276
4. Hertegård S, Larsson H, Wittenberg T. High-speed imaging: applications and development. Logoped Phoniatr Vocol 2003;28:133–139
5. Verdonck-de Leeuw IM, Festen JM, Mahieu HF. Deviant vocal fold vibration as observed during videokymography: the effect on voice quality. J Voice 2001;15:313–322
6. Larsson H, Hertegård S, Lindestad PA, Hammarberg B. Vocal fold vibrations: high-speed imaging, kymography, and acoustic analysis: a preliminary report. Laryngoscope 2000;110:2117–2122
7. Kendall KA. High-speed laryngeal imaging compared with videostroboscopy in healthy subjects. Arch Otolaryngol Head Neck Surg 2009;135:274–281
8. Gelfer MP, Bultemeyer DK. Evaluation of vocal fold vibratory patterns in normal voices. J Voice 1990;4:335–345
9. Yan Y, Ahmad K, Kunduk M, Bless D. Analysis of vocal-fold vibrations from high-speed laryngeal images using a Hilbert transform-based methodology. J Voice 2005;19:161–175
10. Sulter AM, Schutte HK, Miller DG. Standardized laryngeal videostroboscopic rating: differences between untrained and trained male and female subjects, and effects of varying sound intensity, fundamental frequency, and age. J Voice 1996;10:175–189
11. Woo P. Quantification of videostrobolaryngoscopic findings: measurements of the normal glottal cycle. Laryngoscope 1996; 106(3 Pt 2, Suppl 79)1–27
12. Poburka BJ. A new stroboscopy rating form. J Voice 1999;13:403–413
13. Svec JG, Schutte HK. Videokymography: high-speed line scanning of vocal fold vibration. J Voice 1996; 10:201–205
14. Wittenberg T, Tigges M, Mergell P, Eysholdt U. Functional imaging of vocal fold vibration: digital multi-slice high-speed kymography. J Voice 2000;14:422–442

15. Tigges M, Wittenberg T, Mergell P, Eysholdt U. Imaging of vocal fold vibration by digital multi-plane kymography. Comput Med Imaging Graph 1999; 23:323–330

16. Pemberton C, Russell A, Priestley J, Havas T, Hooper J, Clark P. Characteristics of normal larynges under flexible fiberscopic and stroboscopic examination: an Australian perspective. J Voice 1993;7:382–389

17. Linville SE. Glottal gap configurations in two age groups of women. J Speech Hear Res 1992;35: 1209–1215

18. Schuberth S, Hoppe U, Döllinger M, Lohscheller J, Eysholdt U. High-precision measurement of the vocal fold length and vibratory amplitudes. Laryngoscope 2002;112:1043–1049

19. Qiu Q, Schutte HK, Gu L, Yu Q. An automatic method to quantify the vibration properties of human vocal folds via videokymography. Folia Phoniatr Logop 2003;55:128–136

Appendix

Video Clips

1. **Constant Light versus Videostroboscopy.** This video clip demonstrates vocal fold vibration seen with a constant light source and recorded at 30 fps. The vibration of the vocal folds cannot be seen, and the edges of the folds appear blurred. When videostroboscopy is used in the second part of the video clip, the vocal fold vibration is "slowed down" and the viewer has the impression of seeing vocal fold vibration in slow motion. What is actually seen is a composite of images from several cycles of vibration made into a "virtual" movie. Note that the onset of voicing is blurred, even during videostroboscopy. This is because the strobe cannot track during voicing onset when the vibration is aperiodic. Once videostroboscopy is initiated, it is possible to appreciate that the glottic configuration during maximal closure is completely closed. Vibration is periodic and symmetric. The amplitude of vibration and the mucosal wave are normal.

2. **Videostroboscopy in Locked Mode.** This video clip demonstrates the use of the "locked mode" of the videostroboscopy system. By using the locked mode, the strobe is set to flash at the same frequency as vocal fold vibration, and the image recorded appears to be a "still" image because images are captured from the same point in each vibratory cycle recorded. If the locked mode is used to evaluate vocal folds during *aperiodic*

vibration, the resulting recording gives the impression of slight vocal fold movement.

3. **Normal Vibratory Symmetry.** Normal symmetry of vibration requires that both vocal folds begin to move apart at the same time and at the same speed. They move laterally to the same extent. They reach maximal opening at the same time and then begin to close simultaneously, again at the same speed. They reach maximal closure together. The glottic configuration at maximal closure in this example is an anterior glottic chink, with a persistent small opening between the anterior membranous vocal folds. Symmetrical vibration is normally expected to occur for any pitch and loudness.

4. **Videostroboscopy of Falsetto.** During falsetto (ie, using a very high voice), the open phase of the vibratory cycle predominates. In fact, it appears in this example that the vocal fold never completely closes. During the clip, the subject inadvertently begins to use a vibrato technique with rapidly changing pitch, but the examiner prompts her to use "straight" falsetto to eliminate this pitch variability.

5. **The Effect of Pitch Change on Vibratory Characteristics.** This video clip demonstrates normal vibration with changes in pitch. Pitch will affect the amplitude of vibration and the mucosal wave. If vocal volume, or loudness, is stable, then both

amplitude and mucosal wave will diminish in size as the pitch increases. In the middle of this clip, the subject also demonstrates a change in loudness, going from a soft high pitch to a loud high pitch, illustrating that there is also a change in the amplitude of vibration and the mucosal wave with increasing volume. This is seen very well at high pitch, where amplitude and mucosal wave are typically smaller.

6. **The Effect of Volume Change on Vibratory Characteristics.** This video clip demonstrates normal vibration with changes in loudness. Increasing volume while maintaining a stable pitch of phonation will increase the amplitude of vibration and the mucosal wave. During the last segment of the clip, the subject attempts to increase her loudness while maintaining pitch. In this circumstance, she inadvertently begins to use a vibrato. This means that her pitch is unstable, and this is reflected in a sudden loss of tracking with the strobe. The vocal fold margins become blurred, and vibration is no longer clearly visible.

7. **Slow-Motion Assessment of the Normal Mucosal Wave.** In slow motion, the vocal fold vibration can be observed in detail. Note the symmetry of vibration in that the vocal folds begin to open simultaneously, move laterally to the same extent, and begin to close at the same time. The mucosal wave can be appreciated as the difference between the upper and lower lips of the medial edges of the vocal folds and, to some extent, the movement of the wave over the upper surface of the vocal folds. Slow-motion or frame-by-frame analysis is usually the best way to evaluate the mucosal wave.

8. **Videostroboscopy of Rapid Alternating Movements.** Videostroboscopy is unable to visualize the onset and offset of voicing because the frequency of vibration is changing too rapidly for the strobe and camera to track. The result is that the margins of the vocal folds appear blurred, and the vibration is poorly visualized. A common task used to assess vocal fold

movement is the on/off maneuver or the /ee/ /ee/. However, videostroboscopy cannot effectively visualize vocal fold vibration during this task as illustrated by this video clip.

9. **Vibrato.** This video clip shows a normal subject performing vibrato voicing used by singers to produce a throbbing effect by rapidly varying the pitch. The clip illustrates the difficulty with videostroboscopy when there are rapid pitch changes while voicing. The strobe is unable to track the frequency during vibrato, and the margins of the vocal folds are blurred.

10. **Normal Vibration.** This video clip illustrates a videostroboscopic recording through a rigid endoscope of the vibrating vocal folds during a sustained vowel. The pitch is accurately detected to produce slow-motion vocal fold cycles (1.5 cycles per second; 20 frames per period) (subject without vocal pathology).

11. **Poor Tracking Due to Aperiodicity during Videostroboscopy.** This video clip demonstrates a videostroboscopic recording through a rigid endoscope of the vibrating vocal folds during a sustained vowel in a patient who had undergone surgical treatment for glottic cancer. The pitch is not accurately detected, resulting in an unstable depiction of the vocal fold vibration.

12. **High-Speed Imaging of Aperiodic Vibration.** This video clip is a high-speed videoendoscopic recording (rigid endoscope, constant light) demonstrating the true underlying vocal fold tissue motion from the patient in **Video Clip 11**. The image sampling rate ≈ 6006 Hz (sampling period = 166.5 msec).

13. **High-Speed Imaging/Stroboscopy Overlay.** This video clip is a high-speed videoendoscopic recording from a normal subject through a rigid endoscope (constant light) of the vibrating vocal folds during a sustained vowel; image sampling rate = 6250 Hz (sampling period = 160 msec). A second rigid endoscope displayed the strobe flashes locked to the fundamental frequency

($F0 \approx 236$ Hz, strobe frequency ≈ 58.7 Hz), which could be used to create the stroboscopic slow-motion sequence.

14. **"Stroboscopy" Movie from High-Speed Imaging.** This video clip is of the created stroboscopic sequence derived from the high-speed videoendoscopic recording of **Video Clip 13**. The images that were illuminated by the strobe flashes in **Video Clip 13** were extracted to create a simulated stroboscopic sequence; note that the NTSC odd/even field sampling was not simulated.

15. **Posterior Glottic Opening Configuration.** In ~30% of the normal population, the glottic configuration at maximal closure has a posterior glottic chink. There is complete closure between the membranous vocal folds during phonation, but a persistent opening is present between the arytenoid cartilages. This video clip demonstrates an example of a posterior glottic chink. The vibratory characteristics are normal with periodic and symmetric vibration, normal amplitude of vibration, and normal mucosal wave.

16. **Mild Presbyphonia.** Vocal fold "bowing," or presbyphonia, typically results in a spindle-shaped glottic opening at maximal closure. This video clip demonstrates a mild case of presbyphonia. In this instance, the gap between the membranous vocal folds is slight. The vibration is slightly aperiodic so that the tacking of the stroboscopy is not perfectly smooth. The amplitude of vibration may be slightly larger than normal due to increased laxity of the vocal folds, but it is symmetric. The mucosal wave is normal.

17. **Moderate Presbyphonia.** This video clip demonstrates a case of moderate presbyphonia. The glottic configuration is spindle-shaped with a distinct persistent opening between the vocal folds at maximal closure. There is asymmetry of vibration in the first part of the clip when the patient phonates at a high frequency. The right vocal fold begins to move laterally before the left vocal fold. The right fold reaches maximal lateral excursion before the left fold and begins to return toward midline before the left vocal fold. This same pattern of asymmetry is noted at lower pitches as well. The amplitude of vibration is larger than normal due to the laxity of the vocal folds. The mucosal wave may also be slightly larger than normal. To compensate for significant glottic insufficiency during soft phonation, there is squeezing of the supraglottic structures. During loud phonation, the patient is able to achieve complete glottic closure but slips into a higher frequency, likely because it is easier to maintain closure with the vocal folds on stretch.

18. **Mild Nodules.** Patients with vocal fold nodules are often found to have an hourglass glottic configuration as demonstrated in this video clip. During phonation, there is contact between the vocal folds only at the site of mid-membranous vocal fold thickening with a persistent glottic gap anterior and posterior to this region. Despite the nodules, vibration is relatively periodic in this example. In addition, because the nodules are relatively symmetric in size and shape, they affect the vibratory characteristics of each vocal fold equally, and vibration remains symmetric. The nodules "ride" the mucosal wave indicating they are relatively superficial without involvement of the lamina propria. The mucosal wave and amplitude of vibration appear normal in size and symmetry.

19. **Polyp.** Vocal fold polyps are often unilateral and result in an irregular glottic configuration at maximal closure. In this example of a right vocal fold polyp, the patient has difficulty phonating long enough to activate stroboscopy. Phonation duration is shortened because of glottic insufficiency due to air leaking through the vocal folds through persistent glottic openings during voicing. When the strobe is activated, the tracking is poor, indicating aperiodic vibration. The vibration is irregular. The distension of the right vocal fold tissues by the polyp results in a decrease in the amplitude of vibration and the mucosal wave. The vibration on the right is chaotic and irregular. The mucosal wave and amplitude of vibration on the left is relatively normal.

20. **Muscle Tension Dysphonia.** The patient in this video clip suffers from an unusual form of muscle tension dysphonia in which the patient holds the vocal folds open during phonation (as opposed to over-squeezing them together, as in the most common cases of muscle tension dysphonia). The result is an open glottic configuration, even at maximal closure. At lower frequencies, vibration is periodic with stroboscopy producing the impression of smooth vibration. At higher pitches, the vibration becomes aperiodic with poor strobe tracking. During good stroboscopy tracking, the vibration is seen to be asymmetric. Frame-by-frame analysis of vibration reveals that the asymmetry is due to phase asymmetry and asymmetry of the amplitude of vibration. In other words, beginning at a point in the vibratory cycle of maximal closure, the next frames demonstrate that the left vocal fold begins to abduct before the right fold. The left fold also does not travel as far medially as the right vocal fold and begins to move toward the midline before the right vocal fold has reached its maximal lateral excursion. The left fold reaches the midline before the right fold and is actually already beginning to move laterally again at the point of maximal vocal fold closure. In the next few frames, as the left vocal fold continues to move laterally, the right vocal fold continues to move medially. Careful evaluation of each vocal fold separately reveals a normal mucosal wave bilaterally.

21. **Anterior Glottic Gap Configuration.** This video clip demonstrates a glottic configuration with an anterior glottic gap in an individual without voice complaints. The vibration is periodic. Frame-by-frame analysis of vibration symmetry, amplitude of vibration, and mucosal wave reveals slight asymmetry of vibration secondary to a slight phase asymmetry. Beginning with a frame where the vocal folds have reached maximal closure, evaluation of the subsequent frames demonstrates that the left vocal fold reaches maximal lateral excursion before the right vocal fold. The left fold also begins to move back toward and reaches the midline slightly before the left vocal fold. The amplitude of vibration and the mucosal wave are the same for each fold and are normal. The identification of mild asymmetry in a healthy normal individual underscores the need to interpret the examination findings carefully and in the context of the patient's complaints.

22. **Asymmetric Vibration: Shadowing.** The primary finding in this video clip is asymmetry of vibration. The vocal folds are vibrating out of phase. In other words, as the right vocal fold begins to move laterally from the midline, the left vocal fold is moving medially from its most lateral excursion. The second half of the clip is in slow motion and reveals that the folds do touch each other for a short interval as the right fold begins to medialize and the left fold is still moving medially. The glottic configuration at these points of maximal closure is closed, but the open phase predominates during the glottic cycle and allows for increased air loss and breathiness. There are intervals in which there is no closure or there remains a slight anterior gap. The vibration is periodic enough to adequately trigger the strobe for tracking. The amplitude of vibration appears normal for the relatively high pitch of the phonation. Because the vibration is out of phase, it is difficult to evaluate the mucosal wave, although the portion of the wave on the superior surface of the vocal folds appears normal.

23. **Bimodal Vibrations.** The evaluation of this patient's vocal fold margins reveals a soft polyp on the midportion of the left vocal fold. The right vocal fold appears to be slightly thickened in the midportion, just opposite the polyp on the other fold. This may represent a contrecoup lesion as a result of contact at this point with the lesion on the opposite fold. Initially, the vibration is periodic and symmetric. However, at about 7 seconds into the clip, there is a period of bimodal vibration during which the vocal folds alternate between closing anteriorly only and closing posteriorly only. The blurring of the vocal fold margins at the onset of voicing is

expected because of aperiodicity during voice onset and poor strobe tracking due to this aperiodicity. The second half of the clip allows evaluation of the amplitude of vibration and the mucosal wave, which appear normal. Although there is no sound with this clip, the observer is able to tell that the patient is voicing at various frequencies and performs a glissando at the end of the clip. This is a nice example of changes in mucosal wave, amplitude of vibration, and vocal fold length with changes in pitch.

24. **Severe Presbyphonia.** This case illustrates a situation where the patient has difficulty voicing long enough to activate the strobe. Due to severe presbyphonia, the patient's phonation duration is only a few seconds. The glottic configuration is visible only during the early part of the video clip and is spindle-shaped with closure at the vocal processes of the arytenoid cartilages and a persistent opening of the membranous vocal folds. By having the patient voice during inhalation, the clinician is better able to see the shape of the glottis. The patient attempts to compensate for the anterior glottic gap during voicing with squeezing. The arytenoid cartilages overlap as part of this attempt at compensation. There is also narrowing of the glottic inlet in the anterior-posterior direction and closure of the ventricular folds as the patient tries to close the glottis for voicing. The vibration, visible only for a short period at the beginning of the clip, is aperiodic and irregular. The margins of the vocal folds appear smooth, but the mucosal wave cannot really be seen long enough to evaluate because of the aperiodicity of vibration and the supraglottic squeezing that obscures the view of the vocal folds during voicing. The amplitude of vibration is larger than normal because there is less tension of the tissues preventing them from blowing laterally with the force of the exhaled air.

25. **Vocal Fold Paralysis: Using Falsetto.** This patient with right vocal fold paralysis is attempting to improve glottic closure by phonating at a higher-than-normal frequency. The use of this strategy requires an intact superior laryngeal nerve supplying innervation to the ipsilateral cricothyroid muscle. Despite the use of this strategy, this patient demonstrates a persistent glottic gap even at maximal closure, except for a few instances where complete closure is briefly achieved. The ventricular fold on the left is larger than on the right and is active during phonation, indicative of the high level of effort used by the patient in attempting to close the glottis during voicing. Typically, the amplitude of vibration of a paralyzed and thus flaccid vocal fold is larger than normal because there is no muscle contraction to create resistance to airflow, and the tissues vibrate freely with the passage of air. Using a higher pitch tenses the paralyzed vocal fold so that during phonation, there is some resistance to airflow, and the amplitude of vibration of that fold is smaller (although still larger than it would be in a normal vocal fold at that frequency of vibration). In this example, the amplitude of vibration of the right vocal fold is still larger than the nonparalyzed side. This difference in vibration amplitude results in asymmetry of vibration. The mucosal waves are small at this high pitch but appear to be relatively symmetric.

26. **Cyst.** In this video clip, there is a cyst of the left vocal fold. The right vocal fold margin appears slightly thickened at the point where it contacts the cyst in the opposite vocal fold. This may represent a contrecoup lesion. Careful inspection of the right vocal fold reveals a tiny focus of vascular abnormality, perhaps an area of injury. At times, there is complete closure of the glottis, but often, the glottic configuration is hourglass shaped with contact at the location of the cyst and a persistent glottic opening in front and behind the cyst. Glottic insufficiency results in a breathy vocal quality. Vibration is periodic. The amplitude of vibration is decreased at the site of the cyst on the left and is normal on the right. The mucosal wave is also diminished on the left at the site of the cyst. One has the impression that the mucosal wave may be slightly

diminished on the right as well, at the area of mucosal thickening. Further review of this clip in the slow-motion mode would be helpful to clarify this issue.

27. **Vocal Fold Paralysis with Bowing.** This patient with a right vocal fold paralysis has significant glottic insufficiency due to a relatively large persistent glottic opening during voicing. Her phonation duration is so short that the stroboscopy cannot be activated long enough to evaluate the vocal fold vibratory characteristics. The bowed configuration of the paralyzed vocal fold contributes further to the size of the glottic opening and is likely because of vocal fold hypotonia due to denervation. Even at higher frequencies, she demonstrates a large glottic gap during phonation.

28. **Vocal Fold Paralysis with Some Adaption.** Despite a right vocal fold paralysis and the resulting glottic incompetence, the strobe tacking during this example is smooth, indicating periodic vocal fold vibration. At a normal volume, the vocal folds make contact anteriorly. The glottic configuration at maximal closure demonstrates an opening between the vocal processes of the arytenoid cartilages. With attempts at louder voicing, there is almost complete closure of the membranous vocal folds with only a slight gap between the vocal processes of the arytenoid cartilages. Note the prolapsed position of the right arytenoid cartilage and the activity of the left ventricular fold. During phonation, there is asymmetric vibration secondary to the difference in tension between the two vocal folds that becomes less pronounced when the patient tries to phonate at a louder volume. At lower volumes, the right vocal fold moves laterally, reaches maximal excursion, and begins to move back medially before the left vocal fold. The amplitude of vibration and the mucosal waves do not differ substantially between the two vocal folds in this example.

29. **Paralysis with Atrophy.** In cases of long-standing vocal fold paralysis, the vocal fold may become atrophied. The vocal fold margin may appear convex as a result, and the ventricle may appear more open, as it does in this example of left vocal fold paralysis. The left arytenoid cartilage is slightly prolapsed forward so that it is not possible to see the vocal process of the arytenoid cartilage on that side. During phonation, there is a persistent glottic opening in the membranous portion of the vocal folds. The patient is able to phonate long enough to activate the strobe, and the amplitude of vibration on the left is smaller than on the right. The mucosal wave is also smaller on the side of paralysis.

30. **Arytenoid Prolapse.** The prolapsed position of the arytenoid cartilage obscures the view of the posterior part of the paralyzed vocal fold in this example of right vocal fold paralysis. The vocal process and medial aspect of the right arytenoid cartilage cannot be seen even during voicing. This is likely due to a lack of muscular support that keeps the arytenoid cartilage in an upright position. The patient demonstrates severe glottic insufficiency during voicing with a large glottic opening during maximal closure. Stroboscopy cannot be performed because the phonation duration is too short, and thus vocal fold vibratory characteristics cannot be assessed.

31. **After Vocal Fold Augmentation.** In this video clip, the left vocal fold has been augmented to help compensate for a left vocal fold paralysis. The injection has medialized the left vocal fold so that complete glottic closure is achieved during voicing. During sustained voicing, the vibration is periodic (the strobe tracks nicely). The effects of vocal fold differences in tension and mass are apparent during a frame-by-frame analysis of this portion of the recording. There is a slight decrease in the amplitude of vibration and the mucosal wave on the left side, leading to vibratory mild asymmetry.

32. **Vocal Fold Stiffness.** At comfortable and higher pitches, the strobe is able to track well during this video clip, indicating periodic vibration. At lower pitches, however, the strobe is unable to track due to aperiodicity of vibration. This is a good

example of a case where the vocal folds may appear normal on an indirect examination or a flexible exam with a constant light. With videostroboscopy, however, it is clear that this patient has asymmetry of vibration. The amplitude of vibration and the mucosal wave on the right is significantly diminished compared with the left, indicating stiffness, likely due to scar. The mucosal wave and amplitude of vibration seem small on the left as well. This, however, is most likely due to the high frequency of vibration during the examination portion with good stroboscopy tracking.

33. **Vocal Fold Stiffness.** This patient not only has severe scarring of the left vocal fold but also has a lack of bulk on the left, preventing vocal fold closure during voicing. Thus, the glottic configuration at maximal closure is spindle-shaped with closure of the arytenoid cartilages and persistent opening between the membranous vocal folds. There appears to be adequate tracking to evaluate the mucosal wave and amplitude of vibration, but the tracking is not smooth, indicating aperiodic vibration. The mucosal wave is absent on the left with very little amplitude of vibration. The mucosal wave on the right is normal, and the vibration amplitude changes appropriately with changes in pitch and loudness. The difference in the vibratory characteristics between the right and left vocal fold leads to vibration asymmetry.

34. **Submucosal Mass.** In this patient, the margins of the vocal folds appear smooth, but on closer inspection, one can identify fullness in the posterior half of the right membranous vocal fold. There is also a submucosal mass seen in this region through the mucosa on the superior surface of the vocal fold. Although the patient changes pitch during this evaluation, there is periodic vibration during the periods of stable phonation. The glottic configuration at maximal closure reveals a posterior glottic gap. In other words, during voicing, the membranous vocal folds close completely, and there is a gap between the arytenoid cartilages. This configuration is most common in women, observed in up to 30% of healthy females. The evaluation of the vibratory characteristics in this patient gives further clues to the presence of pathology in the posterior aspect of the right membranous vocal fold. At this location, there is a decrease in the mucosal wave and a decrease in vibratory amplitude at all pitches sampled.

35. **Left Vocal Fold Malignancy.** This nonsmoking patient presented with a complaint of hoarseness. The indirect examination revealed a lesion on the posterior aspect of the left true vocal fold and a glottic gap, consistent with vocal fold bowing. The videostroboscopy revealed that the lesion was very firm, with no vibration and complete lack of a mucosal wave. Anterior to the lesion, the vocal fold was also stiff. Direct laryngoscopy and biopsy determined that this lesion was an invasive squamous cell carcinoma.

36. **Polypoid Changes.** This video clip demonstrates the stroboscopy findings with polypoid chorditis, a condition in which the lamina propria becomes distended with gelatinous material. In this example, the left vocal fold is more involved than the right resulting in asymmetry in the mass of the two vocal folds. The glottic closure configuration is irregular. Vibration is, as a result of the asymmetry, mostly chaotic and aperiodic. But there are areas of good stroboscopy tracking in the clip, and vibratory characteristics can be evaluated during these parts of the clip. As expected with asymmetry in the mass of the vocal folds, vibration is asymmetric. On frame-by-frame analysis, the amplitude of vibration of the left cord appears smaller than the amplitude of vibration on the right, likely due to greater involvement with chorditis. The mucosal wave appears symmetric and relatively normal in size bilaterally.

37. **Chronic Inflammation.** Chronic inflammation of the vocal folds causes edema of the lamina propria, making the tissues stiff and less pliable. In this example of chronic inflammation, the vocal fold margins are irregular. The glottic configuration at maximal closure is also irregular. Vibration is

periodic enough to record an impression of smooth vibration. The vibration, however, is asymmetric with the right vocal fold moving laterally before the left. The amplitude of vibration appears to be larger on the right than on the left as well. The mucosal wave is essentially absent bilaterally.

38. **Abnormal Only at High Pitch.** This example illustrates the importance of evaluating the vocal fold vibratory characteristics at various frequencies. This patient demonstrates some mild asymmetry at her comfortable pitch. Frame-by-frame analysis reveals that the amplitude of vibration is slightly decreased on the left compared with the right. Close inspection also reveals a pin-point vascular lesion on the left with a feeding vessel. The mucosal wave is normal bilaterally. If the examination had only been done at this frequency, it would have been difficult to be sure that these mild abnormalities were the cause of vocal complaints. However, at higher pitch, the left vocal fold is very stiff, with essentially no vibration or mucosal wave. With this additional information, it is clear that the left vocal fold is scarred, possibly as the result of previous hemorrhage from the small vascular lesion.

39. **Asymmetry More Pronounced at High Pitch.** This is an example of abnormal vocal fold vibratory characteristics only present during high-pitched phonation. With phonation at a comfortable pitch, vibration is periodic and symmetric. The amplitude of vibration and the mucosal wave are symmetric and normal. At a slightly higher pitch, vibration remains periodic and symmetric with appropriate amplitude of vibration and mucosal wave. However, at the highest pitch, the left vocal fold demonstrates stiffness with a marked decrease in the vibratory amplitude compared with the right vocal fold. This difference in the tissue characteristics leads to asymmetry of vibration.

40. **Nodules with Fibrosis.** In this video clip, the vocal folds are erythematous and their margins are irregular, indicative of chronic inflammation. The mid-membranous portion of both vocal folds is significantly thickened, consistent with nodules. During voicing, the glottic configuration is hourglass with contact occurring only at the location of the nodules. Vibration is periodic during sustained phonation at the beginning of the video clip. Frame-by-frame analysis of this portion of the examination reveals a reduction of the mucosal wave over the nodules and a decrease in the amplitude of vibration at that site as well. This indicates significant involvement of the lamina propria in the pathologic process that is leading to the formation of the nodules, likely recurrent injury.

41. **Thin Right Vocal Fold.** This video clip demonstrates vibration asymmetry secondary to asymmetry of vocal fold bulk. The right vocal fold is "thin" and appears less bulky than the left vocal fold, although the margins of the vocal folds appear smooth, and the tissues demonstrate normal coloration. At low frequencies, the glottic configuration is almost completely closed, but there is a tiny anterior gap and a small gap between the arytenoid cartilages. At higher pitches, however, there is a persistent opening along the entire length of the vocal folds. Vibration symmetry is also almost normal at the lower pitches. At higher pitches, there is significant asymmetry of vibration. Frame-by-frame analysis of vibration reveals that the asymmetry is the result of a difference in the amplitude of vibration between the two vocal folds. The amplitude of vibration on the right is larger than on the left at both low and high frequencies, consistent with a decrease of bulk or tone on that side. The mucosal wave is normal and symmetric indicating a healthy lamina propria.

42. **Thin Left Vocal Fold.** In this video clip, the left vocal fold is atrophic with a significant decrease in size and bulk compared with the right side. The margins of the vocal folds are smooth. The evaluation of glottic closure reveals a persistent gap along the anterior half of the membranous vocal folds and a small gap between the arytenoid cartilages. Likely, the gap between the arytenoid cartilages is premorbid, but the gap at the anterior half of the membranous

vocal folds is due to a change in the bulk of the left vocal fold. The consequences of such glottic insufficiency include a soft and breathy voice, even with attempts at louder phonation. Vibration is adequately periodic for stroboscopy tracking. The vibration is asymmetric and out of phase, however, secondary to asymmetry in vocal fold bulk. This asymmetry makes the evaluation of the amplitude of vibration and the mucosal wave challenging, but on frame-by frame analysis, they appear relatively normal.

43. **Tremor and Scar.** This example illustrates the difficulty in performing videostroboscopy in patients with vocal tremor. Because the frequency of vibration changes rapidly with the tremor, the stroboscopy is unable to track, and the images obtained are not from sequential parts of the vibratory cycle and appear to "jump." Despite this, it is clear from the instances where the strobe can track that there is a difference in the vibratory characteristics between the right and left vocal fold. This patient had a carcinoma removed from the right anterior vocal fold and has scarring in this area as a result. The tissues where the tumor was removed are stiff, and frame-by-frame analysis reveals a decrease in the amplitude of vibration at that location. It is very difficult to assess the mucosal wave in this patient because of poor tracking, but it appears to be diminished on the right compared with the left as well.

44. **Vocal Fold Hemorrhage.** This example of acute vocal fold hemorrhage demonstrates how the distension of the lamina propria with blood prevents vibration of the tissues. During phonation, there is significant squeezing together of the supraglottic tissues. This squeezing makes it impossible to see the right vocal fold during attempts at voicing. Careful evaluation of vibration of the left vocal fold reveals no vibration of the tissues distended by focal hemorrhage, although there is some vibration appreciated of the more posterior parts of the left vocal fold.

45. **Asymmetric Masses.** Vocal fold nodules are usually bilateral and symmetric. This symmetry means that nodules may not impact the vocal fold vibratory characteristics, especially if the nodules are superficial and without associated fibrosis of the tissues in the lamina propria. This example illustrates the impact of bilateral vocal fold nodules that are located asymmetrically on the vocal folds. Vocal fold vibration is asymmetric and even appears bimodal. The amplitude of vibration and the mucosal wave are otherwise normal.

46. **Small Polyp.** This video clip is an example of a soft polyp in the mid-membranous portion of the left vocal fold with an irregularity of the right vocal fold where the right vocal fold makes contact with the polyp on the left. The lesion on the right is probably a contrecoup lesion. Both vocal folds demonstrate evidence of recurrent small hemorrhages, and this is likely the etiology of the polyp. The glottic configuration at maximal closure is hourglass with contact between the polyp and the contrecoup lesion only. Vibration is relatively periodic, as the stroboscopy is able to track reasonably well. Vibration is symmetric indicating that the polyp and the contrecoup lesion impact the characteristics of vibration of each vocal fold equally, allowing them to vibrate symmetrically. The amplitude of vibration is normal bilaterally. The mucosal wave is diminished at the location of the lesions bilaterally but can be appreciated over and lateral to the polyp secondary to its "soft" characteristics.

47. **Chronic Inflammation.** The patient in this example has suffered from severe chronic laryngitis due to inhaler use and chronic cough. During the period of her worse symptoms, videostroboscopy was not really possible because her vocal folds were so inflamed that they really did not vibrate much at all. After a period of treatment, the inflammation improved, and this video clip was made when she felt her voice was almost back to her "normal" voice. The vocal folds remain erythematous, but the margins of the folds are smooth. The vibration has changed from completely chaotic to periodic, so that stroboscopy is possible. The vibration is

relatively symmetric. The amplitude of vibration is slightly less on the right side than on the left, and the mucosal wave is less on that side as well, indicating either the persistence of inflammation in the superficial lamina propria or some early signs of scarring secondary to the injury caused by the inflammation.

48. **High Vagal Nerve Injury.** Supraglottic squeezing during the evaluation makes visualization of the vocal folds during phonation impossible in this case of high vagal nerve injury on the right. Dilation of the right piriform sinus occurs secondary to denervation of the pharyngeal constrictor muscles. The pooling of secretions is made more dangerous by a lack of sensation on the right, increasing the risk of aspiration in these cases.

49. **Vocal Fold Paralysis with Ventricular Hypertrophy.** Clear visualization of the vocal folds during voicing is obstructed by hyperfunction of the ventricular folds in this case of left vocal fold paralysis. Contraction of the contralateral ventricular fold is a natural response to glottic insufficiency and is considered to represent an attempt to improve glottic closure. Despite this effort, the patient demonstrates a persistent significant glottic insufficiency with voicing. The visible portion of the vocal folds appears to be vibrating irregularly. Further evaluation of vocal fold vibratory characteristics in this case is limited by the short phonation duration and limited view of the vocal folds.

50. **After Overinjection.** This videostroboscopy clip reveals why this patient has a poor voice after injection laryngoplasty for medialization of a paralyzed right vocal fold. There has been some overinjection anteriorly that results in a convex vocal fold and contact between the right and left vocal folds even during inspiration. During voicing, there is no passage of air between the vocal folds in this region of overinjection. The vibratory portion of the vocal folds has been effectively shortened to only the posterior half of the vocal folds. In addition, the injected vocal fold is stiff and does not vibrate. On a frame-by-frame analysis, there is a small mucosal wave present on the right but a complete lack of vibratory amplitude, indicating that the injection may have been too superficial, diffusing into the lamina propria.

51. **Persistent Posterior Gap after Medialization.** Despite medialization, the vocal processes of the arytenoid cartilages do not approximate during voicing in this case of left vocal fold paralysis. The result is continued glottic insufficiency due to a persistent posterior glottic gap. An arytenoid adduction procedure can be performed to medialize and elevate the vocal process of the arytenoid cartilage and correct this problem. The analysis of the vibratory characteristics reveals relatively periodic vibration. The amplitude of vibration on the left is less than on the right leading to vibratory asymmetry. The mucosal wave on the right is normal but is obscured on the left secondary to a collection of secretions on the superior surface of the vocal fold. This indicates a possible lack of sensory input from the ipsilateral superior laryngeal nerve.

52. **Medialization Implant Too High.** Fullness of the left ventricle after medialization for left vocal fold paralysis indicates that implant material may have been placed in the ventricular fold during the procedure. The convex shape of the medial aspect of the left vocal fold further indicates possible undercorrection at the level of the true vocal fold. Despite the possible superior placement of the implant, this patient does achieve complete glottic closure during voicing, but the open phase likely still predominates. The malpositioned implant obscures a good view of the superior surface of the left vocal fold during voicing, making the evaluation of the vibratory characteristics difficult on that side. Frame-by-frame analysis reveals mild vibratory asymmetry. A very short phonation duration makes an adequate assessment of amplitude and mucosal wave impossible.

53. **Normal Color High-Speed Imaging.** This video clip is an example of a color HSV playback used in **Fig. 28.1.** The frequency

of vibration of the vocal folds (male subject) is 126 Hz, the HSV frame rate is 4000 fps, and the playback rate is 10 fps.

54. **Digital Kymography.** This video clip demonstrates an example of a DKG playback of sustained phonation. DKG playback is a movie playing from posterior to anterior. The image on the left shows an average image of the vocal folds with the line being scanned across the glottis. On the right, the corresponding kymographic image is shown.

55. **Phonatory Offset: Digital Kymography and High-Speed Imaging.** An example of (a) DKG playback of a phonatory offset and the corresponding (b) HSV playback is shown in this video clip. The image on the left shows an average image of the vocal folds with the line being scanned across the glottis. On the right, the corresponding kymographic image is shown.

56. **Mucosal Wave Playback.** This video clip is an example of an MW playback of sustained phonation. In the MW playback, the color indicates the direction of motion (ie, the opening edges are encoded in green and the closing edges in red). This example demonstrates the effectiveness of the MW playback in emphasizing that in the beginning of the closing phase, when the lower margins are closing, the upper margins of the vocal folds may still be opening. The width of the differential between the upper and lower margins is a measure of the extent of the lateral phase of the mucosal wave.

57. **Mucosal Wave Kymography Playback.** This video clip demonstrates an example of an MKG playback of sustained phonation. This type of display allows for the temporal representation of the dynamics of the mucosal edges during glottal opening and closing in consecutive glottal cycles. The color shows the phase of motion (opening is green, closing is red). The mucosal wave extent appears as a double-edged or thicker red curve during the closing phase.

58. **High-Speed Imaging of Glissando.** High-speed video of normal vocal folds during glissando reveals some aperiodic vibration

and a change in the glottic configuration during the gradual change in pitch.

59. **High-Speed Imaging in Muscle Tension Dysphonia.** This video clip was made from a high-speed imaging of the patient in **Video Clip 19**, who has muscle tension dysphonia. In the videostroboscopy, it appears that the vocal folds never close. The high-speed evaluation reveals that the folds do, indeed, approximate one another, although briefly, and an open phase predominates in the vibratory cycle.

60. **Videostroboscopy of Tremor.** Due to sudden rapid changes in pitch, it is not possible to use videostroboscopy to evaluate the vibratory characteristics of individuals with tremor. Pitch changes occur too rapidly for the stroboscopy to track, and the resulting recording does not show smooth vocal fold movement but gives the impression that the vocal folds "jump" from one position to another. This video clip demonstrates the result of videostroboscopy in a patient with vocal tremor.

61. **High-Speed Imaging of Tremor.** This video clip was made from a high-speed recording in the patient with tremor from **Video Clip 59**. The vibratory characteristics such as symmetry of vibration, amplitude of vibration, and mucosal wave can all be evaluated with high-speed imaging, which was not possible with videostroboscopy. This patient demonstrates a posterior glottic chink configuration at maximal closure. Vibration is symmetric. The amplitude of vibration is normal bilaterally, as is the mucosal wave.

62. **Videostroboscopy Early after Surgery.** During the first few weeks after surgery on the vocal folds, the mucosal wave is absent at the site of the operation. The inflammation of healing likely results in poor vibration. Videostroboscopy typically demonstrates a stiff vocal fold for the first 3 to 4 weeks after a surgical procedure. This video clip demonstrates the videostroboscopy findings in a patient 1 week after the elevation of a mucosal flap and removal of a cyst from the anterior aspect of the left vocal fold. Glottic closure appears incomplete. There is slight amplitude of

vibration visible on the left, but in general, the left vocal fold appears stiff and without a mucosal wave. Most of the acoustic signal in this situation is likely generated from the vibration of the normal right vocal fold. If the left vocal fold is vibrating at a frequency even slightly different than the right vocal fold, it will not be visible with stroboscopy that is being triggered based on the vibration of the right vocal fold.

63. **High-Speed Imaging Early after Surgery.** This video clip shows the results of high-speed imaging from the patient in **Video Clip 61**. Contrary to what is seen with videostroboscopy (see **Video Clip 61**), the glottic configuration at maximal closure is a posterior glottic chink and complete closure between the membranous vocal folds. One week after surgery, it is possible to see some recovery of the mucosal wave on the left side as the inferior lip of the left vocal fold makes contact with the inferior lip of the right vocal fold. The amplitude of vibration remains reduced on the left side, but overall, the vibratory abnormalities are not as severe as they appear with videostroboscopy.

64. **High-Speed Imaging of Polypoid Changes.** Because the onset and offset of vocal fold vibration cannot be seen with videostroboscopy, the details of both functional and physical behaviors during these parts of phonation cannot be observed. This is a high-speed recording from a patient with polypoid changes of the vocal folds whose videostroboscopy can be viewed in **Video Clip 33**. In **Video Clip 33**, there is no evidence of muscle tension or other clues to possible behavioral contributions to the vocal fold pathology observed. With high-speed imaging, however, it is clear that

there is significant squeezing that occurs at vocal onset. Admittedly, the observed muscle tension may, in part, be an adaptation to the pathology, rather than the cause, as it is possible that more subglottic pressure must be generated to set polypoid vocal folds into vibration.

65. **Videostroboscopy of Mild Nodules.** This is a video clip from videostroboscopy recorded in a patient with mild vocal fold nodules. Nodules are considered to be the result of vocal trauma with injury to the vocal fold tissues occurring at the site of maximal closing force along the vocal fold margin. Prolonged voice overuse with repetitive injury results in a thickening of the epithelium at the mid-membranous portion of both vocal folds. Despite the nodules, the glottic configuration at maximal closure in this example is completely closed. The vibration is periodic and symmetric. The amplitude of vibration and the mucosal wave are normal.

66. **High-Speed Imaging of Mild Nodules.** This is the high-speed imaging evaluation from the patient described in **Video Clip 64** with vocal fold nodules. Although closing forces cannot be measured with high-speed imaging, this video clip gives the viewer the impression that the vocal folds in this example are "slamming" together and that vocal fold closing forces are likely higher than in normal individuals. This ability to appreciate some behavioral aspects of phonation that contribute to the formation of nodules in certain individuals with high-speed imaging may also provide a mechanism for tracking the outcome of therapy with the expectation that successful therapy would eliminate this finding on high-speed imaging.

Index

Note: Page numbers followed by f and t indicate figures and tables; *italicized* page numbers indicate video clip descriptions and corresponding clip number, e.g. *284 [11]*.